Pregnancy in the Obese Woman

Pregnancy in the Obese Woman

Clinical Management

EDITED BY

Deborah L. Conway MD

Associate Professor
Division of Maternal-Fetal Medicine
Department of Obstetrics and Gynecology
University of Texas School of Medicine
San Antonio, Texas, USA

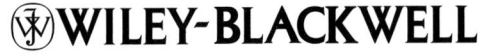

A John Wiley & Sons, Ltd., Publication

This edition first published 2011, © 2011 by Blackwell Publishing Ltd

Blackwell Publishing was acquired by John Wiley & Sons in February 2007. Blackwell's publishing program has been merged with Wiley's global Scientific, Technical and Medical business to form Wiley-Blackwell.

Registered office: John Wiley & Sons Ltd, The Atrium, Southern Gate, Chichester, West Sussex, PO19 8SQ, UK

Editorial offices:
9600 Garsington Road, Oxford, OX4 2DQ, UK
111 River Street, Hoboken, NJ 07030-5774, USA
The Atrium, Southern Gate, Chichester, West Sussex, PO19 8SQ, UK
For details of our global editorial offices, for customer services and for information about how to apply for permission to reuse the copyright material in this book please see our website at www.wiley.com/wiley-blackwell

Library of Congress Cataloging-in-Publication Data

Pregnancy in the obese woman : clinical management / edited by Deborah L. Conway.
       p. ; cm.
   Includes bibliographical references and index.
   ISBN 978-1-4051-9648-2 (alk. paper)
   1. Obesity.   2. Pregnancy–Complications.   I. Conway, Deborah L.
   [DNLM: 1. Obesity.   2. Pregnancy Complications.   3. Pregnancy Outcome.   4. Pregnancy, High-Risk.   5. Risk Factors.   WQ 240]
     RG580.O24P74 2011
     618.2'42–dc22
                    2010038309

ISBN: 978-1-4051-9648-2

A catalogue record for this book is available from the British Library.

This book is published in the following electronic formats: ePDF 9781444391169; Wiley Online Library 9781444391183; ePub 9781444391176

Set in 9.5/13pt Meridien by Toppan Best-set Premedia Limited
Printed and bound in Singapore by Markono Print Media Pte Ltd

1   2011

Contents

v

The color plate section can be found facing p. 214

Preface

As I write in the latter part of 2010, it is no longer newsworthy to declare that the world is experiencing an epidemic of obesity. For many reasons, some well-characterized and others as yet undetermined, overweight and obesity rates have accelerated over recent decades. Recognition of this trend has led to an explosion of research to search for causes and solutions, from the genetic to the population level and all points in between. Strategies to reverse increasing obesity rates and to treat at-risk and affected individuals arrive from many sources: national and international expert panels, government and community agencies, medical researchers, healthcare experts, and others. It can be difficult for a conscientious healthcare provider to stay abreast of it all, and to discern which information is most reliable.

Pregnancy care of obese and overweight women provides a unique set of challenges. Excess weight affects fertility, pregnancy, delivery, and the postpartum period. A specialized knowledge base and skill set are required to provide competent pre-pregnancy, obstetric and postnatal care to obese women. The aim of this book is to supply this knowledge to busy clinicians faced with these challenges. Thus, the reader will find collected in one location information covering every aspect of pregnancy in obese women, beginning with the epidemiological scope of the problem and ending with postpartum care. In addition to the "typical" obstetric topics like prenatal care, fetal surveillance, and delivery, we address bariatric surgery, psychological aspects of obesity in women, nutrition and exercise in obese gravidas, and pre-pregnancy evaluation and preparation.

I am immensely grateful to the phenomenal expert authors who devoted their time and talent to this project. They are not only knowledgeable about their topics, they exemplify dedication to insightful, high quality, evidence-based care of obese patients. I am certain readers will appreciate, as I did, their ability to distill the available data into useful, clear information and recommendations for patient care. My intention as editor has been to maintain a patient-centered focus, and to produce a text that empowers obstetric care providers to do the same for their obese patients.

Deborah L. Conway, MD
San Antonio, TX, USA

Contributor List

Barbara Abrams, DrPH, RD, Professor of Epidemiology, Maternal and Child Health and Public Health Nutrition, School of Public Health, University of California, Berkeley, Division of Epidemiology, California, Berkeley, California, USA

James M. Alexander, MD, Chief of Obstetrics, Parkland Hospital, Professor, Department of Obstetrics and Gynecology, Division of Maternal Fetal Medicine, and Vice Chairman, Institutional Review Board, Department of Obstetrics and Gynecology, University of Texas Southwestern Medical Center at Dallas, Texas, USA

Susan Y. Chu, PhD, MSPH, Senior Epidemiologist, Division of Reproductive Health, National Center for Chronic Disease Prevention and Health Promotion, Centers for Disease Control and Prevention, Atlanta, Georgia, USA

Donald J. Dudley, MD, Vice Chair for Research, Department of Obstetrics and Gynecology, University of Texas Health Science Center at San Antonio, San Antonio, Texas, USA

Anne Lang Dunlop, MD, MPH, Assistant Professor and Preventive Medicine Residency Program Director, Department of Family and Preventive Medicine, Emory University School of Medicine, Atlanta, Georgia, USA

Hugh M Ehrenberg, MD, Associate Professor, Obstetrics and Gynecology, Division of Maternal Fetal Medicine, Ohio State University Medical Center, Columbus, Ohio, USA

Eran Hadar, MD, Senior Attending Physician, Department of Obstetrics and Gynecology, Helen Schneider Hospital for Women, Rabin Medical Center, Petach Tikva and Sackler Faculty of Medicine, Tel Aviv University, Tel Aviv, Israel

C.R. Hall, MD, Clinical Assistant Professor, Division of Minimally Invasive Surgery, Department of Surgery, Ohio State University, Columbus, Ohio, USA

John M. Jakicic, PhD, Chair and Professor, Department of Health and Physical Activity, and Director, Physical Activity and Weight Management Research Center, University of Pittsburgh, Pittsburgh, Pennsylvania, USA

Anatte Karmon, MD, Resident Physician, Department of Obstetrics, Gynecology and Women's Health, Albert Einstein College of Medicine/Montefiore Medical Center, Bronx, New York, USA

Janet King , PhD, Senior Scientist, Children's Hospital Oakland Research Institute and Professor, University of California at Berkeley & Davis, Oakland, California, USA

D. Yvette Lacoursiere, MD, MPH, Assistant Professor and Women's Reproductive and Health Research Scholar, Department of Reproductive Medicine, University of California San Diego Medical Center, San Diego, California, USA

Vita Lam Mayes, MPH, Physician Assistant and Master of Public Health Student, Department of Family and Preventive Medicine, Emory University School of Medicine, Atlanta, Georgia, USA

Divya Narayan, MD, Research Associate, Department of Family and Preventive Medicine, Emory University School of Medicine, Atlanta, Georgia, USA

Bradley J. Needleman, MD, FACS, Director, Bariatric Surgery Program and Associate Professor of Clinical Surgery, Center for Minimally Invasive Surgery, Ohio State University, Columbus, OH, USA

Ashley Parker, MD, Resident, Department of Obstetrics and Gynecology, University of Texas Health Science Center at San Antonio, San Antonio, Texas, USA

Elizabeth Reifsnider, PhD, RN, WHNP, PHCNS-BC, Constance Brewer Koomey Professor of Nursing and Associate Dean for Research, School of Nursing, University of Texas Medical Branch, Galveston, Texas, USA

Krista L Rompolski, MS, Department of Health and Physical Activity, University of Pittsburgh, Pittsburgh, Pennsylvania, USA

Eyal Sheiner, MD, PhD, Professor, Department of Obstetrics and Gynecology, Soroka University Medical Center, Faculty of Health Sciences, Ben-Gurion University of the Negev, Beer-Sheva, Israel

Naomi E. Stotland, MD, Associate Professor, Department of Obstetrics, Gynecology, and Reproductive Sciences, University of California, San Francisco, California, USA

Yariv Yogev, MD, Senior Attending Physician and Associate Professor, Department of Obstetrics and Gynecology, Helen Schneider Hospital for Women, and Rabin Medical Center, Petach Tikva and Sackler Facuylty of Medicine, Tel Aviv University, Tel Aviv, Israel

CHAPTER 1

The Epidemiology of Obesity in Pregnancy

Susan Y. Chu*

National Center for Chronic Disease Prevention and Health Promotion, Centers for Disease Control and Prevention, Atlanta, Georgia, USA

With the rapid increase in the prevalence of obesity in many countries, obesity during pregnancy has become a common high-risk obstetric condition in many populations. The immediate and long-term consequences are considerable. Obesity during pregnancy is associated with several adverse reproductive outcomes, including hypertensive disorders, gestational diabetes mellitus, cesarean delivery, macrosomia, shoulder dystocia, and fetal death [1–7]. Long term, the consequences may be even greater: maternal obesity also is associated with an increased risk for type 2 diabetes mellitus for the mother and child, as well as an increased risk for obesity for the child later in life [8–15].

This chapter will: discuss the definition of overweight and obesity, as well as specific issues concerning the measurement of maternal obesity; present available estimates on the prevalence of maternal obesity in various countries; describe the impact of excessive gestational weight gain on the prevalence of maternal obesity; and summarize studies that have estimated the healthcare costs associated with obesity during pregnancy.

Defining the prevalence of obesity

Estimates of obesity prevalence in populations depend on the definition of obesity. Ideally, obesity should be defined by the amount of excess fat that increases health-related risk factors and associated morbidities; however, in practice, a single, ideal definition of obesity for use in population-based estimates is not possible, for three main reasons. First,

*The findings and conclusions in this article are those of the authors and do not necessarily represent the views of the Centers for Disease Control and Prevention.

an ideal definition requires an exact measurement of excess fat, which involves expensive and complicated methods; second, health risks associated with obesity increase on a continuum, not at a particular defined cut-off point; and third, the impact of excess fat on health varies among individuals and populations.

Historically, the precise measurement of body fat was done using hydrostatic weighing, which involves immersion underwater; currently, the most precise methods for measuring body fat involve the use of computed tomography or imaging techniques such as magnetic resonance imaging [16]. Although these methods most accurately measure body adiposity, the expense, the relative scarcity of the necessary equipment, and the need for an individual clinical visit make these methods impractical for measuring the population prevalence of obesity.

Body mass index (BMI; weight (kg)/height squared (m^2)) is highly, although not perfectly, correlated with fat mass [17,18]. For this reason, as well as the ability to use recorded or self-reported data, BMI is perhaps the most widely used measure to estimate adiposity. One primary limitation of this measurement is that it does not distinguish fat mass from lean mass. For example, BMI would underestimate body fat in older persons, because of their differential loss of lean mass and decreased height [19] and overestimate body fat in persons with a muscular build, such as athletes [20]. Nonetheless, for most clinical and epidemiological studies, BMI is considered an efficient and useful measure for estimating increased health risks related to excess body fat [21,22].

Another issue affecting prevalence estimates of obesity is defining BMI cut-off points. In the USA, one of the earliest suggested criteria for categorizing maternal BMI was included in the 1990 Institute of Medicine (IOM) report *Nutrition during Pregnancy* [23]. The IOM guidelines provided guidance on appropriate pregnancy weight gain levels based on pre-pregnancy BMI primarily to address low-birthweight deliveries related to insufficient nutrition and weight gain during pregnancy. Acknowledging that BMI is a better indicator of maternal nutritional status than is weight alone, the IOM subcommittee suggested the weight-for-height categories shown in Box 1.1. These cut-off points generally correspond to 90%, 120%, and 135% of the 1959 Metropolitan Life Insurance Company weight-for-height standards, standards that were in common use in the USA at that time.

In 1997, the World Health Organization (WHO) proposed a BMI classification based on the risk for co-morbidities (Box 1.1) [24]. These categories of underweight, normal weight, overweight, and obese classes I, II, and III are age-independent and the same for both genders.

Although these standards were developed for adults of European descent, they have been frequently used in many countries and have facilitated international comparisons.

Box 1.1 Body mass index (BMI) categories: World Health Organization (WHO) and Institute of Medicine (IOM; 1990) classifications

BMI category (kg/m^2)	WHO	IOM
Underweight	<18.5	<19.8
Normal weight	18.5–24.9	19.8–26.0
Pre-obese/overweight	25.0–29.9	>26.0–29.0
Obese	≥30.0[a]	>29.0

[a] The WHO/National Heart, Lung, and Blood Institute obese category is sometimes further divided into obese I (30.0–34.9 kg/m^2), obese II (35.0–39.9 kg/m^2), and obese III (≥40.0 kg/m^2), corresponding to moderate, severe, and very severe risk for co-morbidities.

In 1998, the US National Heart, Lung, and Blood Institute (NHLBI) published *Clinical Guidelines on the Identification, Evaluation, and Treatment of Overweight and Obesity in Adults* [25]. The BMI criteria published in this report were essentially the same as those recommended by the WHO, except for a difference in labeling BMI 25.0–29.9 kg/m^2 as "overweight" rather than "pre-obese." As stated by the NHLBI expert panel, this BMI classification was based on available scientific evidence from observational and epidemiological studies of BMI and risk for morbidity and mortality. These guidelines specifically excluded pregnant women with the following statement: "Pregnant women who, on the basis of their prepregnant weight, would be classified as obese may encounter certain obstetrical risks. However, the inappropriateness of weight reduction during pregnancy is well recognized; hence, this guideline specifically excludes pregnant women." Nonetheless, these NBHLI/WHO BMI classifications have been used extensively for prevalence estimates and in etiological studies of pregnant women.

The WHO and the IOM criteria will yield different BMI prevalence estimates in the same population; overall, the WHO criteria will result in higher prevalence estimates of overweight and lower prevalences of obese and underweight than estimates based on the IOM criteria [26]. While the differences in BMI criteria would not affect the ability to monitor trends in obesity of a country or subpopulation, criteria differences can affect international comparisons and etiological studies estimating obesity prevalence and the association with adverse health outcomes.

In 2009, the IOM revised the 1990 guidelines for weight gain during pregnancy, in large part to address the high rates of overweight and obesity in the US population [26]. These new guidelines adopted the WHO BMI cut-off points, recognizing the wider general acceptance of these criteria, which has enabled comparisons between populations, both within countries and internationally. However, these categories were developed using a standard based on adults of European descent, and there is substantial evidence that body fat distribution and the effect of excess body fat on health differ among race and ethnic populations.

BMI does not necessarily describe the same degree of fatness in different populations, partly because of differences in body proportions. For example, Asians have a more centralized distribution of body fat for a given level of BMI compared to people of European descent, and some studies have shown that obesity-related morbidity and mortality among Asians occur at a lower BMI than in other race and ethnic groups [27–29]. This is particularly relevant for gestational diabetes mellitus: Asians have some of the highest rates among all race and ethnic groups, but have a low prevalence of obesity [30]. Thus, visceral fat measurements may be more predictive of risk than BMI. African-Americans tend to have a lower percentage of body fat than people of European descent at the same BMI [31], and there is some suggestion that certain obesity-related conditions (macrosomia, pre-eclampsia) occur at higher BMI levels among black individuals than other race and ethnic groups [32].

Finally, health risks associated with body mass are on a continuum and do not necessarily correspond to rigid cut-off points. For example, an overweight individual with a BMI of 29 does not acquire additional health consequences associated with obesity simply by crossing the BMI threshold of 30 or above. Although health risks generally increase with increasing BMI, these cut-off points may not be as useful as a diagnostic tool [21].

Measuring the prevalence of maternal obesity

In addition to the issues affecting the measurement of obesity prevalence in the general population, there are concerns about the measurement of the prevalence of obesity in pregnant women. First, national reports generally have used the prevalence of obesity among women of reproductive age as an estimate of the prevalence of obesity among pregnant women [33]. While these data are readily available, pregnant women are a distinct subgroup of all women in that age group and estimates based on all women of reproductive age may not accurately reflect estimates among pregnant women.

Second, many prevalence estimates of maternal obesity are clinic rather than population-based. This also can result in inaccurate prevalence estimates, especially if the clinic serves a specific population, selectively excludes healthier women, or does not serve large numbers of women in a particular area.

Finally, information on maternal body mass or weight must reflect status preceding any significant pregnancy weight gain. Because of this, most estimates of maternal obesity based on BMI rely on retrospective self-reported data. These values generally result in underestimates of the prevalence of obesity, as individuals tend to underreport their weight and overreport their height [34], although studies that have examined this error among women who recently delivered have found that, on average, the magnitude of underreporting for overweight women was less than 10lb [35,36].

Worldwide prevalence of obesity during pregnancy

Obesity has reached epidemic proportions globally [37]. Although the prevalence is highest in developed countries, obesity has become an important health issue in many developing countries, often co-existing with undernutrition [38]. Concomitant with the increased rates of obesity in the general population, obesity during pregnancy has also escalated, and it is now a common obstetric high-risk condition. Although data on the prevalence of obesity among pregnant women are limited in most countries, available information demonstrates the extent and range of the problem in many areas in the world. Figure 1.1 displays studies reporting the prevalence of overweight and obesity during pregnancy in various countries; included studies were limited to those that were population-based, used weight or BMI measurements pre-pregnancy or early in pregnancy before substantial weight gain, and included data collected during the year 2000 or after.

In the USA, the reported prevalence of maternal obesity in different cities and states ranged from 10% to 26% [39–42] (Figure 1.1); in part, these disparities reflect differences in populations and years of data collection. In the largest, most recent survey based on data from 26 states and New York City during 2004–05, approximately one in five US women who delivered were obese; in some state, race/ethnicity, and socioeconomic status subgroups, the prevalence was as high as 35% [43]. Race was the strongest predictor of higher obesity prevalence, with black women having an obesity prevalence about 70% higher than white and Hispanic women (black, 29.1%; white, 17.4%; Hispanic, 17.4%). Moreover, these obesity rates are notably higher than in previous years; a previous study of nine US states showed that the prevalence of obesity at the start of pregnancy increased from 13% in 1993–94 to 22.0% in 2002–03, a 70% increase over a 10-year period [44]. The other North American

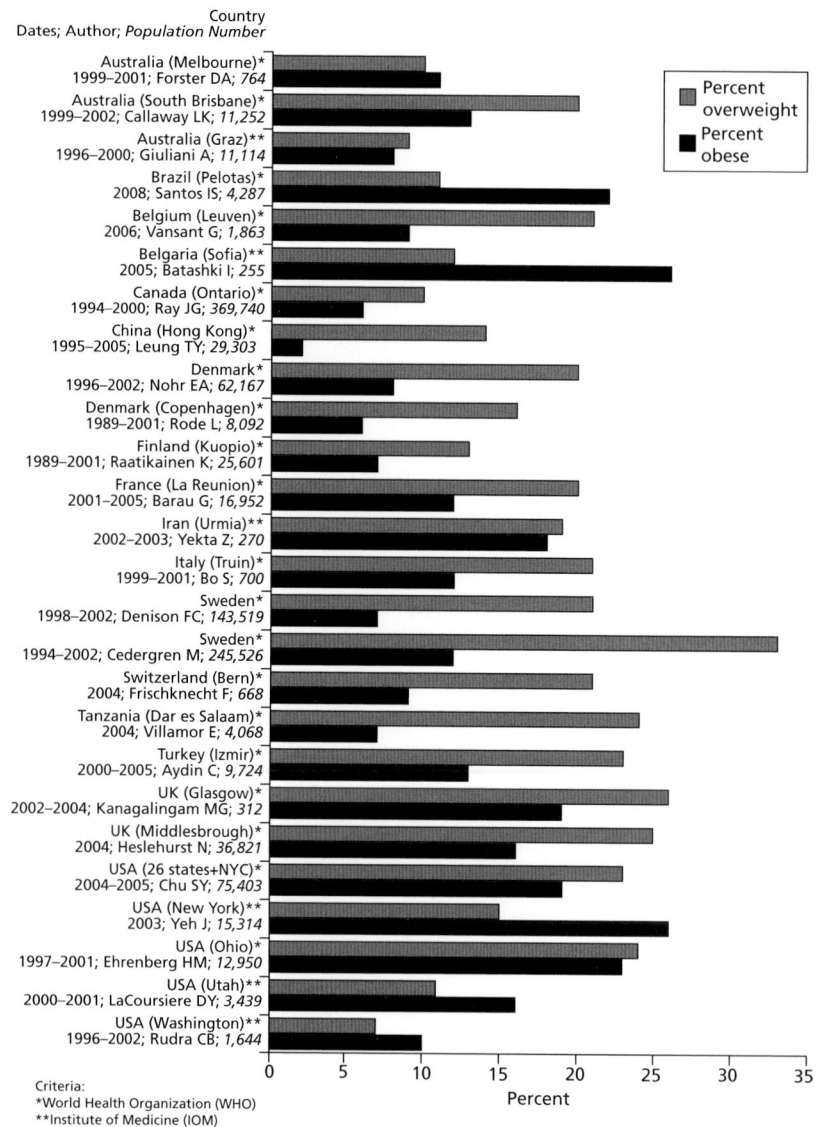

Figure 1.1 Prevalence of overweight and obesity among pregnant women in population-based studies. (Adapted from Guelinckx et al. [6], with permission.)

country with available data, Canada, reported lower prevalence rates of maternal obesity than for the USA (6%) [45], although a direct comparison is difficult given that years of the studies and body weight measures were not equivalent.

The prevalence of obesity among pregnant women in Europe varied considerably by country, with the highest prevalence rates reported in the UK [46,47]. Both UK studies reported a 50% increase in obesity between

1990 and 2002–04, and found that socioeconomic disadvantage or depri-vation was a strong independent predictor of maternal obesity. Race and ethnicity differences were not examined closely as over 90% of the UK study populations were Caucasian. About one in eight pregnant women were obese in studies from France, Italy, and one of the two reports from Sweden [48–51]. Several European countries reported maternal obesity rates below 10% [52–57], although even in the country with the lowest reported prevalence, Denmark, about one in 15 women who are pregnant were obese [55].

Prevalence data on maternal obesity from countries outside the Western hemisphere and Europe are more limited. In one of the more developed countries in the Oceania continent, Australia, prevalence rates of maternal obesity were similar in two east coast areas (Melbourne, 11%; South Brisbane, 13%) [58,59]. Available reports suggest that high levels of maternal obesity are found even in some generally less affluent countries (Bulgaria, 26%; Turkey, 13%; Brazil, 22%; Iran 18%) [60–63]. The preva-lence of maternal obesity was lower in the single African study from Tanzania (7%) [64]; however, the prevalence of overweight among these African pregnant women was as high as in Western countries (24%). China was the exception, with low obesity prevalence (2%) even in a well-developed city, Hong Kong [65]. Direct comparisons among countries cannot be made as the reported obesity prevalence is affected by the cri-teria used (i.e. WHO versus IOM), the size and representativeness of the population surveyed, and the years of the study.

Certain maternal characteristics, such as older maternal age and higher parity, are consistently associated with higher rates of obesity, regardless of culture and geographic location. In the USA, obesity prevalence differs significantly by race and ethnicity, but most studies outside the USA are not able to examine rates by racial and ethnic groups. However, when examined in developed countries (US, UK, Denmark, Sweden), reported maternal obesity was higher in population subgroups with lower socioeco-nomic status; in contrast, in Tanzania, maternal obesity was associated with higher education and more income earned outside the home. This highlights the importance of considering how differences in economic situ-ation and cultural context can affect the patterns of and the risk factors for obesity in various countries or populations.

Impact of gestational weight gain on trends in maternal obesity

In many countries, the current trend of increasing maternal obesity is in part related to excessive levels of weight gain during pregnancy [66,67].

Historically, gestational weight gain guidelines were developed to reduce the well-known adverse impact of inadequate pregnancy weight gain on reproductive outcome [66], with smaller gains recommended for heavier women. However, major changes have occurred in the body weights of pregnant women, prompting discussion to produce new guidelines that consider the short- and long-term adverse impacts of excessive gestational weight gain. Short-term consequences include preterm delivery, neonatal hypoglycemia, and macrosomic infants [67–71]; long term, excessive gestational weight gain increases the risk for weight retention after pregnancy and excessive body weight later in life [70,72–75].

Excessive weight gains during pregnancy have been documented in several developed countries. In a US study of 52,988 underweight, normal, overweight, and obese women who delivered a singleton, full-term infant in 2004–05, approximately 40% of normal-weight and 60% of overweight women gained excessive weight during pregnancy, with the highest rates of excessive gestational weight gains among the youngest and those who were nulliparous [76]. Similar excessive levels of gestational weight gain have been reported among pregnant women in other developed countries, including Belgium [54], Denmark [70], Australia [77], Sweden [51,73,74], Germany [78], and Switzerland [57]. These trends in excessive gestational weight gains predict a further escalation of the problem of obesity among women of reproductive age in many parts of the world.

Economic costs of maternal obesity

Obesity is not only a health issue, but also has economic consequences. Total costs involve both the direct costs related to medical expenditures from obesity-related diseases, including type 2 diabetes, cardiovascular disease, several types of cancer, and musculoskeletal disorders, as well as indirect costs related to absenteeism, reduced productivity, and disability [79]. Many countries have reported on the substantial and increasing economic burden of obesity, including the USA [80,81], Canada [82], Europe [83], Eastern Europe [84], the UK [85], China [86,87], and Japan [88]. A recent projection based on data from the US National Health and Nutrition Examination Survey estimated that, by the year 2030, costs related to overweight and obesity will account for 16–18% of total US healthcare costs [81].

However, precise estimates of the economic costs directly related to maternal obesity are very limited. It is clear that the costs are substantial, because maternal obesity not only increases the risk for adverse pregnancy and infant outcomes, but also may be associated with a higher risk for developing type 2 diabetes mellitus later in life for both mother and child

[8–10]. Moreover, maternal obesity, either independently or through gestational diabetes mellitus, may increase the risk for obesity in offspring [11–15]. The medical care costs related to chronic diabetes and obesity in the mother and her offspring far exceed the immediate costs associated with adverse short-term pregnancy outcomes. So although pregnancy is a time-limited condition in a woman's life, differences in risk during this time can affect the lifelong health of the mother and her offspring.

And although it is recognized that the use of healthcare is increased for pregnant women who are obese, published estimates of the magnitude of that increase are quite limited. Numerous studies have documented the increased risks of adverse outcomes associated with obesity during pregnancy, but few studies have provided quantitative estimates of the associated increase in healthcare utilization. Two papers from Montpellier, France, estimated the complications and costs of obesity during pregnancy based on the same clinic population during two time periods (1980–93 and 1993–94, respectively [88,90]. The authors found that average costs were significantly higher among overweight and obese pregnant women than among normal-weight women; however, these cost estimates were based only on hospitalizations. In a qualitative study from the UK, 33 maternity and healthcare professionals were interviewed on their views of the impact of maternal obesity on maternity services and healthcare resources [91]. There was general consensus that maternal obesity has a major impact on the level of care required for both the mother and the infant, but this study could not provide quantitative estimates of the impact.

Quantitative increases in healthcare services related to maternal obesity were documented in a US study of 13,442 pregnancies among women aged 18 years and older who were participants in a large group practice Health Maintenance Organization [92]. Maternal obesity was associated with significantly greater use of inpatient and outpatient healthcare services, including costly measures such as length of stay during the hospitalization for delivery and use of physician services; mid-level providers were used less during prenatal visits. Almost all of the increase in utilization was related to the increased rates of cesarean delivery and the presence of gestational diabetes, diabetes mellitus, or hypertensive disorders among obese pregnant women. These findings are consistent with a recent systematic review of the literature on the impact of maternal obesity and obstetric care, in which maternal obesity was associated with increased rates of cesarean and instrumental deliveries, hemorrhage, infection, longer hospital stays, and increased use of neonatal intensive care [93]. Because maternal obesity is no longer rare in many countries, even a small increase in healthcare costs associated with obesity can have a substantial economic impact. Understanding the total impact of obesity during pregnancy on the lifetime health of the mother and her children as well as the economic consequences may impel the level of individual and societal changes necessary to control the growing epidemic of obesity.

References

1. American Congress of Obstetricians and Gynecologists. Committee Opinion number 315, September 2005. Obesity in pregnancy. Obstet Gynecol 2005;106:671–5.
2. Catalano PM, Ehrenberg HM. The short- and long-term implications of maternal obesity on the mother and her offspring. BJOG 2006;113(10):1126–33.
3. Garbaciak JA, Jr., Richter M, Miller S, et al. Maternal weight and pregnancy complications. Am J Obstet Gynecol 1985;152(2):238–45.
4. Chu SY, Callaghan WM, Kim SY, et al. Maternal obesity and the risk of gestational diabetes mellitus: a meta-analysis. Diabetes Care 2007;30:2070–6.
5. Chu SY, Kim SY, Schmid CH, et al. Maternal obesity and the risk of cesarean delivery: a meta-analysis. Obes Rev 2007;8:385–94.
6. Guelinckx I, Devlieger R, Beckers K, et al. Maternal obesity: pregnancy complications, gestational weight gain, and nutrition. Obes Rev 2008;9:140–50.
7. Chu SY, Kim SY, Lau J, et al. Maternal obesity and the risk of stillbirth: a meta-analysis. Am J Obstet Gynecol 2007;197(3):223–8.
8. Ben-Haroush A, Yogev Y, Hod M. Epidemiology of gestational diabetes mellitus and its association with type 2 diabetes. Diabet Med 2004;21(2):103–13.
9. Kim C, Newton KM, Knopp RH. Gestational diabetes and the incidence of type 2 diabetes: a systematic review. Diabetes Care 2002;25(10):1862–8.
10. Gillman MW, Rifas-Shiman S, Berkey CS, et al. Maternal gestational diabetes, birth weight, and adolescent obesity. Pediatrics 2003;111(3):e221–6.
11. Plagemann A, Harder T, Kohlhoff R, et al. Overweight and obesity in infants of mothers with long-term insulin-dependent diabetes or gestational diabetes. Int J Obes Relat Metab Disord 1997;21(6):451–6.
12. Schaefer-Graf UM, Pawliczak J, Passow D, et al. Birth weight and parental BMI predict overweight in children from mothers with gestational diabetes. Diabetes Care 2005;28(7):1745–50.
13. Boney CM. Metabolic syndrome in childhood: association with birth weight, maternal obesity, and gestational diabetes mellitus. Pediatrics 2005;115(3):e290–6.
14. Dabelea D, Hanson RL, Lindsay RS, et al. Intrauterine exposure to diabetes conveys risks for type 2 diabetes and obesity: a study of discordant sibships. Diabetes 2000;49: 2208–11.
15. Hillier TA, Pedula KL, Schmidt MM, et al. Childhood obesity and metabolic imprinting. Diabetes Care 2007;30:2287–92.
16. National Heart, Lung, and Blood Institute, National Institute of Diabetes and Digestive and Kidney Diseases. Clinical guidelines on the identification, evaluation, and treatment of overweight and obesity in adults – the evidence report. Bethesda, MD: National Institutes of Health, 1998.
17. Gallagher D, Visser M, Sepulveda D, et al. How useful is body mass index for comparison of body fatness across age, sex, and ethnic groups? Am J Epidemiol 1996;143: 228–39.

18. Deurenberg P, Weststrate JA, Seidell JC. Boyd mass index as a measure of body fatness: age- and sex- specific prediction formulas. Br J Nutr 1991;65:105–11.

19. Sorkin J, Muller D, Andres R. Longitudinal change in height in men and women: implications for interpretation of the body mass index. Am J Epidemiol 1999;150:969–77.

20. Deurenberg P, Deurenberg YM, Wang J, et al. The impact of body build on the relationship between body mass index and percent body fat. Int J Obes Relat Metab Disord 1999;23:537–42.

21. Hubbard VS. Defining overweight and obesity: what are the issues? Am J Clin Nutr 2000;72:1067–8.

22. Kuczmarski RJ, Flegal KM. Criteria for definition of overweight in transition: background and recommendations for the United States. Am J Clin Nutr 2000;72:1074–81.

23. Institute of Medicine, National Academy of Sciences. Nutrition during pregnancy. Part I: Weight gain. Part II: Nutrient supplements. Washington, DC: National Academy Press, 1990.

24. World Health Organization. Report of a WHO consultation on obesity. Obesity: preventing and managing the global epidemic. Geneva: WHO, 1998.

25. NHLBI Obesity Education Initiative Expert Panel on the Identification, Evaluation, and Treatment of Overweight and Obesity in Adults. Clinical guidelines on the identification, evaluation, and treatment of overweight and obesity in adults – the evidence report. Obes Res 1998;6:51S–209S.

26. Institute of Medicine. Weight gain during pregnancy: reexamining the guidelines. Washington, DC: National Academies Press, 2009.

27. Park Y, Allison DB, Heymsfield SB, et al. Larger amounts of visceral adipose tissue in Asian Americans. Obesity Res 2001;9:381–7.

28. Decoda Study Group. BMI compared with central obesity indicators in relation to diabetes and hypertension in Asians. Obesity 2008;16:1622–35.

29. Huxley R, Jamie WPT, Barzi F, et al. Ethnic comparisons of the cross-sectional relationships between measures of body size with diabetes and hypertension. Obes Rev 2009;9(Suppl. 1):53–61.

30. Chu SY, Abe K, Hall L, et al. Gestational diabetes mellitus in the United States: all Asians are not alike. Prev Med 2009;49:265–8.

31. Albu HB, Murphy L, Frager DH, et al. Visceral fat and race-dependent heart risks in obese non-diabetic premenopausal women. Diabetes 1997;46:456–62.

32. Ramos GA, Caughey AB. The interrelationship between ethnicity and obesity on obstetric outcomes. Am J Obstet Gynecol 2005;193:1089–93.

33. Ogden CL, Carroll MD, Curtin LR, et al. Prevalence of overweight and obesity in the United States, 1999–2004. JAMA 2006;295:1549–55.

34. Nawaz H, Chan W, Abdulrahman M, et al. Self-reported weight and height: Implications for obesity research. Am J Prev Med 2001;20:294–8.

35. Schieve LA, Perry GS, Cogswell ME, et al. Validity of self-reported pregnancy delivery weight: an analysis of the 1988 National Maternal and Infant Health Survey. Am J Epidemiol 1999;150:947–56.

36. Lederman SA, Paxton A. Maternal reporting of prepregnancy weight and birth outcome: consistency and completeness compared with the clinical records. Matern Child Health J 1998;2:123–6.

37. World Health Organization. Obesity: preventing and managing a global epidemic. World Health Organ Tech Rep Ser 2000;894:1–4.

38. Misra A, Khurana L. Obesity and the metabolic syndrome in developing countries. J Clin Endocrinol Metab 2008;93:S9–30.

39. LaCoursiere DY, Bloebaum L, Duncan JD, et al. Population-based trends and correlates of maternal overweight and obesity, Utah 1991–2001. Am J Obstet Gynecol 2005;192(3):832–9.

40. Yeh J, Shelton JA. Increasing prepregnancy body mass index: analysis of trends and contributing variables. Am J Obstet Gynecol 2005;193:1994–8.

41. Ehrenberg HM, Dierker L, Milluzzi C, et al. Prevalence of maternal obesity in an urban center. Am J Obstet Gynecol 2002;187(5):1189–93.

42. Rudra CB, Sorensen TK, Leisenring WM, et al. Weight characteristics and height in relation to risk of gestational diabetes mellitus. Am J Epidemiol 2007;165:302–8.

43. Chu SY, Kim SY, Bish CL. Obesity during pregnancy in the United States, 2004–2005. Matern Child Health J 2009;13:614–20.

44. Kim SY, Dietz PM, England L, et al. Trends in prepregnancy obesity in nine states, 1993–2003. Obesity 2007;15:968–73.

45. Ray JG, Nisenbaum R, Singh G, et al. Trends in obesity in pregnancy [letter]. Epidemiology 2007;18:280–1.

46. Kanagalingam MG, Forouhi NG, Greer IA, et al. Changes in booking body mass index over a decade: retrospective analysis from a Glasgow maternity hospital. BJOG 2005;112:1431–3.

47. Heslehurst N, Ells L, Simpson H, et al. Trends in maternal obesity incidence rates, demographic predictors, and health inequalities in 36,821 women over a 15-year period. BJOG 2007;114:187–94.

48. Barau G, Robillard P, Hulsey T, et al. Linear association between maternal pre-pregnancy body mass index and risk of caesarean section in term deliveries. BJOG 2006;113:1173–7.

49. Bo S, Menato G, Signorile A, et al. Obesity or diabetes: what is worse for the mother or for the baby? Diabetes Metab 2003;29:175–8.

50. Denison FC, Price J, Graham C, et al. Maternal obesity, length of gestation, risk of post-dates pregnancy and spontaneous onset of labour at term. BJOG 2008;115:720–5.

51. Cedergren M. Effects of gestational weight gain and body mass index on obstetric outcome in Sweden. Int J Gynecol Obstet 2006;93:269–74.

52. Giuliani A, Tamussino K, Basver A, et al. The impact of body mass index and weight gain during pregnancy on puerperal complications alter spontaneous vaginal delivery. Wien Klin Wochenschr 2002;114:383–6.

53. Vansant G, Guelinckx I, Mullie P, et al. Prevalence of overweight and obesity in pregnant women in Belgium. Int J Obesity 2008;32(Suppl. S1):S104.

54. Nohr EA, Bech BH, Vaeth M, et al. Obesity, gestational weight gain and preterm birth: a study within the Danish National Birth Cohort. Paediatr Perinatal Epidemiol 2007;21:5–14.

55. Rode L, Nilas L, Wojdemann K, et al. Obesity-related complications in Danish single cephalic pregnancies. Obstet Gynecol 2005;105:537–42.

56. Raatikainen K, Heiskanen N, Heinonen S. Transition from overweight to obesity worsens pregnancy outcome in a BMI-dependent matter. Obesity 2006;14:165–71.

57. Frischknecht F, Bruhwiler H, Raio L, et al. Changes in pre-pregnancy weight and weight gain during pregnancy: retrospective comparison between 1986 and 2004. Swiss Med Wkly 2009;139:52–5.

58. Forster DA, McLachlan HL, Lumley J. Factors associated with breastfeeding at six months postpartum in a group of Australian women. Int Breastfeed J 2006;1:18.

59. Callaway LK, Prins JB, Chang AM, et al. The prevalence and impact of overweight and obesity in an Australian obstetric population. Med J Aust 2006;184:56–9.

60. Batashki I, Topalovska D, Milchev N, et al. Obesity and pregnancy. Akush Ginekol (Bulgaria) 2006;45:14–18.

61. Aydin C, Baloglu A, Yavuzcan A, et al. The effect of body mass index value during labor on pregnancy outcomes in Turkish population. Arch Gynecol Obstet 2010;281: 49–54.

62. Santos IS, Barros AJD, Matijasevich A, et al. Mothers and their pregnancies: a comparison of three population-based cohorts in Southern Brazil. Cad Saude Publica 2008;24(Suppl. 3):S381–9.

63. Yekta Z, Ayatollahi H, Porali R, et al. The effect of pre-pregnancy body mass index and gestational weight gain on pregnancy outcomes in urban care settings in Urmia-Iran. BMC Pregnancy Childbirth 2006;6:15.

64. Villamor E, Msamanga G, Urassa W, et al. Trends in obesity, underweight, and wasting among women attending prenatal clinics in urban Tanzania. Am J Clin Nutr 2006; 83(6):1387–94.

65. Leung TY, Leung TN, Sahota DS, et al. Trends in maternal obesity and associated risks of adverse pregnancy outcomes in a population of Chinese women. BJOG 2008;115:1529–37.

66. Institute of Medicine. Influence of pregnancy weight on maternal and child health: workshop report. Washington, DC: National Academies Press, 2007.

67. Viswanathan M, Siega-Ruiz AM, Moos MK, et al. Outcomes of maternal weight gain. Evidence Report/Technology Assessment No. 168. Prepared by RTI International-University of North Carolina Evidence-based Practice Center. AHRA Publication No. 08-E-09. Rockville, MD: Agency for Healthcare Research and Quality, 2008.

68. Hedderson MM, Weiss NS, Sacks DA, et al. Pregnancy weight gain and risk of neonatal complications. Obstet Gynecol 2006;108:1153–61.

69. Stotland NE, Hopkins LM, Caughey AB. Gestational weight gain, macrosomia, and risk of cesarean birth in nondiabetic nulliparas. Obstet Gynecol 2004;104:671–7.

70. Nohr EA, Vaeth M, Baker JL, et al. Combined associations of prepregnancy body mass index and gestational weight gain with the outcome of pregnancy. Am J Clin Nutr 2008;87:1750–9.

71. Dietz PM, Callaghan WM, Cogswell ME, et al. Combined effects of prepregnancy body mass index and weight gain during pregnancy on the risk of preterm delivery. Epidemiology 2006;17:170–7.

72. Rooney BL, Schauberger CW. Excess pregnancy weight gain and long-term obesity: one decade later. Obstet Gynecol 2002;100:245–52.

73. Linne Y, Dye L, Barkeling B, et al. Long-term weight development in women: a 15-year follow-up of the effects of pregnancy. Obes Res 2004;12:1166–78.

74. Amorim AR, Rossner S, Neovius M, et al. Does excess prepregnancy weight gain constitute a major risk for increasing long-term BMI? Obesity 2007;15: 1278–86.

75. Scholl TO, Hediger ML, Schall JI, et al. Gestational weight gain, pregnancy outcome, and postpartum weight retention. Obstet Gynecol 1995;86:423–7.

76. Chu SY, Callaghan WM, Bish CL, et al. Gestational weight gain by body mass among U.S. women delivering live births, 2004–2005: fueling future obesity. Am J Obstet Gynecol 2009;200:271.e1–7.

77. Mamun AA, O'Callaghan M, Callaway L, et al. Associations of gestational weight gain with offspring body mass index and blood pressure at 21 years of age. Circulation 2009;119:1720–7.

78. Schiessl B, Beverlein A, Lack N, et al. Temporal trends in pregnancy weight gain and birthweight in Bavaria 2000–2007: slightly decreasing birth weight with increasing weight gain in pregnancy. J Perinat Med 2009;37:374–9.

79. Trogdon JG, Finkelstein EA, Hylands T, et al. Indirect costs of obesity: a review of the current literature. Obes Rev 2008;9:489–500.

80. Finkelstein EA, Ruhm CJ, Kosa KM. Economic causes and consequences of obesity. Ann Rev Public Health 2005;26:239–57.
81. Wang Y, Beydoun MA, Liang L, et al. Will all Americans become overweight or obese? Estimating the progression and cost of the US obesity epidemic. Obesity 2008;16:2323–30.
82. Birmingham CL, Muller JL, Palepu A, et al. The cost of obesity in Canada. CMAJ 1999;160:483–8.
83. Muller-Riemenschneider F, Reinhold T, Berghofer A, et al. Health-economic burden of obesity in Europe. Eur J Epidemiol 2008;23:499–509.
84. Knai C, Suhrcke M, Lobstein T. Obesity in Eastern Europe: an overview of its health and economic implications. Econ Human Biol 2007;5:392–408.
85. Allender S, Rayner M. The burden of overweight and obesity-related ill health in the UK. Obes Rev 2007;8:467–73.
86. Zhao W, Zhai Y, Hu J, et al. Economic burden of obesity-related chronic diseases in Mainland China. Obes Rev 2008;9(Suppl. 1):62–7.
87. Ko GTC. The cost of obesity in Hong Kong. Obes Rev 2008;9(Suppl. 1):74–7.
88. Nakamura K, Okamura T, Kanda H, et al. Medical costs of obese Japanese: a 10-year follow-up study of National Health Insurance in Shiga, Japan. Euro J Public Health 2007;17:424–9.
89. Galtier-Dereure F, Montpeyroux F, Boulot P, et al. Weight excess before pregnancy: complications and cost. Int J Obes Relat Metab Disord 1995;19(7):443–8.
90. Galtier-Dereure F, Boegner C, Bringer J. Obesity and pregnancy: complications and cost. Am J Clin Nutr 2000;71(5 Suppl.):1242S–1248S.
91. Heslehurst N, Lang R, Rankin J, et al. Obesity in pregnancy: a study of the impact of maternal obesity on NHS maternity services. BJOG 2007;114:334–42.
92. Chu SY, Bachman DJ, Callaghan WM, et al. Increased health care utilization associated with obesity during pregnancy. N Engl J Med 2008;358: 1444–53.
93. Heslehurst N, Simpson H, Ells LJ, et al. The impact of maternal BMI status on pregnancy outcomes with immediate short-term obstetric resource implications: a meta-analysis. Obes Rev 2008;9:635–83.

CHAPTER 2

Psychological Aspects of Obesity in Women

D. Yvette LaCoursiere
University of California San Diego Medical Center, San Diego, California, USA

A growing body of evidence suggests that obese women experience more psychosocial stressors and psychological disorders than normal-weight women (Box 2.1). Numerous factors may co-exist between obesity and psychological problems, including life stressors, early traumatic events, socioeconomic/workforce factors, depression, anxiety, suicidal ideation, and stigmatization. Useful information that is relevant to the practicing obstetrician is limited in two ways: (1) the causal pathways by which obesity is associated with psychosocial stressors and mood disorders need elucidation, and (2) there is a paucity of data during pregnancy. Despite these limitations, inferences from non-pregnant women and emerging pregnancy data are available, and an understanding of the unique psychological challenges faced by obese women is essential to their successful clinical care. The issue of causality is important, but the current lack of a clearly defined causal pathway does not negate the significance or the validity of these associations. Observations that two events co-occur with increased frequency permit targeted and heightened surveillance. Using an anthropometric marker such as increased body mass index (BMI) to screen for associated psychosocial conditions facilitates identification and interventions that have the potential to improve psychological functioning in women and their children.

This chapter will describe the psychosocial aspects of obesity in women outside of and during pregnancy, and will offer pragmatic screening tools for use in clinical assessment during pregnancy.

Pregnancy in the Obese Woman, 1st edition. Edited by Deborah L. Conway.
© 2011 Blackwell Publishing Ltd.

> **Box 2.1 Psychosocial factors and disorders associated with obesity in women**
> - Psychosocial stressors
> - Early traumatic events
> - Socioeconomic/workforce
> - Depression/anxiety/suicide
> - Stigmatization

Psychosocial factors associated with obesity in women

Psychosocial stressors

In mechanics, stress is defined as an action on a body of any system of balanced forces whereby strain or deformation results [1]. Likewise, this definition has applicability in conceptualizing psychological stressors. Psychological stressors are often referred to as psychosocial stressors as they often occur in a social context. Repetitive or chronic events that challenge an individual without an adequate compensatory response have been associated with adverse medical and psychological well-being.

Psychosocial stressors affect health and well-being by eliciting a complex response in the neuroendocrine system. When appropriate, this prioritizes the responses of various organ systems to facilitate a physical or behavioral change that allows the individual to adapt to the stressor [2]. Over time, however, with frequent and chronic insults, a maladaptive response can develop. Chronic stress may tip the energy balance by hyperactivation of the hypothalamic–pituitary axis, leading to increased caloric intake and decreased physical activity, culminating in increased weight. It has been posited that this, in part, is mediated through depression. However, obesity itself may result in stigmatization [3,4], thus impairing an individual's ability to respond to stressful events and/or increasing depressive symptoms. The multiple potential causal pathways between stress, depression, and obesity complicate clinical research. As stressors, depression and obesity frequently co-exist, and it is difficult to study whether, for example, depression causes obesity, obesity causes depression, another factor is responsible for both diagnoses, or obesity and depression exacerbate each other. Attempts to address this cause-and-effect conundrum include using longitudinal designs to assess incidence and multivariable analyses to account for other covariates.

The association between psychosocial stress and weight gain has been reported in women with a baseline elevated BMI. A 9-year longitudinal study among nationally representative adults between age 25 and 74 years demonstrated that, in women who were obese at baseline, the presence of life stressors (such as job-related demands, difficulty paying bills, constraints in life, or relationship strains) were associated with weight gain. These women were also at increased risk for depression and anxiety [5]. These associations were not demonstrable in women who were normal weight or overweight at baseline. In a cohort of black women who were followed for more than a decade, there was an association of perceived stress at baseline and change in BMI. Although BMI went up across time regardless of baseline BMI category, there was a nearly one-third increase in the percentage of change in BMI in those with medium or high baseline stress compared to those with low levels. This association persisted after the inclusion of covariates in the model [6].

Both studies suggest that interventions that target long-term weight management/maintenance in adult women include components that reduce stress or improve coping. Clinicians caring for obese women must recognize the important role that stress can play in their patients' health, and must be ready to acknowledge and address these issues.

History of early traumatic events

Exposure to early traumatic events may predispose some women to obesity in adulthood. Vamosi et al. systematically reviewed the literature and concluded that seven of eight studies supported the hypothesis that abuse, lack of parental support, depression and anxiety disorders, and difficulty in school were correlated with adult obesity [7]. Additionally, in a 30-year cohort study, childhood emotional problems, low level of self-esteem, and external locus of control predicted weight gain in women [8]. Prospectively collected data on female childhood abuse victims showed that 42% of girls exposed to abuse were obese as adults compared to 28% of those not abused [9]. The abused girls exhibited a steeper trajectory of weight gain through childhood and into adulthood. Similarly, sub-threshold and full post-traumatic stress disorder in women predicted subsequent obesity, with an adjusted odds ratio of 3.0 (95% confidence interval 1.3–7.0) [10].

Again, the question of causality can be raised. This association may be mediated through poor psychological functioning, self-protective mechanisms, and hypothalamic–pituitary–adrenal axis dysregulation [11]. An additional possibility is that early trauma results in disordered eating, psychological disturbance, and subsequent obesity. Finally, coping with significant stressors might interfere with one's compliance with physical activity and nutrition recommendations [11].

Clinicians should be aware of the association between obesity and a history of abuse or trauma. Screening for abuse should be incorporated into well woman examinations and obstetric care, especially in obese women. However, given the proportion of women who will screen positive, providers will need to be aware of appropriate referral sources for those with active psychological sequelae from their abuse/trauma history.

Socioeconomic/workforce factors

Psychosocial and socioeconomic risk factors associated with obesity in women include low education level, unemployment, and problems at work [12]. In a population-based study of 73,531 adults, BMI was inversely associated with workforce participation in the week prior to completion of the survey, even after controlling for socioeconomic status and co-morbidities. There was a 6%, 15%, and 34% decrease in participation in adults with obesity class 1, 2, and 3, respectively, and unemployment and absenteeism were increased with obesity [13]. Providers should recognize that unemployment and difficulties at work may be additional stressors faced by obese women, stressing the importance of obtaining a complete psychosocial history.

Depression

Epidemiological data tend to support the association between obesity and depression in women, but not in men [14–17]. The treatment of both obesity and depression is more challenging when they co-exist. Data from an early National Health and Nutrition Examination Survey (NHANES) study demonstrated that obesity was associated with recent (past month) depression in women (Table 2.1). As the degree of obesity increased, the prevalence of major depression in the past month also rose – to over 13% of women with a BMI of greater than $40\,kg/m^2$, compared to 3.8% of normal-weight women [15]. After controlling for multiple covariates, the association remained especially strong in women with class 3 obesity. Recent analysis of the 2005–06 NHANES data supports the previous assessment severe obesity: compromised physical health, low income, young or middle age, and higher education were associated with a greater odds of depression in obese women [18]. Dixon et al. identified a similar trend in depression with increasing BMI, especially in women with poor body image. They also demonstrated a sustained improvement in depression with weight loss after weight-reduction surgery [16].

Extremes of socioeconomic status have been show to be risk factors for depression in obese women [17,18]. A recent study of 1,500 US adults attempted to assess whether the socioeconomic status disparities in diet quality and central adiposity were determined by depressive symptoms. In white women ($n = 396$), there was an inverse effect of socioeconomic status on central adiposity, which was explained in great part by depressive symptoms and unhealthy eating. In black women ($n = 607$), however, there was a positive association between depression and waist:hip ratio that was independent of a woman's socioeconomic status [19].

Table 2.1 Prevalence of DIS[†]/DSM-III[†] major depression in the past month, by relative body weight, in a study of the relation between obesity and depression, Third National Health and Nutrition Examination Survey, 1988–94

Relative body weight‡	No. of participants	% with DIS/DSM-III depression§		
		All respondents	Females	Males
Normal weight (BMI† 18.5–24.9)¶	4,154	2.79	3.82	1.67
Underweight (BMI < 18.5)	301	3.24	3.82	1.82
Overweight (BMI 25.0–29.9)	2,297	2.42	4.01	1.37
Obese (BMI ≥ 30)*	1,658	5.12	6.74	2.85
Obesity class 1 (BMI 30–34.9)	910	3.55	4.97	1.88
Obesity class 2 (BMI 35–39.9)	410	4.8	6.79	0.83
Obesity class 3 (BMI ≥ 40)**	267	12.51	13.03	11.54

*$p < 0.00001$ (x^2 test) for the risk of past-month major depression in the obese (body mass index ≥30) relative to those of normal weight when the four-category definition of relative body weight was used.
**$p < 0.00001$ (x^2 test) for the risk of past-month major depression in persons with class 3 obesity (body mass index ≥40) relative to those of normal weight when the six-category definition of relative body weight was used.
†DIS, Diagnostic Interview Schedule; DSM-III, *Diagnostic and Statistical Manual of Mental Disorders*, Third Edition; BMI, body mass index.
‡Based on body mass index (weight (kg)/height (m)²) and National Heart, Lung, and Blood Institute cutpoints.
§Depression was assessed by means of the Diagnostic Interview Schedule, using the criteria for major depression outlined in the *Diagnostic and Statistical Manual of Mental Disorders*, Third Edition (33).
¶Reference category.

Reproduced from Onyike et al. [15], with permission from Oxford University Press.

Researchers are trying to better understand the complex relationship between obesity and depression. While cross-sectional studies describe a modest univariate association between obesity and depression, this design does not permit an interpretation of causality [20]. One theory suggests that obesity is associated with stressors and stigmatization, which in turn impair one's psychosocial defenses, thus leading to depression. Conversely, depression can lead to uninhibited eating, weight gain, and resultant obesity. Data are available in support of both theories. The Alameda County Study, a prospective study of the association between obesity and depression, demonstrated a temporal relationship between the two, supporting the hypothesis that obesity contributes to the onset of depression [21]. Data exist that also support the opposite causal pathway. In a longitudinal study of women across ages 24, 27, and 30 years, obesity at baseline was associated with depression at the latter time points. Furthermore, depression predicted alcohol use, which was in turn associated with increased obesity in a subgroup of women [21]. More recent data suggest that central obesity increases the risk for depression and anxiety. Adjusting for BMI, activity, somatic disease, and isolation, an increased waist:hip ratio was associated with depression in women [22].

Several studies suggest that poor body image and eating disturbances predispose to depression in women [23,24], and there is preliminary evidence that depression in the obese is partially mediated through body image. Cultural pressures to be thin and stigmatization of obesity could contribute to decreased body satisfaction in the obese, which may lead to dysphoric mood. Friedman and colleagues performed a study of 177 obese men and women in a residential weight-loss facility. In this population of mainly Caucasian subjects, body image was related to BMI and depression. The researches assessed body image using the Multidimensional Body-Self Relations Questionnaire. Of the 14% of the variance in depression accounted for by BMI, half of the effect was due to two subscales: appearance evaluation, which measures the degree of overall satisfaction with one's appearance; and body areas satisfaction, which assesses specific body areas and creates a composite score to assess overall satisfaction [24].

In an interesting study, Murphy et al, set out to determine whether obese adults respond differently to episodes of depression compared to those of normal weight. In adults with a history of major depression, obese subjects were five times more likely than those of normal weight to overeat and gain weight during the depressive episode. They also experienced longer, more frequent events that were associated with increased suicidal ideation [25]. These data should persuade clinicians to heighten surveillance for suicidality and overeating among their depressed obese patients.

Other psychiatric disorders and suicide

Generalized anxiety disorder has likewise been associated with obesity in women. In a study of over 500 women followed for over 30 years, obesity at baseline was associated with a sixfold adjusted odds of meeting *Diagnostic and Statistical Manual of Mental Disorders*, 4th edition (DSM-IV) criteria for generalized anxiety disorder as assessed by a structured interview [26]. Cross-sectional studies also support this association [27].

In addition to depression and anxiety, other psychiatric disorders have been associated with obesity in adults. Mather and colleagues evaluated data from 2002 on nearly 37,000 adults from a cross-sectional nationally representative survey of Canadians. With a response rate of 77%, and 86% of interviews occurring in person, they inquired about mood using the World Mental Health Composite International Diagnostic Interview. This interview is used as a proxy to diagnosis mood, anxiety, and substance abuse disorders based on DSM-IV. After controlling for socioeconomic status and physical illnesses, mania, panic attacks, social phobias, and agoraphobia without panic disorder are all associated with a BMI of over $30\,kg/m^2$. Not surprisingly, this study also demonstrated an increase in suicidal ideation and suicide attempts associated with increased BMI, an association found to be stronger in women than in men [27].

Weight-based stigmatization

A discussion of the psychological aspects of obesity would be incomplete without acknowledging the weight-based stigmatization experienced by overweight and obese individuals. Employment, education, and healthcare are three arenas of reported bias and discrimination [3]. The psychological literature is replete with studies that experimentally alter the weight or image of a job applicant or manager to reveal that overweight and obese adults are viewed less favorably, are less likely to be recommended for hiring, and are seen as having less leadership potential [28,29]. Ten per cent of women aged 25–74 report discriminatory events based on weight and/or height. The percentage of women reporting discrimination increases significantly as BMI rises – normal BMI, 2%; overweight, 8.6%; moderate obesity, 20.6%; and severe obesity, 45.4% – with 60% of the events being associated with employment, followed by provision of services, and education [4]. These events are not without consequences. Poor mental health (including poor body image, depression, phobic anxiety, anxiety, and binge eating) is correlated with frequent stigmatizing events in individuals (mostly women) seeking weight-loss surgery [30]. These data may, however, be subject to recall bias, and further studies are needed to determine the causal pathway.

Healthcare providers, including physicians, exhibit negative biases towards obese patients. These data have been available for years, yet despite increased attention to the issue of obesity, new data continue to describe these stigmatizations. In a 2009 study of 238 patients and 40 physicians, higher patient BMI was negatively associated with physician-reported respect for the patient even after controlling for age and gender [31]. Obesity may also influence a physician's perception of whether a patient is compliant with medications. This association remained after adjusting for patient and physician characteristics [32]. Although we cannot conclude that prescribing practices are altered by these data, it suggests that obesity biases may interfere with patient care.

Pervasive biases in and out of the healthcare arena have the potential to adversely impact public health. Puhl and Heuer conceptualize the potential public health consequences of weight stigma as: (1) disregard for societal and environmental contributors to obesity; (2) impaired obesity prevention efforts; (3) increased health disparities; and (4) social inequalities that, when combined with the stigma experienced at the patient level, may result in increased morbidity and mortality. Collectively, clinicians impact the public's health, and thus should recognize the stigmatization faced by their obese patients from healthcare professionals, reflect on their own biases, and work toward creating a supportive and sensitive environment for obese women.

Special psychosocial considerations during pregnancy

Obesity and depression during pregnancy

Consequences of unrecognized and untreated depression on the mother and fetus include prolonged and more severe maternal symptoms and behavioral disorders in the child, making the identification of risk factors of depression in pregnancy vitally important [33,34]. As obesity and depression tend to co-occur in non-pregnant women, and a history of depression predisposes to depression during pregnancy and the postpartum period, an association between obesity and perinatal depression is plausible. Newer data are emerging in support of this association.

One of the first papers exploring this link evaluated the associations between BMI, eating attitudes, and depression and anxiety during pregnancy and at 4 and 14 months postpartum [35]. They concluded that, at 4 and 14 months postpartum, there is a relationship between BMI and symptoms of depression/anxiety. However, due to the small sample size, there was insufficient power to stratify the subjects by BMI. Furthermore, the use of a measure at 14 months after delivery that associates obesity with postpartum depression more likely reflects the association between obesity and depression rather that than with postpartum depression per se [35]. A study that evaluated depression and weight during pregnancy found that lower self-esteem and greater deviation from medically recommended ideal weight predicted third-trimester dysphoria in white inner-city women [36]. This study was also limited by sample size and did not address the patients' postpartum mood. A recent analysis of the negative psychological states associated with pre-gravid BMI showed depression to be one of six states associated with increasing BMI. The associative trend was seen across all strata (overweight, obese, severely obese), and severe obesity was strongly associated with depressive and anxiety symptoms, locus of control, perceived stress, powerful others, restrained eating and dieting, and weight cycling [37].

A cross-sectional population-based study using the Centers for Disease Control and Prevention's Pregnancy Risk Assessment Monitoring System demonstrated that extremes of pre-gravid BMI conferred a risk for self-reported depressive symptoms [38]. This study was limited in diagnostic precision of the classification of depressive symptoms and in controlling for potential covariates, but exhibited a nearly 50% increase in moderate or greater self-reported depressive symptoms in obese compared to normal-weight women.

With improved validation of the depression measures and controlling for multiple covariates, a study of over 1,000 predominantly Caucasian women, recruited immediately postpartum, demonstrated that pre-pregnancy BMI was associated with depressive symptoms as measured by a score of 12 or more on the Edinburgh Postnatal Depression Screen (EPDS) at 6–8 weeks postpartum [39]. The percentage of women screening positive was 14.4% in normal-weight women, with an increase in all other BMI strata: underweight, 18.0%; overweight, 18.5%; obese class 1, 18.8%; obese class 2, 32.4%; and obese class 3, 40.0%. After controlling for covariates, class 2 and class 3 obesity were strongly associated with screening positive for depression on the EPDS 6–8 weeks after delivery. This study included covariates of history of depression and maternal stressors. Partner-associated stress, both alone and when taken together with traumatic stressors, was also associated with screening positive for depression (adjusted odds ratio 2.6 and 8.5, respectively). Women being treated for depression were excluded from enrollment, but some of the enrolled women may have had antepartum depression that was untreated at the postpartum screen. Thus, the numbers may represent antecedent and postpartum depressive symptoms.

One study was identified showing no association between obesity and postpartum depression. In a secondary analysis of overweight and obese women enrolled in a behavioral trial to increase activity and lose weight, BMI group was not associated with depressed mood. This trial included women interested in participating in an intervention of 24 sessions over 9 months, and may have excluded women experiencing depressive symptoms by virtue of the requirements of the trial [40].

Obesity and quality of life during pregnancy

Publications on the influence of obesity on the quality of life during pregnancy are extremely limited. In 2008, 220 pregnant women were followed across pregnancy with the SF-12 Health Survey, a validated assessment of quality of life that provides a mental and physical summary [41]. The group was equally divided between obese and non-obese women. Whereas all women improved their mental summary score across gestation, obese women reported lower scores and similarly reported lower and worsening physical summary scores compared to normal-weight women [42]. Weight gain was also associated with lower physical summary scores.

Practical tools for the obstetric provider

The American Congress of Obstetricians and Gynecologists recommends that all women be screened for psychosocial risk factors during pregnancy, including assessment of barriers to care, unstable housing, unintended pregnancy, communication barriers, nutrition, tobacco use, substance abuse, depression, safety, intimate partner violence, and stress [43]. Given their increased likelihood of having co-existing psychosocial risk factors, obese women should be screened like all women, but they may benefit from heightened surveillance for abuse, depression, and anxiety during pregnancy and postpartum.

Screening for abuse during pregnancy

As many as one in six pregnant women report having experienced abuse "in the past year." Structured screening results in an increase in the ability to detect and refer women for supportive services [44]. McFarlane and colleagues created the Abuse Assessment Screen for the detection of physical violence against women during pregnancy [45]. It has been used in research and clinical practice, and is presented in Box 2.2.

Screening for depression during pregnancy and postpartum

The DSM-IV defines major depressive disorder (MDD) as the presence of five of the following symptoms (Box 2.3) [46], one of which must be depressed mood or decreased interest or pleasure: appetite disturbance – usually loss of appetite with weight loss; sleep disturbance – most often insomnia and fragmented sleep, even when the baby sleeps; physical agitation or psychomotor slowing; fatigue, decreased energy; feelings of worthlessness or excessive or inappropriate guilt; decreased concentration or ability to make decisions; and recurrent thoughts of death or suicidal ideation.

The definition of MDD is used during pregnancy, and if it occurs in the postpartum period is classified as "MDD with postpartum onset." Only the timing of the symptoms distinguishes the two disorders. In MDD with postpartum onset, symptoms must be present most of the day nearly every day for 2 weeks, and begin within 4 weeks after delivery. Some epidemiological studies use 3 months from delivery to define postpartum depression [47]. The time course and persistence of symptoms differentiate postpartum depression from "postpartum blues." Postpartum blues occurs in the majority of postpartum women. It lasts less than 2 weeks and does not interfere with functioning, whereas untreated postpartum depression can last 6 months [48].

Box 2.2 Abuse Assessment Screen (AAS)

1. Have you ever been emotionally or physically abused by your partner or someone
important to you? .... Yes   No

2. Within the last year, have you been hit, slapped, kicked or otherwise physically
hurt by someone? .... Yes   No

If yes, by whom? (Circle all that apply)

Husband   Ex-husband   Boyfriend   Stranger   Other   Multiple

Total number of times _____

3. Since you have been pregnant, have you been hit, slapped, kicked or otherwise
physically hurt by someone? .... Yes   No

If yes, by whom? (Circle all that apply)

Husband   Ex-husband   Boyfriend   Stranger   Others   Multiple

Number of times _____

Mark the area of injury on a body map

Score the most severe incident to the following scale:

   1 = Threats of abuse, including use of a weapon

   2 = Slapping, pushing; no injuries and/or lasting pain

   3 = Punching, kicking, bruises, cuts and/or continuing pain

   4 = Beaten up, severe contusions, burns, broken bones

   5 = Head, internal, and/or permanent injury

   6 = Use of weapon, wound from weapon

4. Within the past year, has anyone forced you to have sexual
activities? .... Yes   No

If yes, by whom? (Circle all that apply)

Husband   Ex-husband   Boyfriend   Stranger   Others   Multiple

Number of times _____

5. Are you afraid of your partner or anyone you listed above? .... Yes   No

Reproduced from McFarlane et al. [45], with permission from JAMA.

A smaller subgroup of women experience postpartum psychosis. One
or two women in 1,000 births suffer from this severe, debilitating psychiatric emergency [49]. These women experience delusions, hallucinations,
or both, and often have other associated mood disorders [33]. Bipolar
disease may also manifest itself during or after pregnancy, often for the
first time. This can pose a threatening situation if it presents with depressive symptoms, as treatment with antidepressants may exacerbate manic

---

Box 2.3 DSM-IV criteria for major depressive disorder

Five of the following, one of which must be marked*:

- Depressed mood*
- Decreased interest or pleasure*
- Loss of appetite
- Sleep disturbance
- Physical agitation or psychomotor slowing
- Fatigue, decreased energy
- Feelings of worthlessness or excessive or inappropriate guilt
- Decreased concentration or ability to make decisions
- Recurrent thoughts of death, suicidal ideation

---

symptoms. At the antepartum intake visit, any personal or family history of bipolar disorder and history of postpartum psychosis should be elicited. Women endorsing such a history are at increased risk for bipolar disorder in pregnancy. At our institution, we use the following two questions to screen for bipolar disease in women diagnosed with depression: "Have you ever had a time when you felt so happy or excited that you got into trouble, or your family or friends worried about it?" and "Has a clinician ever said you were manic?" Women answering yes to either question are then assessed for suicidal ideation and referred to psychiatry professionals. Women endorsing suicidal intentions are sent to the emergency department.

Several tools have been used to screen for depression in pregnancy including the Beck Depression Inventory, the Center for Epidemiologic Studies – Depression, and the EPDS (Box 2.4). The EPDS was developed in 1987 by Cox et al. to identify women with postpartum depression, and is the only screening test specifically tailored to account for events during pregnancy [50]. The instrument has been validated by the authors and other investigators. When using a scale cut-off of 12 out of 13, the authors report a sensitivity of 86%, a specificity of 78%, and a positive predictive value of 73% for diagnosing clinical depression [51]. Clinically appropriate cut-off points for screening positive are greater than or equal to 10 for mild depression and greater than or equal to 12 for moderate/severe depression. Multiple investigators throughout the world have confirmed the reliability and validity of the EPDS when administered to women of different races or ethnicities [52,53], and its use has also been validated during pregnancy [54].

The EPDS is scored on a 0–30 scale and is presented below. Each response is assigned a score of 0, 1, 2 , or 3. For questions 1, 2, and 4, the scores are

Box 2.4 Edinburgh Postnatal Depression Scale

As you have recently had a baby, we would like to know how you are feeling now. Please <u>underline</u> the answer which best describes how you have felt in the past 7 days, not just how you feel today. Here is an example, already completed:

I have felt happy:

   Yes, most the time

   <u>Yes, some of the time</u>

   No, not very often

   No, not at all

This would mean: "I have felt happy some of the time during the past week". Please complete the other questions in the same way.

In the past 7 days:

1. I have been able to laugh and see the funny side of things:

   As much as I always could

   Not quite so much now

   Definitely not so much now

   Not at all

2. I have looked forward with enjoyment to things:

   As much as I ever did

   Rather less than I used to

   Definitely less than I used to

   Hardly at all

*3. I have blamed myself unnecessarily when things went wrong:

   Yes, most of the time

   Yes, some of the time

   Not very often

   No, never

4. I have been anxious or worried for no good reason:

   No, not at all

   Hardly ever

   Yes, sometimes

   Yes, very often

*5. I have felt scared or panicky for no very good reason:

   Yes, quite a lot

   Yes, sometimes

   No, not much

   No, not at all

(Continued)

Box 2.4 *Continued*

*6. Things have been getting on top of me:

Yes, most of the time I haven't been able to cope at all

Yes, sometimes I haven't been coping as well as usual

No, most of the time I have coped quite well

No, I have been coping as well as ever

*7. I have been so unhappy that I have had difficulty sleeping:

Yes, most of the time

Yes, sometimes

Not very often

No, not at all

*8. I have felt sad or miserable:

Yes, most of the time

Yes, quite often

Not very often

No, not at all

*9. I have been so unhappy that I have been crying:

Yes, most of the time

Yes, quite often

Only occasionally

No, never

*10. The thought of harming myself has occurred to me:

Yes, quite often

Sometimes

Hardly ever

Never

Translations of the scale, and guidance as to its use, may be found in Cox, J.L. & Holden, J. (2003) *Perinatal Mental Health: A Guide to the Edinburgh Postnatal Depression Scale.* London: Gaskell.

assigned in that order, whereas for questions 3 and 5–10, the scores are assigned in reverse order (3, 2, 1, 0). The sum of scores is obtained for assessing risk. Women who screen positive for depression or who endorse suicidality (question 10) should be assessed by their obstetric provider at the time of assessment. Management of postpartum depression is dependent on the training and comfort of the obstetric provider. Providers may consider treating women with depression or referring to a psychiatrist and/or counselor. Women who endorse suicidality require immediate referral to a psychiatrist and may warrant emergency inpatient treatment.

Summary

While all women should be screened for commonly occurring stressors and mood disorders during pregnancy, it is important for the clinician to be aware that obese women have several psychological stressors and conditions that co-occur with greater frequency. Clinicians also should be aware of the existence of bias in the healthcare system and in healthcare providers toward obese patients. This awareness has the potential to improve surveillance and facilitate intervention. The research in this area has many lines of potential inquiry, including: better delineation of the causal pathways between obesity, stressors, and psychological conditions; evaluation of interventions that take into consideration theses covariates; and assessment of the long term outcomes in mother and child germane to these factors.

References

1. Stuebe AM, Oken E, Gillman MW. Associations of diet and physical activity during pregnancy with risk for excessive gestational weight gain. Am J Obstet Gynecol 2009;201(1):58 e1–8.
2. De Vriendt T, Moreno LA, De Henauw S. Chronic stress and obesity in adolescents: scientific evidence and methodological issues for epidemiological research. Nutr Metab Cardiovasc Dis 2009;19(7):511–19.
3. Puhl R, Brownell KD. Bias, discrimination, and obesity. Obes Res 2001;9(12): 788–805.
4. Puhl RM, Andreyeva T, Brownell KD. Perceptions of weight discrimination: prevalence and comparison to race and gender discrimination in America. Int J Obes (Lond) 2008;32(6):992–1000.
5. Block JP, He Y, Zaslavsky AM et al. Psychosocial stress and change in weight among US adults. Am J Epidemiol 2009;170(2):181–92.
6. Fowler-Brown AG, Bennett GG, Goodman MS, et al. Psychosocial stress and 13-year BMI change among blacks: the Pitt County Study. Obesity 2009;17(11):2106–9.

7. Vamosi M, Heitmann BL, Kyvik KO. The relation between an adverse psychological and social environment in childhood and the development of adult obesity: a systematic literature review. Obes Rev 2010;11(3):177–84.

8. Ternouth A, Collier D, Maughan B. Childhood emotional problems and self-perceptions predict weight gain in a longitudinal regression model. BMC Medicine 2009;7:46.

9. Noll JG, Zeller MH, Trickett PK, et al. Obesity risk for female victims of childhood sexual abuse: a prospective study. Pediatrics 2007;120(1):e61–7.

10. Perkonigg A, Owashi T, Stein MB, et al. Posttraumatic stress disorder and obesity: evidence for a risk association. Am J Prev Med 2009;36(1):1–8.

11. D'Argenio A, Mazzi C, Pecchioli L, et al. Early trauma and adult obesity: is psychological dysfunction the mediating mechanism? Physiol Behav 2009; 98(5):543–6.

12. Rosmond R, Bjorntorp P. Psychosocial and socio-economic factors in women and their relationship to obesity and regional body fat distribution. Int J Obes Relat Metab Disord 1999;23(2):138–45.

13. Klarenbach S, Padwal R, Chuck A, et al. Population-based analysis of obesity and workforce participation. Obesity (Silver Spring) 2006;14(5):920–7.

14. Carpenter KM, Hasin DS, Allison DB, et al. Relationships between obesity and DSM-IV major depressive disorder, suicide ideation, and suicide attempts: results from a general population study. Am J Public Health 2000;90(2):251–7.

15. Onyike CU, Crum RM, Lee HB, et al. Is obesity associated with major depression? Results from the Third National Health and Nutrition Examination Survey. Am J Epidemiol 2003;158(12):1139–47.

16. Dixon JB, Dixon ME, O'Brien PE. Depression in association with severe obesity: changes with weight loss. Arch Intern Med 2003;163(17):2058–65.

17. Stunkard AJ, Faith MS, Allison KC. Depression and obesity. Biol Psychiatry 2003;54(3):330–7.

18. Ma J, Xiao L. Obesity and depression in US Women: results from the 2005–2006 National Health and Nutritional Examination Survey. Obesity 2009;18(2):347–53.

19. Beydoun MA, Kuczmarski MT, Mason MA, et al. Role of depressive symptoms in explaining socioeconomic status disparities in dietary quality and central adiposity among US adults: a structural equation modeling approach. Am J Clin Nutr 2009; 90(4):1084–95.

20. Friedman MA, Brownell KD. Psychological correlates of obesity: moving to the next research generation. Psychol Bull 1995;117(1):3–20.

21. McCarty CA, Kosterman R, Mason WA, et al. Longitudinal associations among depression, obesity and alcohol use disorders in young adulthood. Gen Hosp Psychiatry 2009;31(5):442–50.

22. Rivenes AC, Harvey SB, Mykletun A. The relationship between abdominal fat, obesity, and common mental disorders: results from the HUNT study. J Psychosom Res 2009;66(4):269–75.

23. Stice E, Hayward C, Cameron RP, et al. Body-image and eating disturbances predict onset of depression among female adolescents: a longitudinal study. J Abnorm Psychol 2000;109(3):438–44.

24. Friedman KE, Reichmann SK, Costanzo PR, et al. Body image partially mediates the relationship between obesity and psychological distress. Obes Res 2002;10(1):33–41.

25. Murphy JM, Horton NJ, Burke JD, Jr., et al. Obesity and weight gain in relation to depression: findings from the Stirling County Study. Int J Obes (Lond) 2009;33(3): 335–41.

26. Kasen S, Cohen P, Chen H, et al. Obesity and psychopathology in women: a three decade prospective study. Int J Obes (Lond) 2008;32(3):558–66.

27. Mather AA, Cox BJ, Enns MW, et al. Associations of obesity with psychiatric disorders and suicidal behaviors in a nationally representative sample. J Psychosom Res 2009;66(4):277–85.

28. Klassen ML, Jasper CR, Harris RJ. The role of physical appearance in managerial decisions. J Bus Psychol 1993;8:181–98.

29. O'Brien KS, Latner JD, Halberstadt J, et al. Do antifat attitudes predict antifat behaviors? Obesity (Silver Spring) 2008;16(Suppl. 2):S87–92.

30. Friedman KE, Ashmore JA, Applegate KL. Recent experiences of weight-based stigmatization in a weight loss surgery population: psychological and behavioral correlates. Obesity (Silver Spring) 2008;16(Suppl. 2):S69–74.

31. Huizinga MM, Cooper LA, Bleich SN, et al. Physician respect for patients with obesity. J Gen Intern Med 2009;24(11):1236–9.

32. Huizinga MM, Bleich SN, Beach MC, et al. Disparity in physician perception of patients' adherence to medications by obesity status. Obesity 2010 18(10): 1932–7.

33. Miller LJ. Postpartum depression. JAMA 2002;287(6):762–5.

34. Grace SL, Evindar A, Stewart DE. The effect of postpartum depression on child cognitive development and behavior: a review and critical analysis of the literature. Arch Womens Ment Health 2003;6(4):263–74.

35. Carter AS, Baker CW, Brownell KD. Body mass index, eating attitudes, and symptoms of depression and anxiety in pregnancy and the postpartum period. Psychosom Med 2000;62(2):264–70.

36. Cameron RP, Grabill CM, Hobfoll SE, et al. Weight, self-esteem, ethnicity, and depressive symptomatology during pregnancy among inner-city women. Health Psychol 1996;15(4):293–7.

37. Laraia BA, Siega-Riz AM, Dole N, et al. Pregravid weight is associated with prior dietary restraint and psychosocial factors during pregnancy. Obesity (Silver Spring) 2009;17(3):550–8.

38. Anand KJ. Clinical importance of pain and stress in preterm neonates. Biol Neonate 1998;73(1):1–9.

39. LaCoursiere DY, Barrett-Connor E, O'Hara M, et al. The association of obesity and screening positive for postpartum depression. Br J Obstet Gynaecol; 2010;117: 1001–18.

40. Krause KM, Ostbye T, Swamy GK. Occurrence and correlates of postpartum depression in overweight and obese women: results from the active mothers postpartum (AMP) study. Matern Child Health J 2009;13(6):832–8.

41. Ware JE, Kesinski M, Keller SD. 12-item short form health survey: Construction of scales and preliminary test of reliability and validity. Medical Care 1996;34:220–33.

42. Amador N, Juarez JM, Guizar JM, et al. Quality of life in obese pregnant women: a longitudinal study. Am J Obstet Gynecol 2008;198(2):203 e1–5.

43. ACOG Committee Opinion No. 343: psychosocial risk factors: perinatal screening and intervention. Obstet Gynecol 2006;108(2):469–77.

44. Norton LB, Peipert JF, Zierler S, et al. Battering in pregnancy: an assessment of two screening methods. Obstet Gynecol 1995;85(3):321–5.

45. McFarlane J, Parker B, Soeken K, et al. Assessing for abuse during pregnancy. Severity and frequency of injuries and associated entry into prenatal care. JAMA 1992;267(23):3176–8.

46. Society AP. Diagnostic and statistical manual of mental disorders, 4th edn. Washington, DC: American Psychiatric Association, 1994.

47. Kendell RE, Chalmers JC, Platz C. Epidemiology of puerperal psychoses. Br J Psychiatry 1987;150:662–73.

48. Cunningham FG, Gant NF, Leveno KJ, et al. (eds). Williams' Obstetrics, 21st edn. New York: McGraw-Hill, 2001.

49. Gold LH. Women's mental health. Primary Care Clin Office Pract 2002;29(1): 27–41.

50. Cox JL, Holden JM, Sagovsky R. Detection of postnatal depression. Development of the 10-item Edinburgh Postnatal Depression Scale. Br J Psychiatry 1987;150:782–6.

51. Cox J, Holden J. Perinatal mental health: a guide to the Edinburgh Postnatal Depression Scale. London: Gaskell/Royal College of Psychiatrists, 2003.

52. Garcia-Esteve L, Ascaso C, Ojuel J, et al. Validation of the Edinburgh Postnatal Depression Scale (EPDS) in Spanish mothers. J Affect Disord 2003;75(1):71–6.

53. Berle JO, Aarre TF, Mykletun A, et al. Screening for postnatal depression. Validation of the Norwegian version of the Edinburgh Postnatal Depression Scale, and assessment of risk factors for postnatal depression. J Affect Disord 2003;76(1–3):151–6.

54. Murray D, Cox JL. Screening for depression during pregnancy. J Reprod Infant Psychol 1990;8:99–107.

CHAPTER 3

Preparing for Pregnancy: Special Considerations for the Obese Woman

Anne Lang Dunlop, Divya Narayan, and Vita Lam Mayes
Emory University School of Medicine, Atlanta, Georgia, USA

Overweight and obesity impact the probability of conception

Women who are overweight or obese may experience difficulties and delays in conceiving as excess adiposity is associated with reduced fecundity [1,2]. In fact, there is a dose-dependent relationship between increasing body fatness, as measured by increasing body mass index (BMI) and waist:hip ratio, and subfecundity (defined as time to pregnancy of over 12 months) [3,4]. A large-scale prospective study has found that the probability of conceiving in a given cycle is reduced by 8% for overweight and 18% for obese women, with an approximate doubling of these figures for nulliparas [5]. Cumulatively, this translates into approximately 3 months longer for overweight women to become pregnant and 9 months longer for obese women to become pregnant when compared to women of healthy weight.

Obesity decreases fecundity by a variety of mechanisms that disrupt the hypothalamus–pituitary–ovary axis, resulting in irregular menstrual cycles and anovulation. Obesity is characterized by hyperleptinemia, insulin resistance, and consequent hyperinsulinemia. Elevated leptin directly impairs ovarian functioning [6]. Hyperinsulinemia contributes to anovulatory infertility by increasing ovarian androgen secretion and by decreasing sex hormone-binding globulin levels, resulting in elevated concentrations of free estrogen [7,8]. Excess body fat also elevates free estrogen via the increased conversion of androgens to estrogens in peripheral adipose tissue [9].

The obesity-associated reduction in fecundity is not entirely due to anovulation. Reduced fecundity is observed even for obese women with regular menstrual cycles [5,10,11], suggesting the possibility of ova with

Pregnancy in the Obese Woman, 1st edition. Edited by Deborah L. Conway.

low fertilization potential, endometrial abnormalities interfering with implantation, or sociobiological factors. Obese individuals do not have sexual intercourse as frequently as those of healthy body weight, even when co-habiting [12].

The hormonal imbalance brought on by hyperinsulinemia can also contribute to polycystic ovarian syndrome (PCOS). PCOS affects an estimated 4–7% of women of reproductive age, and is a leading cause of infertility due to the chronic anovulation that accompanies the syndrome [13]. Although not all cases of PCOS are obesity-related, the prevalence of obesity is substantially elevated among women with PCOS, with estimates ranging from 30% to 75% in various populations. The measured increase in cases of PCOS in recent years has paralleled the increasing rate of obesity [13–15].

The stage of life during which obesity begins has reproductive consequences. Young adolescents who are obese tend to enter puberty earlier than their normal-weight counterparts. The early initiation of puberty, and its attendant early sexual development, can have psychosocial consequences. Early-maturing girls tend to initiate sexual activity at a younger age, and are more likely to be teased and have body image and self-esteem problems [16–18]. Early puberty has been shown to be a risk factor for self-reported depression in obese adolescents [3]. Obese adolescents also demonstrate increased rates of PCOS and subsequent fertility problems [19].

The negative effect of obesity on fecundity is not limited to natural reproduction, but also impacts the success of assisted reproductive technology (ART). Obese women undergoing ART require substantially higher doses of exogenous gonadotropins and experience retrieval of fewer oocytes and lower implantation and pregnancy rates [3,4,20–22]. Furthermore, the risks of spontaneous abortion and pregnancy complications (such as pre-eclampsia, gestational hypertension, and cesarean section) all progressively increase with severity of obesity among women undergoing ART, underscoring the importance of achieving weight loss prior to fertility treatment [21,23].

Importantly, the adverse effects of obesity on fecundity appear to be reversible. A minimal weight loss of 5–10% of initial body weight can achieve a 30% reduction in visceral adiposity [24], and is effective for induction of ovulation in obese women with and without PCOS [11,25–27]. Furthermore, minimal weight loss in obese women improves the chances of spontaneous conception and conception after fertility treatment [28,29]. In addition, weight loss prior to fertility treatment decreases the occurrence of spontaneous abortion [28]. Obese women who are planning to become pregnant should lose weight to improve their chances of natural conception and their response to fertility treatment should they need it, and to decrease the risk for adverse pregnancy outcomes.

Overweight and obesity impact pregnancy and child health outcomes

Elevated pre-pregnancy body weight is not only associated with numerous pregnancy complications, but also impacts fetal growth and development and the future health of the offspring (Box 3.1). These consequences are addressed in detail in subsequent chapters. In helping an overweight or obese patient prepare for pregnancy, it is essential that healthcare providers know not only the adverse outcomes that can happen, but also the strategies for preventing adverse outcomes from happening.

For example, a population-based cohort study among non-diabetic, obese women indicates that a modest pre-pregnancy weight loss of approximately 10 lb or greater decreases the incidence of gestational diabetes by approximately 37% [35]. Another population-based cohort demonstrates that, compared to women whose BMI changed between −1.0 and +1.0 units, the adjusted odds ratio for adverse pregnancy outcomes for women who gained 3.0 units or more between pregnancies is as follows: pre-eclampsia 1.78 (95% confidence interval [CI] 1.52–2.08), gestational hypertension 1.76 (95% CI 1.39–2.23), gestational diabetes 2.09 (95% CI

Box 3.1 Adverse consequences of maternal obesity [4,20,21,30–34]

Complications of pregnancy

Gestational diabetes

Gestational hypertension

Pre-eclampsia, eclampsia

Shoulder dystocia

Cesarean section

Adverse pregnancy outcomes

Spontaneous abortion

Intrauterine fetal death

Congenital anomalies, including neural tube defects

Indicated preterm birth

Macrosomia

Adverse child and later life health outcomes

Child, adolescent, and adult obesity

High blood pressure

Metabolic syndrome

Cardiometabolic complications later in life

1.68–2.61), cesarean delivery 1.32 (95% CI 1.22–1.44), stillbirth 1.63 (95% CI 1.21–2.21), and large for gestational age 1.87 (195% CI.72–2.04) [36]. These data underscore the importance of preconception weight loss for women who are overweight, as well as postpartum and interconception strategies to reduce postpartum weight retention.

Existing studies do not address women's knowledge of the risks associated with obesity in pregnancy or whether women's knowledge of the reproductive risks of obesity influences their health behaviors. However, there is evidence that a woman's intention to become pregnant is a powerful motivator to change health behaviors such as smoking and illicit drug use, exposure to environmental tobacco smoke, and folic acid supplementation [37]. Healthcare providers should counsel overweight and obese women about the elevated risks of infertility and adverse pregnancy and child outcomes should they become pregnant. Overweight and obese women who are planning to become pregnant may be especially motivated to change their eating and activity behaviors in preparation for pregnancy.

Recommended screening for overweight and obesity in clinical practice

In the USA, many women who are overweight or obese are unaware of their weight status. Misperception of weight status is particularly common among African-Americans, Mexican-Americans, and those of lower socio-economic status [38]. To ensure that overweight individuals are appropriately identified in the clinical setting, a number of organizations recommend regular screening for obesity. The United States Preventive Services Task Force (USPSTF) recommends that clinicians screen all adult patients for obesity using BMI, a summary index calculated by dividing the weight in kilograms by the square of height in meters [39].

BMI has become the accepted method of screening for overweight and obesity because it is easy to measure, non-invasive, highly reliable, and highly correlated with body fat mass [39,40]. BMI is, however, an imperfect proxy of body fatness. BMI can misclassify overweight individuals as being normal weight and vice versa. In particular, BMI does not take into account the higher mass of muscle compared to fat in heavily muscled individuals, which is inversely associated with mortality [39]. Additionally, BMI is age-dependent and does not account for the pattern of body fat distribution, an important independent risk factor for health outcomes. Ethnic origin and puberty also affect body fat distribution and alter the relationship between BMI and body fatness.

The Clinical Workgroup of the Select Panel on Preconception Care recommends that all women of reproductive age have their BMI calculated at least annually, and that overweight and obesity be addressed, whenever possible, prior to conception [41]. The American College of Obstetricians and Gynecologists (ACOG) recommends that healthcare providers measure each woman's BMI at least annually and review other medical, social, and family risks for subsequent mortality [42]. Medical conditions that may be co-morbid with obesity and confer an increased risk for subsequent mortality include coronary heart disease, type 2 diabetes, and sleep apnea. Any three or more of the following risk factors also confer an elevated risk for cardiovascular disease and mortality, and should be ascertained as part of the assessment of obese women: hypertension, cigarette smoking, high low-density lipoprotein level, impaired fasting glucose, and a family history of early cardiovascular disease.

Managing obesity for women of reproductive age

Recommendations for managing obesity
Adults in general
The USPSTF finds fair to good evidence that high-intensity counseling about diet, exercise, or both is an effective strategy for modest, sustained weight loss for those who are obese. A high-intensity intervention is defined as more than one person-to-person (individual or group) session per month for at least the first 3 months of the intervention. Moderate- or low-intensity counseling (defined as monthly intervention and anything less frequent, respectively) with behavioral interventions shows limited evidence for sustained weight loss in obese adults. Although the USPSTF does not find direct evidence that behavioral interventions lower mortality or morbidity from obesity, the modest weight loss resulting from it provides indirect evidence of health benefits [39].

The USPSTF concludes that the most effective interventions for weight loss are intensive interventions that combine nutrition education and diet and exercise counseling with behavioral strategies to help patients change their eating and activity patterns. The USPSTF recommends the "5 As" framework (Box 3.2) as a guide for behavioral counseling for weight loss because it has proved successful in changing health behaviors in other areas [39]. The American Medical Association recommends the stages of change model as adapted for overweight and obesity to help determine patient motivation and interest in weight loss and appropriately target counseling strategies [43]. "Lifestyle case management" approaches that include health education, support, and referrals to registered dietitians have also been shown to be effective and cost-effective [44].

Several key points should be kept in mind when delivering counseling and behavioral strategies to overweight and obese patients in order to

---

Box 3.2 Overview of the "5 As" behavioral intervention framework

Assess: Ask about eating and activity behaviors and factors affecting choices

Advise: Give clear, specific, and personalized behavior change advice, including information about personal health harms/benefits

Agree: Collaboratively select appropriate treatment goals and methods based on the patient's interest in and willingness to change the behavior

Assist: Using behavior change techniques (self-help and/or counseling), aid the patient in achieving agreed-upon goals by acquiring the skills, confidence, and social/environmental supports for behavior change, supplemented with adjunctive medical treatments when appropriate

Arrange: Schedule follow-up contacts (in person or by telephone) to provide ongoing assistance to adjust the treatment plan as needed, including referral to more intensive or specialized treatment

---

optimize results. First, there is a dose–response relationship between the degree of obesity and the risk for adverse health and reproductive consequences [37,45], and even modest weight loss has been shown to decrease health and reproductive risks. Second, the goal of exercise need not be cardiovascular fitness, but rather any type of physical activity where energy is expended to burn calories [45]. Third, an evidence-based review of obesity treatment suggests that we are most successful when treating obesity as a chronic relapsing condition, by using a chronic care model and employing specific behavioral strategies to support changes in eating and activity behaviors. Such strategies include goal-setting and self-monitoring, cognitive restructuring, and rewards for positive behavior [45]. Fourth, structured treatment programs that provide regular follow-up contact with the patient have been demonstrated to support greater patient compliance and long-term weight loss and maintenance [46].

Guidelines from the National Heart, Lung, and Blood Institute (NHLBI) recommend that weight loss therapy be initiated for adults with:

- a BMI greater than $30 \, \text{kg/m}^2$

or

- a BMI of $25–29.9 \, \text{kg/m}^2$ *or* a high-risk waist circumference (more than 35 inches for women and over 40 inches for men) *and* two or more risk factors:
  - hypertension;
  - cigarette smoking;

○ high low-density lipoprotein cholesterol levels;
○ low high-density lipoprotein cholesterol levels;
○ impaired fasting glucose tolerance;
○ a family history of early cardiovascular disease.

The NLHBI guidelines recommend a goal of decreasing body weight by 10% of the baseline weight at a rate of 1–2 lb per week for 6 months in order to have realistic and achievable effects on health outcomes [47]. To achieve this, the NHLBI recommends that obese individuals decrease their caloric intake by 500–1,000 kcal per day from their usual intake. While caloric restriction as low as 800 kcal per day should be part of the weight loss strategy, extreme low-calorie diets of less than 800 kcal per day have not been shown to be any more effective after 1 year, and because of extreme health consequences, they are not recommended [47].

Both the USPSTF and NHLBI recommend that pharmacological treatment of obesity be used only as part of a program that includes intensive dietary and physical activity counseling and behavioral interventions [39,47]. Specifically, NHLBI recommends that the pharmacological management of obesity should only be considered for those with a BMI of 30 kg/m² or over, or one of 27 kg/m² or more with obesity-related diseases (such as cardiovascular disease, type 2 diabetes, or sleep apnea) or risk factors for cardiovascular disease (hypertension, cigarette smoking, high low-density lipoprotein cholesterol, low high-density lipoprotein cholesterol, impaired fasting glucose, family history of early cardiovascular disease). The NHLBI recommend that bariatric surgery be reserved for patients who have a BMI of 40 kg/m² or more, or a BMI of 35–39.9 kg/m² who have at least one other obesity-related illness, and only when all other less invasive options have not been successful [47].

Similarly, the American College of Physicians recommends a doctor–patient discussion weighing the risks and benefits of pharmacotherapy for obese patients who fail to achieve their weight loss goals with lifestyle modifications alone [40]. The American College of Physicians offers an algorithm for the clinical management of obesity for patients with a BMI of 30 kg/m² or over (Figure 3.1) [40].

Recommendations for women of reproductive age

Achieving weight loss and appropriate nutrient intake before pregnancy has been shown in well-designed studies to improve pregnancy outcomes for obese women and their offspring [36,48]. Weight loss during pregnancy is not advisable for women irrespective of pre-pregnancy weight status [42]. Thus, weight loss interventions must occur *prior to* pregnancy to minimize the risks of obesity on pregnancy-related outcomes.

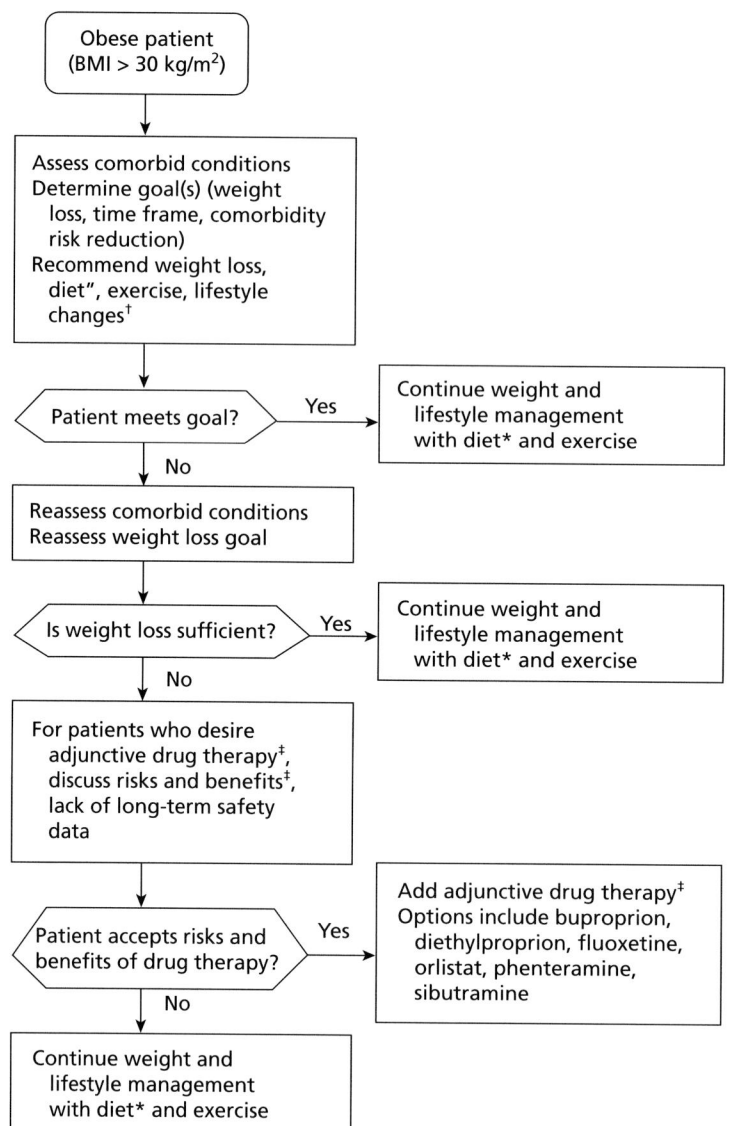

Figure 3.1 Algorithm for managing obesity. (Reproduced from Snow et al. [40] with permission from the American College of Physicians.)

The Clinical Workgroup of the Select Panel on Preconception Care and the ACOG Clinical Practice Bulletin for the care of obese women both recommend that women of reproductive age with a BMI greater than 26 kg/m² receive counseling about the risk being overweight or obese poses to their health, fertility, and pregnancy outcomes [41,42]. The recommendations also stress that women who are overweight or obese should be offered intensive behavioral strategies to decrease caloric intake and increase physical activity, and be encouraged to enroll in structured weight loss programs as these behavioral programs are most likely to result in sustained weight loss [41,42].

Special considerations in managing obesity for women of reproductive age

Post-partum weight retention

Post-partum weight retention is an important contributor to excessive body weight for women of reproductive age. Post-partum weight retention is more likely to occur in minority and low-income women [49,50], especially those who are overweight or obese prior to pregnancy [51]. Additionally, overweight and obese women are less likely to lose pregnancy-related weight without the support of a formal intervention [49,52]. Thus, interconception weight loss interventions may be especially important for overweight women.

Nutrition considerations for women of reproductive age

The lower the caloric content of a diet, the more likely it is to be low in essential nutrients. Diets less than 1,200 kcal per day are likely to require vitamin and mineral supplementation. Even diets with greater than 1,200 kcal per day may necessitate supplementation with calcium, folic acid, and vitamin D for most women of reproductive age, given the difficulty in meeting the recommended dietary intakes for these nutrients through diet alone. Currently, the recommended intake of calcium for women between 19 and 50 years of age is 1,000 mg/day. Overweight and obese women are more likely to be lacking in folic acid and vitamin D, and deficiencies of these vitamins have important reproductive consequences [53–55].

Obese women are less likely to supplement with folic acid prior to pregnancy and ingest less folate through food sources [54]. Even after controlling for intake of folate for women of reproductive age, elevated BMI is associated with lower serum folate concentrations [56,57]. Women who chronically diet are also at increased risk for folic acid deficiency [56]. Deficiency of folic acid during the periconception period is definitively associated with an increased risk for neural tube defects and other congenital anomalies. A recent meta-analysis finds that neural tube defects and other congenital anomalies are twice as common among women who are obese [33]. Existing studies have not evaluated whether the 400 µg dosage of folic supplementation recommended for all women of reproductive age [58] is sufficient to prevent neural tube defects for obese women or whether a higher dosage is needed. Nor have any major US professional organizations issued formal recommendations that focus on the special needs for preconception folic acid among overweight or obese women. Until research to establish the optimum dosage of folic acid for overweight and obese women is available, it is especially important to counsel women of reproductive age who are overweight or obese to achieve the recommendation of 400 μg folic acid daily through supplementation.

Overweight and obese individuals commonly have a poorer vitamin D status than do those of healthy weight [59,60], possibly due to the sequestration of the vitamin in adipose tissue [61] and its lower dietary intake [62]. Pre-pregnancy obesity predicts poor vitamin D status for the woman during her pregnancy and for her birthed infant, with an evident dose–response trend [55]. Poor vitamin D status during the pregnancy is linked with pre-eclampsia [63] and intrauterine growth restriction [64], as well as health problems in the offspring including rickets and other skeletal problems, type 1 diabetes, and asthma [65,66]. The American College of Obstetricians and Gynecologists recommends a daily consumption of 400–800 IU of vitamin D [67]. Existing studies have not evaluated whether this dosage is adequate for overweight and obese women. Furthermore, there are no studies that evaluate whether obese pregnant women and their offspring benefit from screening for vitamin D deficiency and high-dose vitamin D supplementation before or during pregnancy. However, given the increased likelihood of poor vitamin D status among overweight and obese women, clinicians should be aware of other risk factors for vitamin D deficiency (including darkly pigmented skin and low exposure to ultraviolet light) and should pay particular attention to educating overweight and obese women of reproductive age of the importance of achieving 400–800 IU vitamin D daily through dietary or supplement sources [68].

Nutrition during pregnancy for overweight and obese women is discussed in Chapter 9.

Pharmacological considerations for women of reproductive age

The pharmacological treatment of obesity should be part of a program that includes lifestyle modification. Pharmacological treatment of obesity is reserved for those with a BMI of 27.0–29.9 kg/m² or a high waist circumference and two or more risk factors, or those with a BMI of 30 kg/m² or greater regardless of risk factors [40,47]. The American College of Physicians recommends that for obese patients who choose adjunctive drug therapy, options include sibutramine, orlistat, phentermine, diethlpropion, fluoxetine, and bupropion. The choice of agent depends upon the side effect profiles of each drug and the patient's co-morbidities and tolerance for particular side effects [40]. According to a meta-analysis, the pooled amounts of weight loss is 4.45 kg (9.8 lb) at 12 months for sibutramine, 2.89 kg (6.4 lb) at 12 months for orlistat, 3.6 kg (7.9 lb) at 6 months for phentermine, 3.0 kg (6.6 lb) at 6 months for diethylpropion,

Table 3.1 Medications for weight loss

Medication	Mechanism of action	Food and Drug Administration class	Special concerns
Orlistat	Lipase inhibitor that blocks the absorption of fat	B	Potential for reducing the absorption of fat-soluble vitamins
Sibutramine	Norepinephrine and serotonin reuptake inhibitor that suppresses appetite	C	Modest increase in heart rate and blood pressure
Phentermine	Sympathomimetic amine that suppresses appetite	C	Tachycardia, palpitations, elevated blood pressure
Diethylpropion	Sympathomimetic amine that suppresses appetite	C	Tachycardia, palpitations, elevated blood pressure
Fluoxetine	Serotonin reuptake inhibitor that suppresses appetite	C	Agitation, nervousness
Bupropion	Unknown mechanism of action; suppresses appetite	C	Agitation, nervousness

3.15 kg (6.9 lb) at 12 months for fluoxetine, and 2.8 kg (6.2 lb) at 12 months for buproprion. There is no evidence for increased weight loss with combination therapy. There are no data about weight regain after medications are withdrawn [40].

To date, the Food and Drug Administration has approved only two medications for the long-term pharmacological treatment of obesity and morbid obesity: orlistat and sibutramine (Table 3.1). Both of these drugs have been evaluated in multiple randomized controlled trials, which have shown that, combined with lifestyle modification, they are more effective than placebo with lifestyle modification in promoting and maintaining weight loss [69,70]. Orlistat is a pancreatic lipase inhibitor that inhibits absorption of up to 30% of dietary fat. Steatorrhea, bloating and distention, and anal leakage are all potential side effects if dietary intake of fat is not restricted. Vitamin deficiencies, particularly of the fat-soluble vitamins (A, D, E, and K), are also of concern. Sibutramine is a centrally acting serotonin and adrenergic reuptake inhibitor. Hypertension and increased heart rate are risks of sibutramine, which is contradicted in individuals with known heart disease, uncontrolled hypertension, heart failure, stroke, and arrhythmias. Sibutramine is also contradicted in those who are taking monoamine oxidase inhibitors and other serotonin uptake inhibitors, including medications for depression and migraines.

Two drugs that are approved by the FDA for up to 3 months are phentermine and diethylpropion, which are sympathomimetic anorexogenic agents [69]. Side effects include insomnia, constipation, dry mouth, and hypertension, and thus these agents are contraindicated in people with cardiovascular disease, uncontrolled hypertension, hyperthyroidism, glaucoma, and agitated states. Prolonged use followed by abrupt withdrawal of sympathomimetics such as these may be cause for extreme fatigue and depression.

Orlistat is a pregnancy category B drug; controlled animal studies do not indicate risks to the fetus, but no adequate studies have been performed on pregnant women. Sibutramine, phentermine, and diethylpropion are pregnancy category C drugs, and generally should not be used in pregnancy [69]. Women who are attempting to lose weight with these medications should use an appropriate form of contraception while taking the medications to avoid exposure of the conceptus during the embryonic period when they might not even realize they are pregnant.

Insulin-sensitizing drugs such as metformin, although not approved for weight loss, can be a useful adjunct to lifestyle modification in achieving weight loss, particularly for women who anticipate becoming pregnant. Substantial data support the safety of metformin use in the first trimester of pregnancy [71,72]. Studies of large numbers of women with and without PCOS demonstrate a consistent and long-standing beneficial effect of metformin upon weight loss [73–76]. Metformin also seems to have a positive effect upon lipid profiles and insulin levels [76,77]. Studies support that high-dose metformin [2,550 mg per day) results in more pronounced reductions in BMI when compared to low-dose metformin (<1500 mg per day) without increased drop-out rates from gastrointestinal side effects [76].

Metformin also has documented beneficial effects upon fertility for women with PCOS. A systematic review confirms that metformin is effective for ovulation induction in women with PCOS [77,78]. An RCT comparing metformin and placebo, metformin and clomiphene, and clomiphene and placebo in women with PCOS showed more weight loss in women treated with metformin [79].

Two antidepressants, fluoxetine and bupropion, although not approved as weight loss adjuvants, also show some evidence for effectiveness in improving weight loss outcomes. Overweight and obese women with depressive symptoms may be especially appropriate for treatment with these medications. However, both fluoxetine and bupropion are pregnancy category C medications, so relative benefits and risks as well as the ideal timing of a pregnancy should be discussed with patients [40].

Surgical considerations for women of reproductive age

Bariatric surgery has become an increasingly common treatment option for morbidly obese women (BMI > 40 kg/m^2) whose obesity is refractory to medical management. A more complete discussion of bariatric surgery can be found in Chapters 4 and 5.

Contraceptive considerations for obese women of reproductive age

Given the benefits of achieving weight loss prior to conception, it is important to provide overweight women with safe and effective contraceptive methods to help them delay pregnancy until weight reduction has been achieved. For overweight and obese women, there are three principle considerations in selecting a contraceptive method. First, the efficacy of some hormonal contraceptive methods is adversely affected by elevated BMI. Second, some hormonal methods of contraception are linked with weight gain, with the potential to decrease fecundity and increase risks of adverse pregnancy outcomes. Third, obesity increases the risks of adverse health effects associated with some contraceptive methods [80]. Because of the associated risk for thromboembolism with combined hormonal contraceptive methods, the decreased efficacy and potential risks of weight gain for some hormonal contraceptive methods, and potential delays in return to ovulation with depot preparations, barrier methods may be a good choice during the preconception period. A discussion of contraceptive considerations for obese women is found in Chapter 14.

Barriers to physician management of obesity

Given that obesity is a chronic condition requiring ongoing management, and that obese individuals are at increased risks for weight-related co-morbidities, access to quality healthcare is essential. Unfortunately, substantial research finds numerous barriers to the receipt of healthcare services by obese individuals, including the lack of adequately trained healthcare providers, effective obesity treatments and approaches, and health insurance coverage of treatments as well as attitudes and beliefs of healthcare professionals [81]. Identifying and addressing barriers to the receipt of appropriate healthcare services by obese individuals, as well as the attitudes of healthcare providers, is essential for patients to make the necessary lifestyle changes for achieving and sustaining weight loss.

Surveys document that healthcare providers feel a sense of futility in treating obese patients and that their advice and counseling are unlikely to contribute to improvements in eating and activity behaviors and body weight [82,83]. Also, numerous studies document that healthcare providers possess negative stereotypes about and attitudes toward obese patients, including that obese patients are non-compliant, lazy, undisciplined, and have low will power [84].

The negative perceptions of healthcare providers about obesity translate into suboptimal healthcare services. Healthcare providers spend less time with overweight and obese patients [85,86]. These attitudes do not go unnoticed by obese patients, who indicate that they feel disrespected by providers, perceive that they will not be taken seriously due to their weight, and report that their weight is blamed for all of their medical problems, and that they are reluctant to address their weight concerns with their healthcare providers [87–89]. In fact, healthcare-seeking behavior for other health services and conditions is also affected by obesity. For example, obese women are less likely to undergo routine gynecological cancer screening [89] and age-appropriate preventive cancer screenings [90–93].

Importantly, it is established that physicians who are better prepared to counsel their patients about weight management may be more likely to provide effective obesity prevention and management services [82]. Effective approaches to weight management counseling include assessing a patient's readiness to change by investigating reasons and motivations for weight loss, previous weight loss attempted, expected social support, attitudes toward diet and activity, and potential barriers and limitations. Additionally, patients' chances of succeeding in their weight loss attempts are increased by physicians being sensitive and empathic to patients' concerns, conveying confidence that the patient can succeed, providing advice regarding specific steps the patient can make in the attempt to lose weight, and writing lifestyle prescriptions for physical activity and eating behaviors [39,47,94]. In fact, research supports that when physicians show empathy, patients are more likely to increase their levels of physical activity in an attempt to lose weight, and that the use of motivational interviewing as part of the encounter also increases patients' attempts to lose weight [95].

References

1. Franks S. Genetic and environmental origins of obesity relevant to reproduction. Reprod Biomed Online 2006;12:5526–31.
2. Pasquali R, Gambineri A. Metabolic effects of obesity on reproduction. Reprod Biomed Online 2006;12:5542–51.
3. Lash MM, Armstrong A. Impact of obesity on women's health. Fertil Steril 2009;91: 1712–16.
4. Siega-Riz AM, King JC, Siega-Riz AM, et al. Position of the American Dietetic Association and American Society for Nutrition: obesity, reproduction, and pregnancy outcomes. J Am Diet Assoc 2009;109:918–27.
5. Gesink Law D, Maclehose R. Obesity and time to pregnancy. Hum Reprod 2007;22: 313–16.
6. Mosochos S, Chan J. Leptin and reproduction: a review. Fertil Steril 2002;77: 433–44.
7. Pasquali R, Pelusi C. Obesity and reproductive disorders in women. Hum Reprod Update 2003:9;359–72.

8. Haslam D, James W. Obesity. Lancet 2005;366:1197–209.

9. Pralong F, Castillo E. Obesity and the reproductive axis. Ann Endocrinol 2002;63: 129–34.

10. Yilmaz N, Kilic S, Kanat-Pektas M, et al. The relationship between obesity and fecundity. J Womens Health 2009;18:633–6.

11. Jensen T, Scheike T. Fecundability in relation to body mass and menstrual cycle patterns. Epidemiology 1999;10:422–8.

12. Brody S. Slimness is associated with greater intercourse and lesser masturbation frequency. J Sex Marital Ther 2004;30:251–61.

13. Ehrmann DA. Polycystic ovary syndrome. N Engl J Med 2005;352:1223–36.

14. Gambineri A, Pelusi C, Vicennati C, et al. Obesity and the polycystic ovary syndrome. Int J Obes Relat Metab Disord 2002;26:883–96.

15. Cnattinguis S, Bergstrom R, Lipworth L, et al. Prepregnancy weight and the risk of adverse pregnancy outcomes. N Engl J Med 1998;338:147–52.

16. Phinney VG, Jensen LC, Olsen JA, et al. The relationship between early development and psychosexual behaviors in adolescent females. Adolescence 1990;25:321–32.

17. Sonis WA, Comite F, Blue J, et al. Behavior problems and social competence in girls with true precocious puberty. J Pediatr 1985;106:156–60.

18. Graber J, Lewinsohn PH, Seeley JR, et al. Is psychopathology associated with the timing of pubertal development? J Am Acad Child Adolesc Psychiatry 1997;36:1768–76.

19. Schuster DP. Changes in physiology with increasing fat mass. Semin Pediatr Surg 2009;18:126–35.

20. Yogev Y, Visser GH, Yogev Y, et al. Obesity, gestational diabetes and pregnancy outcome. Semin Fetal Neonatal Med 2009;14:77–84.

21. Arendas K, Qiu Q, Gruslin A, et al. Obesity in pregnancy: pre-conceptional to postpartum consequences. J Obstet Gynaecol Can 2008;30:477–88.

22. Grainger DA, Frazier LM, Rowland CA, et al. Preconception care and treatment with assisted reproductive technologies. Matern Child Health J 2006;10:S161–4.

23. Dokras A, Baredziak L, Blaine J, et al. Obstetric outcomes after in vitro fertilization in obese and morbidly obese women. Obstet Gynecol 2006;108:61–9.

24. Despres JP, Lemieux I, Prud'homme D. Treatment of obesity: need to focus on high risk abdominally obese patients. Br Med J 2001;322:716–20.

25. Moran L, Norman R. The obese patient with infertility: a practical approach to diagnosis and treatment. Nutr Clin Care 2002;5:6290–7.

26. Norman R, Naokes M, Wu R, et al. Improving reproductive performance in overweight/obese women with effective weight management. Hum Reprod Update 2004;10:3267–80.

27. Saleh AM, Khalil HS. Review of non-surgical and surgical treatment and the role of insulin-sensitizing agents in the management of infertile women with polycystic ovarian syndrome. Acta Obstet Gynecol Scand 2004;83:614–21.

28. Clark AM, Thornley B, Tomlinson L, et al. Weight loss in obese infertile women results in improvement in reproductive outcome for all forms of fertility treatment. Hum Reprod 1998;13:1502–5.

29. Clark AM, Ledger W, Galletly C, et al. Weight loss results in significant improvement in pregnancy and ovulation rates in anovulatory obese women. Hum Reprod 1995;10:2705–12.

30. Goldenberg RL, Culhane JR, Iams JD, et al. Epidemiology and causes of preterm birth. Lancet 2008;371:75–84.

31. Salihu HM, Lynch O, Alio AP, et al. Obesity subtypes and risk of spontaneous versus medically indicated preterm births in singletons and twins. Am J Epidemiol 2008;168: 13–20.

32. Stotland NE, Stotland NE. Obesity and pregnancy. Br Med J 2008;337:a2450.

33. Stothard JJ, Tennant PW. Maternal overweight and obesity and the risk of congenital anomalies: a systematic review and meta-analysis. JAMA 2009;301:636–50.

34. Oken E, Gillman MW. Fetal origins of obesity. Obes Res 2003;11:496–506.

35. Glazer NL, Hendrickson AF, Schellenbaum GD, et al. Weight change and the risk of gestational diabetes in obese women. Epidemiology 2004;15:733–7.

36. Villamor E, Cnattingius S. Interpregnancy weight change and risk of adverse pregnancy outcomes: a population-based study. Lancet 2006;368:1164–70.

37. Dott M, Rasmussen SA, Hogue CJ, et al. Association between pregnancy intention and reproductive health related behaviors before and after pregnancy recognition, National Birth Defects Prevention Study, 1997–2002. Matern Child Health J 2010;14:373–81.

38. Dorsey RR, Eberhardt MS, Ogden CL. Racial/ethnic differences in weight perception. Obesity 2009;17:790–5.

39. US Preventive Services Task Force. Screening and interventions for obesity in adults: Summary of the evidence for the U.S. Preventive Services Task Force. Ann Intern Med 2003;139:933–40.

40. Snow V, Barry P, Fitterman N, et al. Pharmacologic and Surgical Management of Obesity in Primary Care: a clinical practice guideline from the American College of Physicians. Ann Intern Med 2005;142:525–31.

41. Moos MK, Dunlop AL, Jack BW, et al. Healthier women, healthier reproductive outcomes: recommendations for the routine care of all women of reproductive age. Am J Obstet Gynecol 2008;199:S280–9.

42. The role of the obstetrician–gynecologist in the assessment and management of obesity. ACOG Committee Opinion No. 319. American College of Obstetricians and Gynecologists. Obstet Gynecol 2005;106:895–6.

43. Kushner RF. Roadmaps for clinical practice: Case studies in disease prevention and health promotion assessment and management of adult obesity: a primer for physicians. Chicago: American Medical Association, 2003.

44. Wolf AM, Siadaty M, Conaway MR, et al. Effects of lifestyle intervention on health care costs: improving control with activity and nutrition (ICAN). J Am Diet Assoc 2007;107:1365–73.

45. Orzano AJ, Scott JG. Diagnosis and treatment of obesity in adults: an applied evidence-based review. J Am Board Fam Med 2004;17:359–69.

46. Perri MG, Sears SF, Clark JE. Strategies for improving maintenance of weight loss: toward a continuous care model of obesity management. Diabetes Care 1993;16: 100–9.

47. National Institutes of Health, National Heart, Lung, and Blood Institute. Clinical guidelines on the identification, evaluation, and treatment of overweight and obesity in adults: the evidence report. Obes Res 1998;6:51S–209S.

48. Atalah E, Castro R. Maternal obesity and reproductive risk. Rev Med Chil 2004;132: 923–30.

49. O'Toole ML, Sawicki MA, Artal R. Structured diet and physical activity prevent postpartum weight retention. J Womens Health 2003;12:991–8.

50. Chang MW, Nitzke S, Guilford E, et al. Motivators and barriers to healthful eating and physical activity among low-income overweight and obese mothers. J Am Diet Assoc 2008;108:1023–8.

51. Krummel DA. Postpartum weight control: a vicious cycle. J Am Diet Assoc 2007;107: 37–40.

52. Gore SA, Brown DM, West DS. The role of postpartum weight retention in obesity among women: a review of the evidence. Ann Behav Med 2003;26:149–59.

53. Shepherd AA, Shepherd AA. Nutrition through the life-span. Part 1: Preconception, pregnancy and infancy. Br J Nurs 2008;17:1261–8.

54. Case AP, Ramadhani TA, Canfield MA, et al. Folic acid supplementation among diabetic, overweight, or obese women of childbearing age. J Obstet Gynecol Neonatal Nurs 2007;36:335–41.

55. Bodnar L, Simhan H, Powers R, et al. High prevalence of vitamin D insufficiency in black and white pregnant women residing in the northern United States and their neonates. J Nutr 2007;137:447–52.

56. Ortega RM, Lopez-Sobaler AM, Andres P, et al. Changes in folate status in overweight/obese women following two different weight control programmes based on increased consumption of vegetables or fortified breakfast cereals. Br J Nutr 2006;96:712–18.

57. Mojtabai R. Body mass index and serum folate in childbearing age women. Eur J Epidemiol 2004;19:1029.

58. Agency for Healthcare Research and Quality. Folic acid supplementation to prevent neural tube defects. US Preventive Services Task Force. Rockville, MD: Agency for Healthcare Research and Quality, 2008.

59. McGill AT, Stewart JM, Lithander FE, et al. Relationships of low serum vitamin D3 with anthropometry and markers of the metabolic syndrome and diabetes in overweight and obesity. Nutr J 2008;7:4.

60. Arunabh S, Pollack S, Yeh J, et al. Body fat content and 25-hydroxyvitamin D levels in healthy women. J Clin Endocrinol Metab 2003;88:157–61.

61. Wortsman J, Matsuoka LY, Chen TC, et al. Decreased bioavailability of vitamin D in obesity. Am J Clin Nutr 2000;72:690–3.

62. Rajakumar K, Fernstrom JD, Holick MF, et al. Vitamin D status and response to Vitamin D(3) in obese vs. non-obese African American children. Obesity 2003;16:90–5.

63. Bodnar LM, Catov JM, Simhan HS, et al. Maternal vitamin D deficiency increases the risk of preeclampsia. J Clin Endocrinol Metab 2007;92:3517–22.

64. Morley R, Carlin JB, Pasco JA, et al. Maternal 25-hydroxyvitamin D and parathyroid hormone concentrations and offspring birth size. J Clin Endocrinol Metab 2006;91: 906–12.

65. Holick MF. Resurrection of vitamin D deficiency and rickets. J Clin Invest 2006; 116:2062–72.

66. McGrath J. Does "imprinting" with low prenatal vitamin D contribute to the risk of various adult disorders? Med Hypotheses 2001;56:367–71.

67. American College of Obstetricians and Gynecologists. Osteoporosis. ACOG Practice Bulletin 50. Washington, DC: American College of Obstetricians and Gynecologists, 2004.

68. Gardiner PM, Nelson L, Shellhaas CS, et al. The clinical content of preconception care: nutrition and dietary supplements. Am J Obstet Gynecol 2008;199:S345–56.

69. Li Z, Magione M, Tu W, et al. Meta-analysis: pharmacologic treatment of obesity. Ann Intern Med 2005;142:532–46.

70. Avenell A, Broom J, Brown TJ, et al. Systematic review of the long-term effects and economic consequences of treatments for obesity and implications for health improvement. Health Technol Assess 2004;8:1–182.

71. Practice Committee of the American Society for Reproductive Medicine. Obesity and reproduction: an educational bulletin. Fertil Steril 2008;90:S21–9.

72. Gilbert C, Valois M, Koren G. Pregnancy outcome after first trimester exposure to metformin: a meta-analysis. Fertil Steril 2006;86:658–63.

73. Lilja AE, Mathiesen ER. Polycystic ovary syndrome and metformin in pregnancy. Acta Obstet Gynecol Scand 2006;86:861–8.

74. Knowler WC, Barrett-Connor E, Fowler SE, et al. Diabetes Prevention Program Research Group. Reduction in the incidence of type 2 diabetes with lifestyle intervention or metformin. N Engl J Med 2002;346:393–403.

75. Harborne L, Fleming R, Lyall H, et al. Descriptive review of the evidence for the use of metformin in polycystic ovary syndrome. Lancet 2003;361:1894–901.

76. Harborne L, Sattar N, Norman J, et al. Metformin and weight loss in obese women with polycystic ovary syndrome: comparison of doses. J Clin Endocrinol Metab 2005;90:4593–8.

77. Lord JM, Flight IH, Norman RJ. Metformin in polycystic ovary syndrome: systematic review and meta-analysis. Br Med J 2003;327:951–3.

78. Lord JM, Flight IH, Norman RJ. Insulin-sensitising drugs (metformin, troglitazone, rosiglitazone, pioglitazone, D-chiro-inositol) for polycystic ovary syndrome. Cochrane Database Syst Rev 2003;CD003053.

79. Legro RS, Barnhart HX, Schlaff WD, et al. Clomiphene, metformin, or both for infertility in the polycystic ovary syndrome. N Engl J Med 2007;356:551–66.

80. Hatcher RA, Trussell J, Nelson AL, et al. Contraceptive technology, 19th edn. New York: Ardent Media, 2007.

81. Mauro M, Taylor V, Wharton S, et al. Barriers to obesity treatment. Eur J Intern Med 2008;19:173–80.

82. Foster GD, Wadden TA, Makris AP, et al. Primary care physicians' attitudes about obesity and its treatment. Obes Res 2003;11:1168–77.

83. Puhl RM, Brownwell KD. Bias, discrimination, and obesity. Obes Res 2001;9: 788–805.

84. Puhl RM, Heuer CA. The stigma of obesity: a review and update. Obesity 2009;17: 941–64.

85. Hebl MR, Xu J. Weighing the care: physicians' reaction to the size of a patient. Int J Obes Relat Metab Disord 2001;25:1246–52.

86. Bertakis KD, Azari R. The impact of obesity on primary care visits. Obes Res 2005;13: 1615–22.

87. Anderson DA, Wadden TA. Bariatric surgery patients' views of their physicians: weight-related attitudes and practices. Obes Res 2004;12:1587–95.

88. Brown I, Thompson J, Tod A, et al. Primary care support for tackling obesity: a qualitative study of the perceptions of obese patients. Br J Gen Pract 2006;56:666–72.

89. Amy NK, Aalborg A, Lyons P, et al. Barriers to routine gynecological cancer screening for White and African-American obese women. Int J Obes 2006;30:147–55.

90. Ferrante JM, Ohman-Strickland P, Hudson SV, et al. Colorectal cancer screening among obese versus non-obese patients in primary care practices. Cancer Detect Prev 2006;30:459–65.

91. Ostbye T, Taylor DH, Jr., Yancy WS, Jr., et al. Associations between obesity and receipt of screening mammography, Papanicolaou tests, and influenza vaccination: results from the Health and Retirement Study (HRS) and the Asset and Health Dynamics Among the Oldest Old (AHEAD) Study. Am J Public Health 2005;95:1623–30.

92. Wee CC, McCarthy EP, Davis RB, et al. Screening for cervical and breast cancer: is obesity an unrecognized barrier to preventive care? Ann Intern Med 2000;132: 697–704.

93. Mitchell RS, Padwal RS, Chuck AW, et al. Cancer screening among the overweight and obese in Canada. Am J Prev Med 2008;35:127–32.

94. Poston WS, Foreyt JP. Successful management of the obese patient. Am Fam Physician 2000;61:3615–22.

95. Pollak KI, Ostbye T, Alexander SC. Empathy goes a long way in weight loss discussions. J Fam Prac 2007;56:1031–36.

CHAPTER 4

Bariatric Surgery: A Primer for the Obstetric Care Provider

C.R. Hall and Bradley J. Needleman
Center for Minimally Invasive Surgery, Ohio State University, Columbus, Ohio, USA

Morbid obesity presents a special challenge to all healthcare providers as it can then be difficult to provide even the most basic and routine care to the patient. The lack of adequately sized equipment, the limited mobility of the individual, and the multiple co-morbid conditions complicate any treatment plan. Obesity itself is an independent risk factor for developing medical problems that include but are not limited to type 2 diabetes [1], hypertension, obstructive sleep apnea, non-alcoholic steatohepatitis, degenerative joint disease, infertility, and an increased risk for cancers, including ovarian and breast in women. Obesity is a life-shortening disease, as individuals with a body mass index (BMI) of $30 \, kg/m^2$ or more have a 1–2 times increased risk for death from all causes in any given year compared to normal-weight individuals (BMI $\leq 25 \, kg/m^2$), mostly due to cardiovascular causes [2]. It is estimated that white women between 20 and 30 years of age with a BMI of $45 \, kg/m^2$ or more could lose up to 8 years of life, and African-American women in the same age range can lose up to 5 years [3].

Despite the prevalence of obesity and the large number of diets and commercially available weight loss programs, the medical treatments for obesity are met with discouraging results. In 1991, the National Institutes of Health (NIH) Consensus Development Conference report found that approximately 95% of people who participated in weight loss programs, with or without behavior modification, regained their weight within 2 years of their maximal weight loss. It was this NIH Conference that recommended only two treatments for the durable control of excess body weight, both operative – the vertical banded gastroplasty and the Roux-en-Y gastric bypass (RYGB). Candidacy for weight loss surgery was determined to be individuals with a BMI of $40 \, kg/m^2$ or over who have failed conventional weight loss attempts, who have been properly educated, and who are motivated for surgery; or patients that have a BMI over $35 \, kg/m^2$ with

Pregnancy in the Obese Woman, 1st edition. Edited by Deborah L. Conway.
© 2011 Blackwell Publishing Ltd.

co-morbidities related to their obesity that are imminently life-threatening and/or cause severe lifestyle limitations. These recommendations continue to be the guidelines that help most insurance companies and surgery programs to determine the medical necessity of bariatric surgery [4].

These NIH findings, the feasibility of a minimally invasive approach to weight loss surgery, and the media exposure of celebrity successes have all led to the markedly increased popularity of bariatric surgery as a way to treat severe obesity and its metabolic consequences. In addition, there is now an abundance of medical literature, much of which investigates women after undergoing either a RYGB or an adjustable gastric band. These papers clearly demonstrate the positive effects that weight loss surgery has on an individual's general health, including several studies in which overall quality of life, body image, and sexual function were all significantly improved [5–8]. Recent studies confirm a decrease in the rates of breast, endometrial, and colon cancer following weight loss surgery [9,10]. The positive effects that occur after bariatric surgery increase fertility and decrease amenorrhea, as well as resulting in the resolution of polycystic ovarian syndrome in many patients [11–14]. A decrease in gestational complications and an improvement in neonatal health have also been demonstrated [15]. Finally, it has been shown that pregnancy is not only feasible, but may also be safer and associated with fewer complications when compared to unoperated obese populations [16,17].

Bariatric surgery programs

In 2004, the American Society for Bariatric Surgery, now the American Society for Metabolic and Bariatric Surgery (ASMBS), published a consensus statement that all patients undergoing bariatric surgery need to be well informed and motivated, be compliant with lifestyle changes, and participate in long-term follow-up [18]. Therefore, a multidisciplinary team approach to patient evaluation and selection is deemed essential. Bariatric surgery programs should include medical, dietary, and psychological evaluations by specialists with experience in the care of obese individuals and knowledge about the different weight loss operations. Preoperative counseling and educational programs are indicated to prepare the patient for the multitude of physical and psychological changes that occur in the postoperative period. This multidisciplinary approach is required by the organizations that credential bariatric programs as "Centers of Excellence": the American College of Surgeons and the ASMBS via the Surgical Review Corporation.

As there is no gold standard operation, the procedures that are offered to a patient should reflect an understanding of that patient's dietary and psychological history, medical and surgical history, and surgeon's experience, along with the patient's comfort and expectations. Algorithms to match a patient with a specific operation, such as one proposed by Buchwald, are based upon multiple patient factors including BMI, gender, race, age, body habitus, and presence of major co-morbidities [19]. Although most programs do not employ a specific algorithm, most bariatric surgeons select a weight loss operation for an individual based upon an understanding of all of these factors.

Patients today are considerably knowledgeable regarding their options for bariatric surgery and can readily obtain information from television, magazines, support groups, and the Internet, where they have access to medical websites, online support groups, chat rooms, and even scientific literature and videos of operations. Therefore, physicians are encouraged to understand the criteria for candidacy for weight loss surgery and the surgical options, as well as the basic risks and benefits, so that they may be able to dispel common misconceptions. It is generally recognized that there is not one operation that is best for all patients and that most operations can be performed safely by minimally invasive approaches. These factors should be kept in mind when choosing a program to which to refer patients.

In addition to the extensive preoperative evaluation and counseling that is commonly done, the importance of after-surgery care cannot be overemphasized. Obesity and weight loss should be considered lifelong problems regardless of the operation performed and the amount of weight loss achieved. Patients should be encouraged to participate in lifetime follow-up that may include dietary assessments, checking laboratory values, participating in support groups, maintaining an active lifestyle, and getting mental health support if needed. The resumption of bad habits and non-compliance with optimal eating behaviors can lead to weight gain after even the best of operations, and patients should be encouraged to seek help if they are gaining weight or participating in self-destructive behaviors.

Bariatric surgery can be performed safely and is a highly effective means of producing meaningful weight loss that has a profound effect on obesity-related co-morbidities and often leads to their amelioration and even remission. In 1993, there were approximately16,500 weight loss operations performed in the USA, and that number increased to over 200,000 by 2008. These weight loss operations include the most commonly performed procedures: the RYGB and the laparoscopic adjustable gastric band (LAGB). In addition, the biliopancreatic diversion with duodenal switch (BPD/DS) and more recently the sleeve gastrectomy (SG) are also commonly performed. Each of these operations has its own advantages and complications, which can occur in a myriad of clinical scenarios.

The laparoscopic Roux-en-Y gastric bypass

The RYGB was first described in 1966 in Iowa by Mason and Ito [20] and has since become the most commonly performed weight loss operation in the USA. The typical time required to perform a laparoscopic operation averages 2–2.5 hours, with an average hospital stay of between 2 and 4 days. When performing an RYGB, the stomach is completely divided, beginning at the lesser curve and continued towards the angle of His, leaving a small, proximal gastric pouch that is typically less than 30 ml in volume. The small bowel is divided some distance distal to the ligament of Treitz, and the distal end of the divided end is anastomosed to the gastric pouch, creating a gastrojejunostomy of approximately 1 mm in diameter. The Roux limb, which is the limb of small bowel traveling from the gastric pouch, is then measured to a length of 60–250 cm or more and is anastomosed to the biliopancreatic limb. The biliopancreatic limb is in continuity with the remnant stomach (residual, non-functioning stomach) and carries the secretions from the stomach, liver, and pancreas to mix with ingested materials at the small bowel anastomosis. After the Roux limb and the biliopancreatic limb are joined, they empty into the "common channel," the small bowel distal to this small bowel anastomosis, where the absorption of nutrients occurs in normal fashion.

There are data to suggest that for a BMI of over $50 \, \text{kg/m}^2$, a 150 cm Roux limb may impart greater weight loss than a 75 cm limb, without increased metabolic consequences. When the BMI is below 50, there is no significant weight loss difference between a Roux limb of 75 and 150 cm. A longer Roux limb, therefore, may be chosen for patients who have more than 200 lb of excess body weight [21].

The RYGB is a restrictive operation that imparts a change in appetite and a feeling of early satiety, resulting in the consumption of significantly less food at any given time. Patients must make changes in their eating habits to comply with their new anatomy; these include chewing their food well, eating slowly, and stopping when they sense their new feeling of being "full" – otherwise they may encounter symptoms such as discomfort, nausea, and vomiting. The operation may also impact food tolerances and the potential for dumping syndrome, the reaction to foods high in sugar content, by causing cramping abdominal pain and diarrhea, diaphoresis, and light-headedness. As a result, some studies suggest that an RYGB may be better than purely restrictive operations for patients identified as "sweet-eaters" [22], but more recent studies have not been able to demonstrate this result [23].

The RYGB is not typically considered a malabsorptive operation because, other than the response to food with a high sugar content, most proteins and fats, as well as medications, are absorbed normally. Therefore, as long as individuals consume the daily required amount of protein or take medications as prescribed, these should be digested and absorbed normally. The RYGB, however, does put the patient at risk for certain vitamin and mineral deficiencies as food no longer passes through the majority of the stomach, duodenum, and first portion of the jejunum. These patients will then be at risk for developing deficiencies. Specifically, deficiencies can occur with vitamin B_{12}, due to the exclusion of intrinsic factor, which is produced in the bypassed portion of the stomach, and with iron, calcium, folate, and thiamine, which are absorbed primarily in the duodenum or proximal small bowel. Other potential deficiencies include vitamins A and D, selenium, copper, and zinc. Multivitamins, iron, and calcium citrate supplements are the only medications that individual should need to take for the rest of their life as a result of having this operation for weight loss.

The advantages of RYGB include known long-term results, the permanence of the operation, and the multiple factors that impart weight loss. Diet is restricted immediately, and therefore weight loss is also immediate and may continue for 18–24 months after operation. Mean excess body weight loss (EBWL) is estimated to be between 60% and 75% during this time, with improvements in, or even remission of, many weight-related co-morbidities [24]. This improvement is well documented after gastric bypass operations and includes the amelioration of diabetes, as well as improvements in insulin resistance and glucose tolerance. Bypassing the antrum, duodenum, and jejunum with an RYGB may provide additional benefits to the treatment of diabetes by altering gut signaling mechanisms that are beneficial to treating insulin resistance and/or glucose intolerance compared to restrictive operations alone [25]. Additional beneficial effects have been seen by reducing other cardiovascular risk factors and mortality [26].

Disadvantages of RYGP may be related to short-term and long-term complications related specifically to the procedure, such as leakage at the gastrojejunal anastomosis, pouch, remnant stomach, or jejunojejunostomy. Overall mortality from all causes in the immediate perioperative period ranges between 1% and 2%, and may be from cardiopulmonary complications, pulmonary embolism, or sepsis from gastrointestinal leak. Other late-onset complications include gastrojejunal stricture, marginal ulceration, and internal hernias.

Gastrojejunal strictures and the associated marginal ulceration occur at the staple or suture line of the gastrojejunal anastomosis. Strictures generally occur between 3 weeks and 2 months after operation and are a narrowing of the anastomosis that may make it difficult for the patient to tolerate solid foods. Typically, these patients report progressive symptoms of vomiting and food feeling "stuck." With severe strictures, vomiting may also include liquids. Stricture are generally successfully treated with endoscopy and dilatation, taking care not to overdilate the anastomosis, which might allow patients to eat too much and not lose weight.

A marginal ulcer may occur at any time after operation, and patients typically have nausea with or without emesis with moderate to severe epigastric pain, especially related to eating, the opposite of what is seen in typical
peptic ulcer disease. A high index of suspicion should be maintained in
the setting of a post-RYGB patient having the above symptoms, particularly if the patient is a smoker, is taking non-steroidal anti-inflammatory
medications (NSAIDs), or drinks alcohol.

Internal hernias, which can result in catastrophic small bowel necrosis,
occur when any one of several openings in the mesentery created during
the RYGB cause the bowel to become incarcerated and potentially stran-
gulate. These patients may complain of intermittent signs and symptoms
of bowel obstruction with sharp pain often boring though their abdomen
and into their back. The typical findings on computed tomography include
"swirling" of the mesenteric vessels, but it is not uncommon for the films
to appear normal. If there is clinical suspicion for internal hernia, the
treatment of choice is diagnostic laparoscopy or laparotomy.

An important consideration when choosing an RYGB should be the loss
of access to the distal stomach and duodenum, making the diagnosis of
pathology and the performance of endoscopic retrograde cholangiopan-
creatography (ERCP) difficult without undergoing additional surgical
intervention. Patients at high risk for future gastric and duodenal pathology, those requiring the chronic use of NSAIDs or other ulcerogenics, and
those at highest risk for vitamin and mineral deficiencies may not be ideal
candidates for RYGB.

Weight gain after maximal weight loss may occur between 2 and 5 years
postoperatively and lead to failure as judged by not maintaining more than
50% EBWL. Ten years after RYGB, the rate of failure to maintain over
50% EBWL may be as high as 20.4% for morbidly obese patients and
34.9% for "super-morbidly obese" patients (patients with a BMI greater
than 50kg/m^2) [27].

The laparoscopic adjustable gastric band

The LAGB was approved by the Food and Drug Administration in the USA
in June 2001 and has been increasing in popularity. It had already been
a popular operation outside the USA since first being described in 1993
by Belachew and colleagues [28]. Two types of band are currently available in the USA: the Lap-Band adjustable gastric banding system distributed by Allergan, Inc. (Irvine, CA, USA) and the Realize Personalized
Banding Solution distributed by Ethicon Endo-Surgery, Inc. (Cincinnati,
OH). The relative ease of laparoscopic placement, short operative times
(<1 hour), low morbidity and mortality (<0.1%), and short hospital stays

(<1 day) make this an attractive option for patients and surgeons that has essentially replaced the vertical banded gastroplasty as the most commonly performed purely restrictive operation.

During the procedure, an inflatable silicone band is placed around the stomach to create a small gastric pouch (usually <20 ml). Tubing connects the band to a port that is implanted in the subcutaneous tissue within the abdominal wall. Access to this port, which is placed with or without radiological guidance by a non-coring needle, allows adjustment of the band. The instillation of saline will tighten the stoma between the proximal pouch and distal stomach, thereby creating earlier satiety. Negative symptoms caused by overeating or a band that is too tight may include food intolerances, symptoms of reflux, and pain. These symptoms can be treated by aspirating fluid, thereby opening the stoma. Adjustments can be made as often as needed to optimize weight loss, injecting enough fluid into the band to achieve a prolonged sensation of satiety. In addition, after this operation a patient should be able to tolerate a variety of healthful foods, does not have any adverse symptoms, and is losing weight in the range of 0.5–1 kg (1–2 lb) per week. Loss of excess weight may occur over a period of 3–5 years or longer [29].

Weight loss results seen with the band may vary. Without malabsorption or dumping syndrome, it is generally accepted that food selection plays a greater role in the success of restrictive operations such as the LAGB, although there is evidence suggesting the presence of behaviors like sweet-eating before surgery will not predict failure after band placement [30]. A systematic review and meta-analysis of the large body of data describing the Swedish adjustable gastric band and Lap-Band was published in 2008 by Cunneen et al. These data showed a 3-year mean EBWL for the Lap-Band system of 50.2% and a BMI reduction of 11.81 kg/m^2 from baseline. A resolution of co-morbidities after banding was found for diabetes (60.29% reduction) and hypertension (43.58% reduction) [31].

In an attempt to profile the best candidates for LAGB, one nationwide survey in France found that the most successful gastric banding patients were around 40 years old with an initial BMI of below 50 kg/m^2. They were willing to change their eating habits and to recover or increase their physical activity after surgery, and they were operated on by a team usually performing more than two bariatric procedures per week. This study emphasized that obesity surgery, and LAGB specifically, requires significant experience on the part of the surgical team and a multidisciplinary approach to improve behavioral changes [32]. Patients with a lower excess body weight who improve especially their eating behavior after surgery have the highest chance of success after LAGB [33].

Complications at the time of band placement are infrequent and could include injury to the stomach and esophagus, bleeding, splenic injury, and poor placement of the band. Complications from the LAGB may be unique, and reoperations may be required 10–13% of the time due to port displacements, infection, gastric slippage, erosion, and removal due to intolerance or significant esophageal complaints [34]. In a study of 573 patients in Italy followed for 5 years after LAGB, complications included migration of the band (4.1%), erosion (2.1%), mortality (0.87%), and conversion to other bariatric procedures (1.9%). Band removal was performed in 5.7% of patients due to gastric pouch dilation and band erosion [35]. In another study from Portugal of 591 patients with a 10 year follow-up, the percentage of EBWL at 10 years was 82.7% (range ± 4.2%), with band failure in 9.3%, slippage in 5.3%, and erosion 4.6% [36].

Patients who may benefit from LAGB are those with co-morbidities that put them at the highest risk for perioperative and surgical complications but who would reap significant benefit from meaningful weight loss. Extremes of age, prior abdominal operations with extensive adhesive disease, a history of inflammatory bowel disease, (such as Crohn's disease, in which an anastomosis may not be desired), patients in whom any malabsorption would be disadvantageous, and the potential for future medical conditions including pregnancy or interventions that would benefit from an adjustable operation may be considered better candidates for LAGB over RYGB or BPD/DS.

LAGB may not be the most desirable operation for patients in whom the presence of a foreign body would be contraindicated or who are not able to participate in follow-up enough to have the necessary adjustments for optimal success. It is also not the preferred operation in patients with a large hiatal or paraesophageal hernia. In addition, those patients with super-morbid obesity (BMI > 50 kg/m^2) or who are unable or unwilling to make lifestyle changes related to their diet and activity may benefit more from a more aggressive weight loss intervention such as RYGB.

Biliopancreatic diversion with duodenal switch

BPD, a malabsorptive procedure, was first described by Scopinaro in 1976 as an operation that included a partial gastrectomy [37], leaving a 250–500 ml gastric pouch emptying into a 250 cm Roux limb with a 50 cm common channel for absorption. In order to decrease the incidence of marginal ulceration and metabolic derangements, Marceau and Hess both described a modification of the BPD termed the duodenal switch (BPD/DS), creating a gastric sleeve and preserving the pylorus [38,39]. The BPD/DS is currently being performed by minimally invasive techniques. This operation creates a gastric sleeve 100–200 ml in volume with the pylorus preserved, which is anastomosed to an alimentary limb of 200–300 cm in length, and a common channel between 50–100 cm in length. The lengthening of the limb from 50 to 100 cm in BPD/DS seems to decrease the incidence of metabolic complications such as iron deficiency anemia and protein malnutrition.

Long-term results after BPD/DS reported by Marceau et al. show that 82% of patients lost more 50% of their excess body weight, with a mean EBWL of 73% (range ± 19%). Thirty-day mortality was reported as 1.1%, and 90-day mortality as 1.3%. BPD/DS may have more success in patients who have a higher starting BMI. In those patients with a BMI of less than 50 kg/m^2, 92% achieve a BMI of below 35, while 83% of those who start with a BMI of over 50 achieve these same results. In addition, the resolution of co-morbidities is also exceptional after BPD/DS. Medications were able to be discontinued in 92% of diabetic patients, continuous positive airway pressure ventilation was able to be discontinued in 90% of those with sleep apnea, and the prevalence of those with a cardiac risk index of greater than 5 was decreased by 86% [40]. The excellent weight loss seen in BPD/DS, especially given the consistency of results in patients with a BMI greater than 50 kg/m^2, makes this a more attractive operation for the super-obese population, especially if the risks from a large abdominal incision can be ameliorated by performing the operation using a minimally invasive approach.

Malabsorptive procedures such as the BPD/DS have the advantage of providing excellent weight loss with fewer patient-related factors influencing weight loss. The preservation of the pylorus in these patients means they are less likely to experience the dumping syndrome when eating sweets, which may influence the surgeon's decision in offering this as a choice of operation. The overall flexibility in diet is what may make this option more attractive for some patients. However, despite the decreased absorption, the gastric reservoir is large enough to eventually allow the patients to consume larger amounts of foods. This may be detrimental to weight loss, especially when foods high in fat content are ingested. This carries an increased risk and frequency of abdominal bloating and foul-smelling stool and gas, which may ultimately alter patient satisfaction as well as comfort.

Long-term complications are mostly related to the short common channel and absorption, and include the potential for protein malnutrition and a deficiency of fat-soluble vitamins and minerals, and may place the individual at risk for metabolic bone disease. In Marceau's study of long-term results, 10% presented with hypoalbuminemia, 5% were hospitalized at least once for malnutrition, and revision was required for malnutrition in 0.7% of patients. Commonly seen was the risk for anemia, decreased vitamin A, increased vitamin D, and decreased calcium levels, with 20% of patients having below normal levels and 1.3% serious deficiencies. The incidence of kidney stones was also significantly increased after surgery [40].

There is a lack of studies that prospectively compare BPD/DS with other weight loss operations. However, BPD/DS appears to be a considerably effective operation for patients that are super-obese (BMI > 50 kg/m^2) compared to the other procedures, and results in a significant reduction in co-morbidities related to obesity, especially diabetes. Because the stomach remains intact, surveillance continues to be possible and makes this a good choice for patients who may be at risk for developing gastric pathology. Yet, as with the RYGB, the ampulla will not be readily accessible to endoscopy. ERCP, even with operative access, will be very difficult and may not be possible. Patients who are considered at too high an operative risk to undergo this operation, and those who may have difficulty complying with long-term follow-up and the required daily dietary supplements may be more suitable for one of the less invasive, less aggressive procedures.

Laparoscopic sleeve gastrectomy

The laparoscopic SG is a relatively newer, purely restrictive procedure that is the gastric portion of the BPD/DS but without completing the remainder of the operation. This operation has the unique features of providing restriction with relatively normal gastrointestinal continuity without the presence of a foreign body. It can be considered as a bridge procedure that can later be converted to a more definitive operative, that is, an RYGB or duodenal switch, or as its own primary weight loss operation. Although this operation is currently gaining in popularity, it is not yet seen as a conventional operation by insurance providers.

The SG is commonly performed laparoscopically and requires division of the vasculature along the greater curve of the stomach to the angle of His to facilitate complete resection of the gastric fundus. Division of the stomach generally begins 6–10 cm proximal to the pylorus, leaving an antral remnant of 150–200 ml in volume to facilitate gastric emptying. The gastric sleeve is then fashioned by placing a sizing tube inside the stomach along the lesser curve and stapling out the fundus along the tube up to the angle of His. The size of the tube can vary greatly, but it is likely that a smaller tube optimizes weight loss when SG is offered as a definitive procedure, by resulting in the creation of a gastric tube of lesser volume. It is generally accepted that some reinforcement of the staple line is recommended, either by oversewing, using buttressing material, or utilizing a fibrin sealant [41].

Using the SG component as a bridge to a more definitive weight loss operation was first described by Chu in higher risk, super-morbidly obese patients [42]. As a operation that is technically easier to perform laparoscopically than the BPD/DS or RYGB, its performance allows the patient to have a safer operation, lose weight, and then undergo a secondary, more definitive procedure in more favorable circumstances. Most commonly, the second procedure is the BPD/DS, but it can also be easily converted to an RYGB or LAGB. On the other hand, another indication proposed for SG is in patients with a lower BMI who do not have as much weight to lose and may not need a more aggressive operation, or malabsorption, to achieve the desired weight loss goals. In one study from Korea, patients with a preoperative BMI of below $35\,kg/m^2$ maintained an EBWL of 85% 3 years after surgery, with diabetes resolving in all patients [43].

Given the prior experiences of bariatric surgery with stapled gastroplasties, it was assumed that these operations, although initially effective for weight loss, would ultimately fail to be able to maintain this loss. Therefore the weight loss curves of these patients were followed, and when maximal weight loss was achieved, evidenced by a prolonged plateau and the beginning of weight regain, the patient would then undergo the second stage of the procedure. It was observed that there was a subset of the super-obese population that had an SG as a staged procedure but, despite never undergoing the second stage of the procedure, were nevertheless able to successfully maintain weight loss. In one multicenter study of SG performed on 163 patients, the percentage of EBWL at 1 and 2 years postoperatively was 59.45% and 61.52%, respectively [44]. In another study, by Lee et al. in 2007, 216 patients with 2-year follow-up data demonstrated an EBWL of 59% (range ± 17%) in patients with a preoperative mean BMI of $49\,kg/m^2$ (range ± $11\,kg/m^2$) [45]. At the First International Consensus Summit for SG in New York in October 2007, 87 surgeons completed questionnaires regarding the SG and reported that 93.8% of them performed SG as a primary weight loss procedure achieving 56.3% (range ± 21.6%) EBWL at 3 years.

Co-morbidities also improve after SG. In one report, 193 patients underwent SG: 66% of the patients with type 2 diabetes resolved and 20% improved, 88% of patients with hypertension resolved, and 87% of patients' sleep apnea resolved [45]. Five-year data presented by Crookes showed that 23 of 49 diabetics resolved their diabetes after SG, and another 11 reduced their medications [46,47].

Complications of SG can be related to the staple line and include leaks, which can be difficult to manage and have been reported to occur in up to 5.52% of cases [44], as well as bleeding and strictures. Metabolic complications of SG should be rare due to preservation of the continuity of the gastrointestinal tract, allowing for a relatively normal absorption of nutrients, yet most surgeons treat patients with postoperative supplements and proton pump inhibitors [41].

Although more studies are needed to evaluate the long-term data, it is clear that there are advantages to the SG either as a bridge operation or as a definitive weight loss procedure. It is a technically easier operation to perform than either the RYGB or BPD/DS, offering patients a greater chance of success to undergo a minimally invasive operation performed with lower morbidity due to the avoidance of performing two additional anastomoses. Weight loss seems to be better with the SG than the LAGB in the short term (up to 3 years after surgery). It has the advantage of being able to be easily converted to other operations, due to the success in weight loss, allowing the secondary operations to be performed at a lower subsequent BMI. In addition, absorption is unchanged, and therefore there is minimal risk for nutritional deficiencies and dumping syndrome. SG has the advantage of not involving foreign bodies, eliminating the risk for complications requiring future operations due to slip, prolapse, erosion, device malfunction, and infection, and it may be utilized as a preferred operation in patients who are at risk for these complications with a band. Disadvantages include irreversible resection of normal gastric tissue and the lack of long-term data, especially given the history of gastroplasties in bariatric surgery; complications of the staple lines include leak and fistula, which can be difficult to manage.

Future considerations

As more becomes known about the physiological effects that bariatric surgery has on obesity and its co-morbidities, the more the field continues to evolve. Surgeons who perform these operations have become very familiar with the positive benefits of weight loss: improvements in quality of life indicators, and improvements in the medical sequelae of obesity (diabetes, hypertension, hyperlipidemia, and obesity-related hypoventilation syndromes). As a result, the field is undergoing a paradigm shift in which the target of surgery is remission of the co-morbid conditions and weight loss is a secondary benefit. Recent studies are geared towards breaking down the components and physiological alterations produced by each procedure to identify what specific changes in gastrointestinal anatomy produce a desired effect on a specific disease state. Effects may be through weight loss, a change in gut hormonal response, or some combination of both. Once these processes are better known, specific operations can be tailored for a particular metabolic disease that may change the indications for surgery irrespective of a patient's BMI.

In addition, there is a tremendous amount of industry resources being put towards developing weight loss procedures that can be performed entirely by an endoscopic approach. Whether it is a procedure that alters gastric anatomy to impart early satiety or an endoluminal device that separates food from digestive enzymes to impart some degree of malabsorption, there is a great deal of excitement surrounding the ability to perform a procedure without incisions – and perhaps without general anesthesia – on an outpatient basis. Although still several years away, there are currently several Food and Drug Administration and other clinical trials underway evaluating these new techniques.

References

1. National Institute of Diabetes and Digestive and Kidney Diseases. Diabetes Prevention Program Meeting Summary. Diabetes Mellitus Interagency Coordinating Committee, Bethesda, MD, August 2001.
2. Clinical Guidelines on the Identification, Evaluation, and Treatment of Overweight and Obesity in Adults – the evidence report. National Institutes of Health. Obes Res 1998;6 (Suppl., 2):51S–209S.
3. Fontaine KR, Redden DT, Wang C, et al. Years of life lost due to obesity. J Am Med Assoc 2003;289(2):187–93.
4. Gastrointestinal surgery for severe obesity: National Institutes of Health Consensus Development Conference statement. Am J Clin Nutr 1992;55:615S–19S.
5. Van der Beek ES, Te Riele W, Specken TF, et al. The impact of reconstructive procedures following bariatric surgery on patient well-being and quality of life. Obes Surg 2010;20(1):36–41.
6. Myers JA, Clifford JC, Sarker S, et al. Quality of life after laparoscopic adjustable gastric banding using the Baros and Moorehead–Ardelt quality of life questionnaire II. JSLS 2006;10(4):414–20.
7. Song AY, Rubin JP, Thomas V, et al. Body image and quality of life in post massive weight loss body contouring patients. Obesity 2006;14(9):1626–36.
8. Assimakopoulos K, Panayiotopoulos S, Iconomou G, et al. Assessing sexual function in obese women preparing for bariatric surgery. Obes Surg 2006;16(8):1087–91.
9. Christou NV, Lieberman M, Sampalis F, et al. Bariatric surgery reduces cancer risk in morbidly obese patients. Surg Obes Relat Dis 2008;4(6):696–7.
10. McCawley GM, Ferriss JS, Geffel D, et al. Cancer in obese women: potential protective impact of bariatric surgery. J Am Coll Surg 2009;208(6):1093–8.
11. Maggard MA, Yermilov I, Li Z, et al. Pregnancy and fertility following bariatric surgery: a systematic review. JAMA 2008;300(19):2286–96.
12. Teitleman M, Grotegut CA, Williams NN, et al. The impact of bariatric surgery on menstrual patterns. Obes Surg 2006;16(11):1457–63.
13. Stroh C, Hohmann U, Lehnert H, et al. PCO syndrome – is it an indication for bariatric surgery? Zentralbl Chir 2008;133(6):608–10.
14. Escobar-Morreale HF, Botella-Carretero JI, Alvarez-Blasco F, et al. The polycystic ovary syndrome associated with morbid obesity may resolve after weight loss induced by bariatric surgery. J Clin Endocrinol Metab 2005;90(12):6364–9.
15. Weintraub AY, Levy A, Levi I, et al. Effect of bariatric surgery on pregnancy outcomes. Int J Gynaecol Obstet 2008;103(3):246–51.
16. Ducarme G, Revaux A, Rodrigues A, et al. Obstetric outcome following laparoscopic adjustable gastric banding. Int J Gynaecol Obstet 2007;98(3):244–7.
17. Dixon JB, Dixon ME, O'Brien PE. Birth outcomes in obese women after laparoscopic adjustable gastric banding. Obstet Gynecol 2005;106(5 Pt 1):965–72.
18. Buchwald H. Consensus Conference Statement. Bariatric surgery for morbid obesity: health implications for patients, health professionals, and third-party payers. Surg Obes Relat Dis 2005;317–18.

19. Buchwald H. A bariatric surgery algorithm. Obes Surg 2002;12:733–46.

20. Mason EE, Ito C. Gastric bypass in obesity. Surg Clin N Am 1967;47:1345–51.

21. Brolin RE, Kenler HA, Gorman JH, et al. Long-limb gastric bypass: a five-year prospective randomized study. Ann Surg 1992;215:123–43.

22. Sugerman H, Starkey J, Birkenhauer R. A randomized prospective trial of gastric bypass versus vertical banded gastroplasty for morbid obesity and their effects on sweets versus non-sweets eaters. Ann Surg 1987;205:613–24.

23. Hudson SM, Dixon JB, O'Brien PE. Sweet eating is not a predictor of outcome after Lap-Band placement. Can we finally bury the myth? Obes Surg 2002;12:789–94.

24. Buchwald H, Avidor Y, Braunwald E, et al. Bariatric surgery: a systematic review and meta-analysis. JAMA 2004;292:1724–37.

25. Rubino F, Gagner M. Potential of surgery for curing type 2 diabetes mellitus. Ann Surg 2002;236(5):554–9.

26. Sjostrom L, Narbro K, Sjostrom C, et al. Effects of bariatric surgery on mortality in Swedish obese subjects. NEJM 2007;357:741–52.

27. Sjostrom L, Lindroos AK, Peltonen M, et al. Lifestyle, diabetes, and cardiovascular risk factors 10 years after bariatric surgery. NEJM 2004;351(26):2683–93.

28. Belachew M, Legrand MJ, Defechereux TH, et al. Laparoscopic adjustable silicone gastric banding in the treatment of morbid obesity: a preliminary report. Surg Endosc 1994;8:1354–56.

29. Favretti F, O'Brien P, Dixon J. Patient management after Lap-Band placement. Am J Surg 2002;184(6):S38–41.

30. Dixon J, O'Brien P, Playfair J, et al. Adjustable gastric banding and conventional therapy for type 2 diabetes: a randomized controlled trial. JAMA 2008;299(3):341–3.

31. Cunneen S, Phillips E, Gielding G, et al. Studies of Swedish adjustable gastric band and Lap-Band: systematic review and meta-analysis. Surg Obes Relat Dis 2008;4(2):174–85.

32. Chevallier J, Paita M, Rodde-Dunet M, et al. A nationwide survey on the role of center activity and patients' behavior. Ann Surg 2007;246(6):1034–9.

33. Ren C, Horgan S, Ponce J. US experience with the Lap-Band system. Am J Surg 2002;184(6B):46S–50S.

34. Angrisani L, Di Lorenzo N, Favretti F, et al. The Italian group for Lap-Band: predictive value for initial body mass index for weight loss after 5 years of follow-up. Surg Endosc 2004;18(10):1524–7.

35. Biagini J, Karam L. Ten years experience with laparoscopic adjustable gastric banding. Obes Surg 2008;18:573–7.

36. Scopinaro N, Gianetta E, Civaller D, et al. Biliopancreatic bypass for obesity. Initial experience in man. Br J Surg 1979;66:618–20.

37. Hess DW, Hess DS. Biliopancreatic diversion with a duodenal switch. Obes Surg 1998;8:267–82.

38. Marceau P, Biron S, Bouroque R, et al. Biliopancreatic diversion with a new type of gastrectomy. Obes Surg 1993;3:29–35.

39. Marceau P, Biron S, Hould F, et al. Duodenal switch: long-term results. Obes Surg 2007;17:1421–30.

40. Carmichael AR, Sue-Ling HM, Johnston D. Quality of life after the Magenstrasse and Mill procedure for morbid obesity. Obes Surg 2001;11:708–15.

41. Chu CA, Gagner M, Quinn T, et al. Two-stage laparoscopic biliopancreatic diversion with duodenal switch: an alternative approach to super-super morbid obesity [abstract]. Surg Endosc 2002;16:s069.

42. Nocca D. A prospective multicenter study of 163 sleeve gastrectomies: results at 1 and 2 years. Obes Surg 2008;18:560–5.zxz.

43. Himpens J, Dapri G, Cadière GB. A prospective randomized study between laparo-scopic gastric banding and laparoscopic isolated sleeve gastrectomy: results after 1 and 3 years. Obes Surg 2006;16(11):1450–6.
44. Lee CM, Cirangle PT, Jossart GH. Vertical gastrectomy for morbid obesity in 216 patients: report of two-year results. Surg Endosc 2007;21(10):1810–16.
45. Silecchia G, Boru C, Pecchia A, et al. Effectiveness of laparoscopic sleeve gastrectomy (first stage of biliopancreatic diversion with duodenal switch) on comorbidities in super-obese high-risk patients. Obes Surg 2006;16:1138–44.
46. Almogy G, Crookes PF, Anthone GJ. Longitudinal gastrectomy as a treatment for the high-risk super obese patient. Obes Surg 2004;14:492–7.
47. Hamoui N, Anthone GJ, Kaufman HS, et al. Sleeve gastrectomy in the high-risk patient. Obes Surg 2006;16:1445–9.

CHAPTER 5

Pregnancy After Bariatric Surgery

Anatte Karmon[1] and Eyal Sheiner[2]

[1]Albert Einstein College of Medicine/Montefiore Medical Center, Bronx, New York, USA
[2]Medical Center, Faculty of Health Sciences, Ben-Gurion University of the Negev, Beer-Sheva, Israel

The impact of obesity on worldwide health has resulted in its definition as the second leading cause of death in the West [1,2]. Obese women who become pregnant are at higher risk for reproductive and fetal complications such as infertility, gestational diabetes mellitus (GDM), macrosomia, pre-eclampsia, and cesarean section [3–6]. Bariatric surgery, a highly effective treatment for obesity, has also been shown to decrease obesity-related medical complications [7–9]. In addition, the majority of bariatric surgery is performed on women, a large percentage of whom are of reproductive age [10].

Recent research has put the spotlight on two different aspects of pregnancy after bariatric surgery: safety of the mother and fetus, and the procedure's effectiveness in preventing the complications surrounding reproduction and pregnancy that are often seen in the obese woman. Series documenting surgical complications and poor perinatal outcomes following post-bariatric surgery pregnancies (hereafter referred to as post-operative pregnancies) do exist [11–15], although larger systematic studies have failed to demonstrate high rates of such complications during post-operative pregnancies, especially when compared to pre-bariatric surgery pregnancies (hereafter referred to as preoperative pregnancies) [16–20]. By reviewing the available data on pregnancy and bariatric surgery, this chapter attempts to elucidate the reproductive benefits and complications associated with weight loss surgery. Areas requiring further research will be identified, and clinical recommendations will be provided.

Fertility

Infertility is a known potential complication of obesity, likely related to anovulatory cycles and disorders such as polycystic ovarian syndrome [3,21,22]. In addition, the literature suggests that weight loss through non-surgical means can improve fertility in women [3,21,22]. Although

---

bariatric surgery is a proven effective treatment for obesity, data on post-surgery fertility are limited and ambiguous [2,9].

One major limitation of studies investigating fertility and bariatric surgery is that many of the data come from deliveries, and therefore only women successfully becoming pregnant are included in the subject pool. Information about infertility is obtained by history regarding the use of infertility treatments and preoperative infertility. Those women who failed to become pregnant altogether either pre- or post-bariatric surgery are not sampled. Information comparing the number of failed and successful attempts at pregnancy is also not available from the majority of studies on the subject.

Reports exist citing both improved and worsened fertility after bariatric surgery. A number of small-series document improvements in fertility post-weight loss surgery, although most of their findings are not statistically significant due to small sample sizes [23–26]. Sheiner et al. [18], however, report an increased rate of infertility treatment after bariatric surgery compared to the general population, persistent even after controlling for confounders such as obesity (adjusted odds ratio [OR] 2.3; 95% confidence interval [CI] 1.6–3.8, $p < 0.001$). In addition, some women undergoing bariatric surgery may choose to do so because of a prior history of infertility, entering selection bias into studies that compare postoperative women with the general population [2]. A more recent study by Weintraub et al. [19] comparing preoperative with postoperative deliveries reports no difference in the rate of infertility treatment before and after surgery (6.6% and 7.5%, respectively; $p = 0.38$).

Bariatric surgery may increase the chance of unintended pregnancy through changes in gastrointestinal uptake of oral contraceptive pills (OCPs), with one study reporting low plasma levels of OCP hormones among post-malabsorptive procedure patients [27]. It is not known how differences in procedure type (malabsorptive versus restrictive; see Chapter 4) might affect OCP absorption, or whether low levels of plasma OCP translate to decreased OCP effectiveness. However, the suggestion has been made to avoid OCPs in patients who have undergone bariatric surgery [28].

Until more is known about whether or not bariatric surgery improves fertility, patients should not be counseled to undergo a weight loss procedure solely to increase their chances of becoming pregnant [29,30].

Pregnancy-related complications

A number of pregnancy-related complications and maternal outcomes in post-bariatric surgery pregnancies have been studied, including diabetes, hypertension, mode of delivery, and intrapartum complications [4,17,18, 20,25,31–33]. Results reported in the literature regarding these parameters vary according to study design. Of particular importance in evaluating these studies is attention to the control group chosen for comparison. Whereas some series comparing postoperative pregnancies with those in the general population have found higher rates of certain co-morbidities and complications among cases [18], studies using unoperated obese women as the control group often found the opposite or no difference in complication rates among cases and controls [19]. This is likely a reflection of the relationship between body mass index (BMI) and these parameters, indicating that bariatric surgery may decrease the incidence of these obesity-related complications [19] but not bring rates down to general population levels, perhaps because BMI remains elevated in postoperative women compared to the general population [18]. Indeed, controlling for BMI in studies using the general population as controls often, although not always, causes differences among groups to disappear [18].

Hypertensive disorders of pregnancy

Hypertensive diseases, including chronic hypertension and hypertensive disorders of pregnancy, are positively associated with obesity [6,34]. Studies comparing postoperative women with the general population reveal higher rates of hypertension during pregnancy in patients who have undergone bariatric surgery [18,20]. However, controlling for BMI via multivariate analysis reveals no significant difference in adjusted OR for hypertensive disorders among postoperative and control women [18,20]. These data suggest that although crude rates of hypertensive disorders may be higher among postoperative women than controls, this difference is attributable to elevated BMI among cases and not post-bariatric surgery status.

Not only is bariatric surgery safe in terms of future risk for hypertension during pregnancy, it may also decrease risk for the disease in those women who undergo the operation prior to becoming pregnant. In a study by Weintraub et al. [19] comparing 301 deliveries before bariatric surgery (of any type) with 507 deliveries after bariatric surgery, the rates of hypertension (chronic and pregnancy-induced) and of severe pre-eclampsia were significantly lower in the postoperative group compared to the preoperative group. In addition, a logistic regression model controlling for diabetes mellitus, fetal macrosomia, and maternal age demonstrated hypertensive disorders to be independently associated with bariatric surgery status (OR 0.38; 95% CI 0.25–0.59, $p < 0.001$).

Another study comparing first post-surgery pregnancy with last pre-surgery pregnancy, as well as with a cohort who were obese, revealed lower rates of pregnancy-induced hypertension and pre-eclampsia among postoperative women compared to both their own preoperative deliveries and the obese cohort [16]. The authors report that the postoperative pregnancy-induced hypertension rate was similar to their community rate. Similarly, a recent study by Ducarme et al. [17] reports a decreased rate of pre-eclampsia among postoperative women, although rates of pregnancy-induced hypertension and labor induction were similar. Interestingly, there is no statistically significant difference in BMI among their post-bariatric surgery women compared to their obese controls. These data suggest that there may be an independent effect of bariatric surgery on pre-eclampsia, regardless of reduction in BMI. A more likely explanation is that the study power was not sufficient to detect differences in BMI, although a significant difference in gestational weight gain was noted (5.5 kg [12.1 lb] in postoperative pregnancies versus 7.1 kg [15.7 lb] in obese controls, $p < 0.05$).

It appears as though the growing body of literature on this subject supports the premise that, by treating obesity, bariatric surgery may lower risk for hypertension in subsequent pregnancies.

Gestational diabetes mellitus

GDM is another obesity-related disease [6] that can theoretically be prevented via weight loss methods such as bariatric surgery. Ducarme et al. [17] describe a lower rate of GDM in postoperative women versus obese controls (0% and 22.1%, respectively; $p < 0.05$), although their sample size is small and includes only 13 postoperative women. In a study of 301 pre-bariatric surgery pregnancies and 507 pregnancies following surgery, Weintraub et al. [19] found a lower rate of total diabetic disorders but no difference in the rate of GDM specifically (11.6% among preoperative pregnancies versus 8.7% among postoperative pregnancies, $p = 0.11$). A logistic regression model controlling for maternal age, fetal macrosomia, and hypertensive disorders suggests that diabetes mellitus (all disorders including pre-gestational and gestational diabetes) is independently associated with bariatric surgery status. The lack of a significant difference in rate of GDM among postoperative and preoperative women in the abovementioned study [19] may be a reflection of decreased study power, which increased once the authors combined all forms of diabetes mellitus. Similarly, Dixon et al. [16] found postoperative women to have a lower rate of GDM compared to their obese controls, but the same rate of GDM in comparison to their own preoperative pregnancies, despite an average pre-pregnancy weight loss of 28.3 kg (62.4 lb) among postoperative women. This may indicate differences in power or it may reflect interactions with unknown confounders [2,16].

Procedure type may also affect GDM rate in postoperative women. The malabsorptive procedures appear to increase insulin secretion and inhibit glucagon production, theoretically making them more likely to prevent GDM. However, when comparing outcomes of pregnancies complicated by GDM in women after restrictive procedures versus malabsorptive ones, Sheiner et al. [31] did not observe any significant differences in fasting glucose or hemoglobin A1C levels.

Studies comparing bariatric surgery patients with the general population often report no difference in the rate of GDM or increased rates of GDM in postoperative patients versus controls. In their study comparing 298 postoperative pregnancies with 158,912 pregnancies in the general population, Sheiner et al. [18] found a higher prevalence of GDM in postoperative parturients (9.4% in women post-bariatric surgery and 5.0% in all other women; $p = 0.001$) but no difference in prevalence of pre-GDM among all subjects. However, in a logistic regression model controlling for a number of factors including maternal BMI, the relationship between bariatric surgery status and diabetes mellitus was no longer significant [18].

Even if the increased GDM rate among postoperative patients (8–16%) [18,35,36] is solely due to their elevated BMI despite bariatric surgery, the fact remains that crude rates of diabetes mellitus during pregnancy are elevated in this population. However, testing for GDM can be challenging in post-bariatric surgery patients, especially in those women who have undergone a malabsorptive procedure. Cases have been reported of dumping syndrome, a condition stemming from malabsorption and osmotic fluid shifts, after the administration of the a 50 g glucose challenge test [37]. Some authors recommend avoiding this test altogether in postoperative women. Instead, 1–2 weeks of fasting and 2-hour postprandial fingerstick monitoring can be performed at 26–28 weeks of gestation [38].

An increased prevalence of GDM along with altered glucose metabolism in postoperative women raises the concern that GDM treatment or perinatal outcome may be different in postoperative GDM patients versus GDM patients who did not undergo bariatric surgery. Sheiner et al. [31] investigated this question in a study comparing characteristics of pregnancies and their outcomes among postoperative GDM patients and GDM patients who did not undergo surgery for obesity. The authors found no significant differences in hemoglobin A1C, obstetric characteristics, or perinatal outcomes among the two groups, suggesting that although the prevalence of GDM may be higher in postoperative women, disease features and prognoses are similar in GDM patients who have or have not had bariatric surgery.

Cesarean section

A number of studies have noted increased rates of cesarean section in women who have undergone bariatric surgery [18,19], although others report rates similar to their respective community levels [25,35]. The issue of caregiver bias influencing the decision to counsel for cesarean delivery was raised by Sheiner et al. [18] in their study comparing postoperative patients with the general population. The authors demonstrated an increased risk for cesarean section in post-bariatric surgery patients, persistent even after controlling for confounders such as obesity, previous cesarean section, and labor induction. In addition, rates of labor dystocia were similar among the two study groups, eliminating this factor as a possible cause of the difference in cesarean section rate. Although bias may play a role in increasing postoperative risk for cesarean section, postoperative women studied by Sheiner et al. [18] were significantly older and more obese than the general population, two independent risk factors for cesarean delivery. Although the authors did control for these factors in their multivariate analysis, residual confounding cannot be excluded.

Weintraub et al. [19] found higher rates of cesarean section among postoperative deliveries compared to deliveries in obese women before they had undergone bariatric surgery. However, this difference was no longer significant when previous cesarean section was controlled for. The authors suggest that it is the previous status of postoperative women, namely history of obesity and its known association with cesarean delivery, that puts postoperative women at higher risk for cesarean section [19]. The study also demonstrated a decreased rate of cesarean delivery for fetal macrosomia among post-bariatric surgery patients.

The effect of bariatric surgery on mode of subsequent deliveries remains unclear. Providers need to be aware of caregiver bias and avoid operating on postoperative women without a clear indication [2]. In addition, postoperative women should be counseled that although overall rates of cesarean section may be higher for them in comparison to the general population, their personal risk is heavily dependent on factors such as current BMI, age, and previous cesarean section.

Intrapartum complications

The few studies that have reported on intrapartum complications in postoperative women generally reveal no difference in rates of such complications among postoperative patients and controls [17,18,20]. Sheiner et al. [18] report similar rates of placental abruption, labor dystocia, and meconium-stained amniotic fluid among post-bariatric surgery women versus the general population, although the rate of packed-cell transfusion was higher in postoperative deliveries (3.4% versus 1.6%, respectively; $p =$ 0.017), while rates of anemia (hemoglobin < 10 g/dl) were similar. In comparing indication for cesarean section among postoperative deliveries versus deliveries prior to bariatric surgery, Weintraub et al. [19] noted no difference in the rate of first-stage dystocia as an indication for cesarean delivery.

Other labor characteristics and complications, such as postpartum hemorrhage, operative vaginal delivery, and third- or fourth-degree lacerations appear to be similar among postoperative patients and controls [17,20].

Bariatric surgery and fetal complications

Malformation

The state of relative nutritional deficiency created by bariatric surgery could theoretically put a developing fetus at risk for malformations, particularly neural tube defects (NTDs). Although malabsorptive procedures have traditionally been associated with vitamin deficiencies, women who have undergone restrictive procedures may also suffer from similar micronutrient deficiencies [16].

In their study on 301 deliveries before bariatric surgery and 507 deliveries after bariatric surgery, Weintraub et al. [19] found a higher rate of fetal malformations in postoperative deliveries versus preoperative controls (7.9% versus 3.3%; $p = 0.006$). Unfortunately, type of procedure could not be identified in their retrospective study and included both malabsorptive and restrictive categories. This relationship disappeared, however, in a multivariate model constructed using fetal malformation as the outcome variable. Once maternal age and preterm delivery were controlled for, there was no significantly increased risk for fetal malformation in women who had undergone bariatric surgery versus women who had not yet undergone the surgery (OR 1.9; 95% CI 0.88–4.12, $p = 0.089$). Women delivering after bariatric surgery were significantly older than preoperative women, a known risk factor for fetal malformation (mean maternal age 31.3 and 26.5, respectively; $p < 0.001$), although the relationship between preterm delivery and bariatric surgery was not mentioned.

In a prior study by Sheiner et al. [18] comparing 298 deliveries in postoperative women with 158,912 other deliveries, no difference in congenital malformation rate was observed (5.0% and 4.0%, respectively; $p = 0.355$). Of note, mean age was higher in postoperative women in comparison to the general population, but only by 1 year (mean maternal age 29.1 and 28.3 years, respectively; $p = 0.026$). Another more recent study comparing women who underwent gastric bypass with women who had not undergone weight loss surgery also demonstrated no significant difference in the rates of birth defects among the two groups [20].

Despite the fact that systematic studies have failed to report an association between bariatric surgery and fetal malformations including NTDs, micronutrient deficiencies do appear to occur in post-bariatric surgery patients [16,37], with some patients requiring parenteral nutrition [25,39]. One study observed elevated levels of homocysteine in pregnant post-bariatric surgery patients, theoretically putting their fetuses at risk for NTD, although no control homocysteine levels were provided [16]. Case reports documenting fetuses with NTDs born to post-bariatric surgery women exist in the literature [12], but to date the risk remains theoretical as larger studies have not confirmed a causal link [17,18]. In addition, obesity itself appears to increase the risk for NTD [40], further confounding the picture when considering that postoperative women are more likely to be obese compared to the general population [18].

It is important to note that post-bariatric surgery patients are often monitored for nutritional deficiencies and are encouraged to take nutritional and multivitamin supplements. Indeed, the theoretical risk for NTD in postoperative deliveries may be counteracted by the supplements these women receive. It is not known whether postoperative women should take higher than the recommended amount of folic acid supplementation, and current recommendations suggest daily supplementation with 400 μg of folic acid [37,41].

Birthweight

Obesity is a well-known risk factor for large-for-gestational-age and macrosomic babies [42,43]. A number of studies have demonstrated that bariatric surgery, an effective treatment for obesity, may lower the incidence of fetal macrosomia in those women who choose to undergo the procedure [19,25,44]. On the other hand, some studies have suggested that weight loss surgery may be associated with small-for-gestational-age (SGA) babies, likely due to the expected state of malnourishment these women experience postoperatively and the micronutrient deficiencies they may develop [25,39].

Studies comparing preoperative and postoperative women or postoperative patients and obese controls have generally shown a decreased incidence of macrosomic infants born to post-bariatric surgery women [16,17,19]. In their study of 301 pre-bariatric surgery deliveries and 507 deliveries after surgery, Weintraub et al. [19] observed a significantly lower rate of macrosomia among postoperative women compared to controls (3.2% and 7.6%, respectively; OR 0.4; 95% CI 0.2–0.8, $p = 0.004$). In addition, this risk reduction remained significant even when controlling for diabetes, maternal age, and hypertension (adjusted OR 0.45; 95% CI 0.21–0.94, $p = 0.033$). Other studies describe similar results [16,17], suggesting that bariatric surgery is an effective intervention for the prevention of macrosomia in obese patients.

Studies comparing women post-bariatric surgery with women in the general population do not always reveal a decrease in rate of macrosomia [18]. However, this is to be expected given that mean BMI tends to be higher in postoperative patients compared to the general population

[18,20]. Wax et al. [20] demonstrate no difference in rate of macrosomia among postoperative parturients and control parturients matched for maternal age and prior cesarean section. By comparing 298 postoperative women with 158,912 control women from the general population, Sheiner et al. [18] demonstrated an increased risk for fetal macrosomia in women who had undergone bariatric surgery compared to controls. This risk was persistent even after controlling for confounders such as obesity (adjusted OR 2.1; 95% CI 1.4 – 3.0, $p < 0.001$), although caution must be exercised when interpreting these results as complex, and residual confounding may be involved, especially since postoperative patients were significantly more obese (BMI > 30) than controls (10.7% and 1.2%, respectively, $p < 0.001$).

The therapeutic state of malnutrition caused by bariatric surgery raises concerns regarding fetal growth and specifically the theoretical risk for increased incidence of SGA, low birthweight (LBW), and intrauterine growth restriction (IUGR). Although a few series have reported high rates of IUGR and LBW babies born to patients who have undergone bariatric surgery [25,39], many systematic studies have not confirmed these findings. Interestingly, Ducarme et al. [17] found a higher rate of LBW babies in obese women compared to those who had received laparascopically assisted gastric banding. Weintraub et al. [19] observed no difference in rates of IUGR and LBW among 301 preoperative and 507 postoperative women. In a systematic study comparing 298 post-bariatric surgery patients with 158,912 members of the general population, a higher rate of IUGR was noted among postoperative women, although no elevated risk for IUGR was observed in multivariate analysis controlling for confounders such as hypertensive disorders [18].

Larger systematic studies are needed to elucidate the effect of bariatric surgery on birthweight in pregnancies following surgery. However, current studies have consistently demonstrated no association between bariatric surgery and adverse perinatal outcomes including fetal malformation, perinatal mortality rates, and low Apgar scores at 1 and 5 minutes [2,16,18,31].

Interval to pregnancy after bariatric surgery

Little is known about the influence of pregnancy timing on post-bariatric surgery complications. Some authorities have recommended waiting at least 12 postoperative months before becoming pregnant [45], although this recommendation remains based on largely theoretical risks. Rapid weight loss characterizes the first few months after bariatric surgery, potentially leading to a malnourished fetus and complications such as IUGR and malformation [44]. Although few systematic studies have investigated pregnancies specifically in the first postoperative year, the available data do not support such complications [16,32,33,46].

Another theoretical concern regarding pregnancy during the rapid weight loss phase post-bariatric surgery is the potential adverse effect of maternal ketosis on fetal outcome. Antepartum ketosis may negatively affect parameters such as child intelligence [47], although this topic has been studied among diabetic mothers and not in postoperative women. Furthermore, it is unclear how significant ketosis is in the first few months after various types of bariatric procedure. Maternal metabolism is affected by some weight loss surgeries, with one small series documenting a greater degree of starvation ketosis in two study subjects 3 months after jejunoileal bypass compared to similar conditions prior to the surgery [48]. To the best of our knowledge, studies investigating long-term perinatal outcomes after bariatric surgery, such as child intelligence, have not been carried out.

Studies by Dao et al. [33] and Patel et al. [32] compared early (defined as less than 12 months postoperatively in both studies) versus late (defined as over 18 months postoperatively by Patel et al. and over 12 months postoperatively by Dao et al.) post-bariatric surgery pregnancies and found no differences in major or minor pregnancy complications including oligohydramnios, pregnancy-induced hypertension, preterm delivery, and IUGR. Mean birthweight also does not appear to be affected [16,32,33]. Mean maternal weight gain, however, was significantly lower among women with early postoperative pregnancies as demonstrated by Dixon et al. [16] and Dao et al. [33]. Although Dixon et al. [16] reported similar birthweights among early and late postoperative pregnancies based on univariate analysis, the authors observed a direct positive correlation between maternal weight change and birthweight after controlling for gestational age. It is unclear what the clinical significance of this finding is, since higher complication rates among early postoperative pregnancies have not been reported [26,32,33].

In addition, a series following 18 postoperative pregnancies reported weight loss in five pregnancies, all of which occurred in the first or second postoperative years, with no obvious effects on fetal parameters [26]. Similarly, a study comparing 20 pregnancies conceived 18 months or less after Roux-en-Y gastric bypass (RYGB) with 32 post-RYGB pregnancies conceived more than 18 months after delivery observed no differences in adverse obstetric or fetal outcomes such as gestational diabetes, IUGR, neonatal Apgar score below 7 at 5 minutes, neonatal intensive care unit admission, or birth defect [46].

Interestingly, the type of bariatric procedure may affect the time interval to pregnancy post-procedure. A study by Sheiner et al. [49] demonstrated a shorter mean time to conception in post-restrictive procedure pregnancies compared to post-malabsorptive pregnancies (36.2 months versus 57.4 months; $p < 0.001$). A number of factors could be responsible for this, including differences in postoperative fertility or variables related to the procedure itself, such as postoperative complication rate (higher among malabsorptive pregnancies although not significantly so) or recovery time.

To date, studies comparing early and late post-bariatric surgery pregnancies are small, and some do not mention statistical significance. Future research should address whether or not early postoperative pregnancy is safe compared to late postoperative pregnancy, whether or not it has a lower risk for obesity-related complications compared to cohorts who are obese, and whether or not type of bariatric procedure affects perinatal outcome among such pregnancies [50]. No strict consensus has been reached regarding how to best counsel patients about early postoperative pregnancies, with the American College of Obstetricians and Gynecologists recommending a closer surveillance of maternal nutritional status and ultrasound for the serial monitoring of fetal growth if conception does occur before 12–24 postoperative months [41].

Type of bariatric procedure

Weight loss can be successfully achieved by a variety of bariatric procedures that can be broadly categorized into restrictive procedures, including adjustable gastric banding (AGB), or mixed procedures with some malabsorptive and restrictive components, including RYGB and biliopancreatic diversion (BPD). Studies have investigated pregnancies after both categories of procedure, although more research is needed comparing pregnancies after restrictive surgery with those after malabsorptive or mixed surgery. Moreover, some studies do not distinguish between these categories but combine subjects who may have undergone very different procedures [18,19]. Since medical and surgical complications vary by procedure type, theoretical risks and advantages to the pregnant woman and her fetus may also differ based on what type of bariatric surgery she underwent prior to conception. A recent study by Sheiner et al. [49] compared 394 pregnancies after restrictive procedures with 55 pregnancies after malabsorptive procedures. Although differences were reported among a few variables of interest such as maternal weight gain and birthweight, fetal outcomes including Apgar score, perinatal mortality, LBW, and macrosomia were similar among the two groups.

Restrictive procedures such as AGB are the most common bariatric procedures performed in Europe [51]. A major advantage of AGB is band adjustability, allowing for alleviation of nausea and appropriate weight gain [16,26]. Conversely, one potential complication of AGB is band slippage [35], although this has not been widely observed in systematic studies. In a study comparing 79 postoperative pregnancies with those same patients' penultimate preoperative pregnancies, Dixon et al. [16] found that women who were not managed early during their pregnancy with band adjustments when necessary were less likely to meet the gestational weight gain guidelines set by the Institute of Medicine. However, the authors did not clarify how many patients underwent band adjustment and for what reasons specifically, and in addition it is unclear whether the band adjustment alone affected weight gain or whether some other aspects of early pregnancy monitoring could have been involved [2,16]. Another series presenting descriptive statistics on 23 post-AGB pregnancies reports normal-birthweight babies (mean birthweight 3,676 g; range 2,381–3,912 g) without band adjustment, although a few bands were adjusted due to nausea, vomiting, or patient request [26]. Nevertheless, it appears that band adjustment is often necessary to control nausea and vomiting [16,17,26], with one study reporting a 60% rate of band adjustment for the prevention and/or treatment of first-trimester nausea and vomiting [17].

RYGB is the predominant bariatric procedure performed in the USA [52]. Surgeries such as RYGB may lead to deficiencies in nutrients such as vitamin B_{12} and folate in women who undergo them [25,37]. This raises concern surrounding the nutritional status of post-RYGB pregnant women and their fetuses, theoretically leading to complications such as fetal malformation and LBW babies. In their study of women post-BPD, Marceau et al. [25] report a higher rate of SGA babies in postoperative pregnancies compared with preoperative pregnancies (9.6% and 3.1%, respectively), although the authors claim the higher rate is within the normal range of their community levels. In a recent study comparing patients who had undergone RYGB with control women matched for age and prior cesarean section, Wax et al. [20] report no significant differences in birthweight or babies born at birthweights below the 10th percentile among groups. Sheiner et al. [49] also observed a higher mean birthweight for post-malabsorptive procedures compared to restrictive ones, although no difference was noted in LBW (<2,500 g) or macrosomia (>4,000 g) between the two groups.

Deficiency in serum albumin is also a concern specific to pregnancy after malabsorptive procedures, with one study documenting a decrease in mean serum album concentration in pregnancies after BPD (from 40.4 g/l to 35.7 g/l; $p < 0.001$), including four out of 251 postoperative pregnant patients requiring hospitalization for this complication [25]. Another study on post-restrictive procedure pregnancies reported no differences in mean plasma protein concentration among preoperative and postoperative pregnancies [16].

Finally, late surgical complications, including bowel ischemia and internal hernia formation, have been reported in post-malabsorptive procedure pregnancies [53,54]. However, systematic studies have not demonstrated high rates of such complications [20,25,49].

Surgical complications such as band slippage after AGB or internal hernia formation after RYGB are often difficult to diagnose secondary to their non-specific symptoms, which are often similar to those seen in a number of other conditions. Band slippage, for example, can result in stomach herniation through the band, with resultant gastric pouch dilation and ischemia [55]. Severe epigastric pain and failure to tolerate food are the usual presenting symptoms. Right upper quadrant pain may be present, and acute cholecystitis should also be considered in the differential diagnosis. Band position can usually be assessed with abdominal plain films, with a gastrograffin swallow assisting in the diagnosis of gastric pouch dilation and obstruction. Patients presenting with symptoms consistent with band slippage should be evaluated by a general surgeon in the emergency room. If band deflation does not relieve symptoms, surgeons should have a low threshold for surgical exploration [55]. On the other hand, post-RYGB patients suffering from internal hernia formation may have very mild complaints such as intermittent abdominal pain and vomiting, although vomiting is often not present. In addition, computed tomography scan or upper gastrointestinal series are not always diagnostic [53]. The definitive diagnosis and management of internal hernia formation often requires surgical exploration and correction.

Conclusions and recommendations

Pregnancy after bariatric surgery appears to be safe [18] and, regarding certain complications, is safer for both mother and fetus than pregnancy in the obese [19]. Table 5.1 summarizes the findings of select systematic studies regarding postoperative pregnancies. It is important for the clinician to note, however, that data on this subject were collected from women who received prenatal care consisting of excellent monitoring and intervention when necessary [2]. Therefore, providers should be aware of potential complications in their postoperative pregnant patients and manage them accordingly.

Systematic studies have not shown an association between bariatric surgery and fetal malformation [16,18], although study subjects were likely to have received supplements and close monitoring for nutritional deficiencies. All postoperative women should be observed for deficiencies

Table 5.1 Summary of select studies on pregnancy after bariatric surgery

Authors	Type of procedure	Number of postoperative pregnancies	Comparison groups	Findings
Dixon et al. [16]	AGB	79	Pregnancies after surgery and penultimate preoperative pregnancies	No difference in birthweight. Pregnancy-induced hypertension lower in postoperative pregnancies. Stillbirth, preterm delivery, low-birthweight, and high-birthweight rates were similar to community levels
Ducarme et al. [17]	AGB	13	Pregnancies after surgery and pregnancies in obese women	Rates of pre-eclampsia, gestational diabetes mellitus, low birthweight, and fetal macrosomia were lower in the postoperative group. No differences in birthweight, preterm birth, Apgar score < 7 at 5 minutes, or umbilical pH < 7.20
Marceau et al. [25]	BPD	251	Pregnancies before and after surgery	Lower rate of fetal macrosomia in postoperative pregnancies. High rate of miscarriage before and after surgery. Increase in small-for-gestational-age infants in postoperative pregnancies. Lower mean serum albumin concentration in postoperative pregnancies
Patel et al. [32]	RYGB	26	Pregnancies after RYGB and pregnancies to the general population stratified by BMI	Higher rate of small-for-gestational-age infants in post-surgery pregnancies. No difference in mean birthweight. Two postoperative patients required abdominal exploration during pregnancy for small bowel obstruction. No differences in complication rates among pregnancies conceived less than 12 months postoperatively compared to those conceived over 18 months postoperatively
Sheiner et al. [18]	Mixed	298	Pregnancies after bariatric surgery and pregnancies to the general population	Higher rates of fertility treatments, macrosomia, obesity, and cesarean section in postoperative pregnancies. No differences in fetal outcomes such as perinatal death, Apgar score, or non-reassuring heart rate pattern

Table 5.1 (*Continued*)

Authors	Type of procedure	Number of postoperative pregnancies	Comparison groups	Findings
Sheiner et al. [49]	Mixed	449	Post-restrictive procedure pregnancies and post-malabsorptive procedure pregnancies	Higher mean birthweight in post-malabsorptive procedure patients. No differences in low-birthweight infants, macrosomia, low Apgar scores, or perinatal mortality
Wax et al. [46]	RYGB	52	Postoperative pregnancies 18 months or less and postoperative pregnancies over 18 months	No differences in preterm premature rupture of membranes, gestational diabetes mellitus, oligohydramnios, intrauterine growth restriction, preterm or post-term deliveries. No differences in fetal outcomes such as low 5-minute Apgar score, neonatal intensive care admission, or birth defect
Weintraub et al. [19]	Mixed	507	Pregnancies before and after bariatric surgery	Lower rates of diabetes mellitus, hypertensive disorders, and fetal macrosomia in postoperative pregnancies. No differences in low Apgar score and perinatal mortality. Higher crude rate of fetal malformation in postoperative pregnancies; no difference on multivariate analysis controlling for maternal age, preterm delivery, diabetes mellitus, and birthweight

AGB, adjustable gastric banding; BMI; body mass index; BPD, biliopancreatic diversion; RYGB, Roux-en-Y gastric bypass.

in folate, vitamin B_{12}, and albumin. Screening for malformation and growth restriction using ultrasound may also be beneficial, along with careful attention to maternal weight gain. In addition, surgeons should be consulted for those women who underwent AGB regarding the possibility of band adjustment, especially if excessive nausea and vomiting occurs. Consultation with a nutritionist soon after conception may also be considered [41].

As previously discussed, obese women should not be counseled to undergo bariatric surgery solely to improve fertility. However, postoperative patients should be warned that they may experience increased fertility after surgery. In addition, providers may choose to recommend contraception other than the OCP due to the possible changes in its absorption [28].

There is no consensus on guidelines for interval to conception after bariatric surgery. Some authorities have recommended waiting at least 12–24 months after a weight loss procedure before attempting to conceive, although this may not be necessary considering that higher rates of poor outcomes have not been seen in such early pregnancies [32,46]. More research in this area is needed.

Although larger, prospective studies are needed to better elucidate some of the risks and benefits of pregnancy after bariatric surgery, it appears that, with appropriate prenatal care, postoperative women are at lower risk for perinatal complications than their obese counterparts.

References

1. Allison DB, Fontaine KR, Manson JE, et al. Annual deaths attributable to obesity in the United States. JAMA 1999;282(16):1530–8.
2. Karmon A, Sheiner E. Pregnancy after bariatric surgery: a comprehensive review. Arch Gynecol Obstet 2008;277(5):381–8.
3. Pasquali R, Pelusi C, Genghini S, et al. Obesity and reproductive disorders in women. Hum Reprod Update 2003;9(4):359–72.
4. Weiss JL, Malone FD, Emig D, et al. Obesity, obstetric complications and cesarean delivery rate – a population-based screening study. Am J Obstet Gynecol 2004; 190(4):1091–7.
5. Young TK, Woodmansee B. Factors that are associated with cesarean delivery in a large private practice: the importance of prepregnancy body mass index and weight gain. Am J Obstet Gynecol 2002;187(2):312–18.
6. Burstein E, Levy A, Mazor M, et al. Pregnancy outcome among obese women: a prospective study. Am J Perinatol 2008;25(9):561–6.
7. Buchwald H, Avidor Y, Braunwald E, et al. Bariatric surgery: a systematic review and meta-analysis. JAMA 2004;292(14):1724–37.
8. Tice JA, Karliner L, Walsh J, et al. Gastric banding or bypass? A systematic review comparing the two most popular bariatric procedures. Am J Med 2008;121(10):885–93.
9. Maggard MA, Yermilov I, Li Z, et al. Pregnancy and fertility following bariatric surgery: a systematic review. JAMA 2008;300(19):2286–96.

10. Davis MM, Slish K, Chao C, et al. National trends in bariatric surgery, 1996–2002. Arch Surg 2006;141(1):71–4.

11. Granstrom L, Granstrom L, Backman L. Fetal growth retardation after gastric banding. Acta Obstet Gynecol Scand 1990;69(6):533–6.

12. Haddow JE, Hill LE, Kloza EM, et al. Neural tube defects after gastric bypass. Lancet 1986;1(8493):1330.

13. Huerta S, Rogers LM, Li Z, et al. Vitamin A deficiency in a newborn resulting from maternal hypovitaminosis A after biliopancreatic diversion for the treatment of morbid obesity. Am J Clin Nutr 2002;76(2):426–9.

14. Martin L, Chavez GF, Adams MJ, Jr., et al. Gastric bypass surgery as maternal risk factor for neural tube defects. Lancet 1988;1(8586):640–1.

15. Ramirez MM, Turrentine MA. Gastrointestinal hemorrhage during pregnancy in a patient with a history of vertical-banded gastroplasty. Am J Obstet Gynecol 1995; 173(5):1630–1.

16. Dixon JB, Dixon ME, O'Brien PE. Birth outcomes in obese women after laparoscopic adjustable gastric banding. Obstet Gynecol 2005;106(5 Pt 1):965–72.

17. Ducarme G, Revaux A, Rodrigues A, et al. Obstetric outcome following laparoscopic adjustable gastric banding. Int J Gynaecol Obstet 2007;98(3):244–7.

18. Sheiner E, Levy A, Silverberg D, et al. Pregnancy after bariatric surgery is not associated with adverse perinatal outcome. Am J Obstet Gynecol 2004;190(5): 1335–40.

19. Weintraub AY, Levy A, Levi I, et al. Effect of bariatric surgery on pregnancy outcome. Int J Gynaecol Obstet 2008;103(3):246–51.

20. Wax JR, Cartin A, Wolff R, et al. Pregnancy following gastric bypass surgery for morbid obesity: maternal and neonatal outcomes. Obes Surg 2008;18(5):540–4.

21. Clark AM, Thornley B, Tomlinson L, et al. Weight loss in obese infertile women results in improvement in reproductive outcome for all forms of fertility treatment. Hum Reprod 1998;13(6):1502–5.

22. Crosignani PG, Colombo M, Vegetti W, et al. Overweight and obese anovulatory patients with polycystic ovaries: parallel improvements in anthropometric indices, ovarian physiology and fertility rate induced by diet. Hum Reprod 2003;18(9): 1928–32.

23. Bilenka B, Ben-Shlomo I, Cozacov C, et al. Fertility, miscarriage and pregnancy after vertical banded gastroplasty operation for morbid obesity. Acta Obstet Gynecol Scand 1995;74(1):42–4.

24. Deitel M, Stone E, Kassam HA, et al. Gynecologic–obstetric changes after loss of massive excess weight following bariatric surgery. J Am Coll Nutr 1988;7(2):147–53.

25. Marceau P, Kaufman D, Biron S, et al. Outcome of pregnancies after biliopancreatic diversion. Obes Surg 2004;14(3):318–24.

26. Martin LF, Finigan KM, Nolan TE. Pregnancy after adjustable gastric banding. Obstet Gynecol 2000;95(6 Pt 1):927–30.

27. Victor A, Odlind V, Kral JG. Oral contraceptive absorption and sex hormone binding globulins in obese women: effects of jejunoileal bypass. Gastroenterol Clin North Am 1987;16(3):483–91.

28. Merhi ZO. Challenging oral contraception after weight loss by bariatric surgery. Gynecol Obstet Invest 2007;64(2):100–2.

29. Merhi ZO. Weight loss by bariatric surgery and subsequent fertility. Fertil Steril 2007;87(2):430–2.

30. Merhi ZO, Pal L. Effect of weight loss by bariatric surgery on the risk of miscarriage. Gynecol Obstet Invest 2007;64(4):224–7.

31. Sheiner E, Menes TS, Silverberg D, et al. Pregnancy outcome of patients with gestational diabetes mellitus following bariatric surgery. Am J Obstet Gynecol 2006 Feb;194(2):431–5.

32. Patel JA, Patel NA, Thomas RL, et al. Pregnancy outcomes after laparoscopic Roux-en-Y gastric bypass. Surg Obes Relat Dis 2008;4(1):39–45.

33. Dao T, Kuhn J, Ehmer D, et al. Pregnancy outcomes after gastric-bypass surgery. Am J Surg 2006;192(6):762–6.

34. Sibai BM, Ewell M, Levine RJ, et al. Risk factors associated with preeclampsia in healthy nulliparous women. The Calcium for Preeclampsia Prevention (CPEP) Study Group. Am J Obstet Gynecol 1997;177(5):1003–10.

35. Bar-Zohar D, Azem F, Klausner J, et al. Pregnancy after laparoscopic adjustable gastric banding: perinatal outcome is favorable also for women with relatively high gestational weight gain. Surg Endosc 2006;20(10):1580–3.

36. Skull AJ, Slater GH, Duncombe JE, et al. Laparoscopic adjustable banding in pregnancy: safety, patient tolerance and effect on obesity-related pregnancy outcomes. Obes Surg 2004;14(2):230–5.

37. Wax JR, Pinette MG, Cartin A, et al. Female reproductive issues following bariatric surgery. Obstet Gynecol Surv 2007;62(9):595–604.

38. Wax JR. Risks and management of obesity in pregnancy: current controversies. Curr Opin Obstet Gynecol 2009;21(2):117–23.

39. Friedman D, Cuneo S, Valenzano M, et al. Pregnancies in an 18-year follow-up after biliopancreatic diversion. Obes Surg 1995;5(3):308–13.

40. Blomberg MI, Kallen B. Maternal obesity and morbid obesity: the risk for birth defects in the offspring. Birth Defects Res A Clin Mol Teratol 2010;88(1):35–40.

41. ACOG Practice Bulletin No. 105: bariatric surgery and pregnancy. Obstet Gynecol 2009;113(6):1405–13.

42. Ehrenberg HM, Mercer BM, Catalano PM. The influence of obesity and diabetes on the prevalence of macrosomia. Am J Obstet Gynecol 2004;191(3):964–8.

43. Jensen DM, Damm P, Sorensen B, et al. Pregnancy outcome and prepregnancy body mass index in 2459 glucose-tolerant Danish women. Am J Obstet Gynecol 2003;189(1):239–44.

44. Wittgrove AC, Jester L, Wittgrove P, et al. Pregnancy following gastric bypass for morbid obesity. Obes Surg 1998;8(4):461–4.

45. ACOG Committee Opinion No. 315, September 2005. Obesity in pregnancy. Obstet Gynecol 2005;106(3):671–5.

46. Wax JR, Cartin A, Wolff R, et al. Pregnancy following gastric bypass for morbid obesity: effect of surgery-to-conception interval on maternal and neonatal outcomes. Obes Surg 2008;18(12):1517–21.

47. Rizzo T, Metzger BE, Burns WJ, et al. Correlations between antepartum maternal metabolism and child intelligence. N Engl J Med 1991;325(13):911–16.

48. Al Shamma GA, Fell GS, Joffe SN. Response to starvation before and after a jejuno-ileal bypass operation for morbid obesity. Scott Med J 1979;24(3):206–10.

49. Sheiner E, Balaban E, Dreiher J, et al. Pregnancy outcome in patients following different types of bariatric surgeries. Obes Surg 2009;19(9):1286–92.

50. Karmon A, Sheiner E. Timing of gestation after bariatric surgery: should women delay pregnancy for at least 1 postoperative year? Am J Perinatol 2008;25(6):331–3.

51. Buchwald H, Williams SE. Bariatric surgery worldwide 2003. Obes Surg 2004;14(9):1157–64.

52. Santry HP, Gillen DL, Lauderdale DS. Trends in bariatric surgical procedures. JAMA 2005;294(15):1909–17.

53. Kakarla N, Dailey C, Marino T, et al. Pregnancy after gastric bypass surgery and internal hernia formation. Obstet Gynecol 2005;105(5 Pt 2):1195–8.
54. Charles A, Domingo S, Goldfadden A, et al. Small bowel ischemia after Roux-en-Y gastric bypass complicated by pregnancy: a case report. Am Surg 2005;71(3):231–4.
55. Kirshtein B, Lantsberg L, Mizrahi S, Avinoach E. Bariatric emergencies for non-bariatric surgeons: complications of laparoscopic gastric banding. Obes Surg 2010 Jan 15 [Epub ahead of print].

CHAPTER 6

The Impact of Maternal Obesity on Fetal and Neonatal Outcomes

Donald J. Dudley
University of Texas Health Science Center at San Antonio, Texas, USA

Obesity in general is associated with a number of adverse health consequences. These well-known complications, such as heart disease and early death, have drawn much attention in the scientific and lay press, and the impact of obesity on health overall and on the healthcare system (both delivery and cost) is under great scrutiny. Less well known are the effects of maternal obesity on the fetus and baby. Early reports from the 1970s [1] and 80s [2] were mere harbingers of several studies regarding adverse pregnancy outcomes in the 1990s until now. The purpose of this chapter is to review the impact of maternal obesity on fetal and neonatal outcomes, but it is not intended to be a meta-analysis. Several perinatal complications associated with obesity have been studied using meta-analytic techniques, and these will be highlighted in this review.

Spontaneous abortion

Obese women are at increased risk for spontaneous abortion, with an overall odds ratio (OR) of 1.2–1.7 [3–5]. Moreover, one report noted a greater risk for recurrent spontaneous losses (OR 3.5). Obese women who undergo some form of fertility treatment, for example *in vitro* fertilization or sperm injection, also have a greater risk for miscarriage than normal-weight control women [4]. A recent meta-analysis by Metwally et al. [6] summarized 16 studies, the authors reporting an overall OR of 1.67 for miscarriage in obese women regardless of whether the conception was spontaneous or assisted. Moreover, the risk for miscarriage after oocyte donation (OR 1.52) or ovulation induction (OR 5.1) was also statistically significant. However, in this study, no increase in miscarriage was evident after intracytoplasmic sperm injection.

Pregnancy in the Obese Woman, 1st edition. Edited by Deborah L. Conway.
© 2011 Blackwell Publishing Ltd.

A potential pathophysiological cause for miscarriage in obese women is that these women are more prone to metabolic syndrome and polycystic ovarian syndrome, with associated elevations in insulin and androgen levels, thus leading to an elevation in circulating estrogens and a relative deficiency in luteal phase and early gestational progesterone. Progesterone deficiency in this setting may lead to inadequate support of early pregnancy, thus leading to spontaneous pregnancy loss.

Clinical implications

Currently, there are no specific recommendations to prevent pregnancy loss in obese women, aside from the customary recommendations to lose weight and improve nutrition. Standard therapy for the prevention of recurrent pregnancy loss, based on a standard evaluation, remains the same in women with obesity, with specific targeting of known causes of recurrent pregnancy loss based on the best available evidence [7]. However, there are no specific recommendations to supplement progesterone during early pregnancy in obese women unless progesterone levels are decreased. Ovulation induction with clomiphene citrate also serves to supplement progesterone, but it can lead to other consequences such as multiple gestation.

Fetal anomalies

Maternal obesity is associated with an increased risk for a variety of fetal structural anomalies [8]. Perhaps the most comprehensive meta-analysis of birth defects in association with maternal obesity was recently completed by Stothard et al. [9]. Among the many birth defects associated with maternal obesity, neural tube defects had the highest OR (1.87; 95% confidence interval [CI] 1.62–2.15). In this report, they found an even higher OR for spina bifida alone (OR 2.24; 95% CI 1.86–2.69). A different meta-analysis by Ramsussen et al. [10] focused exclusively on the association of maternal obesity with neural tube defects. They noted an increased risk for neural tube defects with increasing maternal weight, with the highest risk being seen in morbidly obese women (BMI > 40 kg/m^2; OR 3.11; 95% CI 1.75–5.46). The association of neural tube defects with maternal obesity has been noted in women from a variety of locations, including the USA (the National Birth Defects Registry [11]), Texas, USA [12,13], Ontario, Canada [14], Atlanta, USA [15], and California, USA [16].

A common theme from these studies is that there is a dose-dependent response of the risk for fetal neural tube defects with maternal weight. Also, supplementation with folic acid did not decrease the risk for neural tube defects in obese women [14]. Moreover, the incidence of most types of neural tube defect, including spina bifida, anencephaly, and isolated hydrocephaly, is increased in obese women. In one study [12], the risk for fetal holoprosencephaly was not increased in obese women. Similarly, Shaw and Carmichael [17] were unable to find an association of neural tube defects and maternal obesity in a case-control study of California births from 1999–2004.

One speculation about the pathophysiological causes of this association is that women who are obese often have undiagnosed type 2 diabetes and that elevated plasma glucose levels result in the interruption of closure of the neural tube [18]. In addition, obese women have a poorer nutritional status than normal-weight women, particularly with regard to folic acid, and obese women appear to have less benefit from folic acid supplementation [19]. Along with abnormalities in folic acid level, obese women are at increased risk for deficiencies in other micronutrients that may be essential for closure of the neural tube [20].

The second most common birth defect associated with maternal obesity involves congenital heart defects. In the meta-analysis by Stothard et al. [9], the OR for congenital heart defects was 1.3 (95% CI 1.12–1.51). Septal anomalies alone carried an OR of 1.20. Waller et al. [11] found a similar association, but only in obese women with a body mass index (BMI) of $30 \, kg/m^2$ or more (OR 1.33; 95% CI 1.17–1.52). In the Atlanta study [15], underweight women had a lower risk for infants with congenital heart defects, while the OR for overweight and obese women was 1.36. In this study, the most common heart defects in the offspring included septal defects, outflow tract defects, and right-sided defects. Similarly, Cedergren and Kallen [21] found a weight-dependent association of congenital heart defects, with morbidly obese women having the greatest risk (OR 1.40; 95% CI 1.22–1.64). Septal defects were the most common defects noted.

However, other reports have not reported this association. Neither Khalil et al. [22], in an Arab population, nor Shaw and Carmichael [17], in a Californian population, detected an association of obesity with congenital heart defects. These differences might be explained by different study designs and different populations under study. One confounder that might explain some of the differences is the presence or absence of gestational or type 2 diabetes. Martinez-Frias et al. [23], in a Spanish population, found that obese women with gestational diabetes had on OR of 2.78 for congenital birth defects, whereas obese women with normal glucose tolerance had no increased risk for infants with congenital heart defects. This finding may explain the overall pathophysiology of heart defects with maternal obesity, but the data to prove this are incomplete. As with neural tube defects, there may be nutritional defects in folic acid and other micronutrients that might be a pathophysiological link for the association [24]. However, there are few data to confirm these suspicions.

In addition to neural tube defects and congenital heart defects, maternal obesity is associated with an increased risk for orofacial clefts [9,25], hypospadias [9,26], anorectal atresia [9], and limb reduction anomalies [9]. A clear pathophysiological cause or sequence leading to these anomalies is not clear.

Notably, the risk for fetal gastroschisis is reduced in women who are obese [9] (OR 0.17; 95% CI 0.10–0.30). Siega-Riz et al. [27] reported on data from the National Birth Defects Prevention Study, noting that a woman with a BMI of $17 kg/m^2$ at age 15 has an OR of 7 of having an offspring with gastroschisis compared to a 23-year-old woman with a normal BMI. Young, thin women are at much greater risk for gastroschisis than older women of normal weight, and young obese women are at less risk than those who are underweight. For example, a 19-year-old woman with a BMI of $17 kg/m^2$ has an adjusted OR for gastroschisis of 3.9, while a 19-year-old woman with a BMI of 30 has an adjusted OR of 1.1. This study provides compelling evidence for the interrelation of maternal age and weight in determining the risk for fetal gastroschisis. The pathophysiological basis for this association is not clear, although speculation is that young women with low body weight do not offer the same hormonal support during a critical embryonic developmental stage [27].

Table 6.1 summarizes recent reports regarding the association of common birth defects with obesity. Neural tube defects, congenital heart disease, orofacial clefts, hypospadias, and limb reduction defects have all been associated with obesity, although the studies listed in this table show conflicting results. For example, the study by Oddy et al. [28] found no such associations in an Australian population. However, there appears to be a consensus that birth defects are more common in obese and morbidly obese pregnant women.

Clinical implications

Although folate supplementation clearly prevents neural tube defects in a normal-weight population, this may not be the case for the obese pregnant woman. Careful attention to the nutritional status of obese women is recommended, although there are no studies to show that this will lead to a lower risk for birth defects. Antenatal detection of fetal structural anomalies is limited in obese women due to the technical limitations of sonography in these patients (see Chapter 8). Overall, there are no specific interventions to improve these outcomes in obese women.

Stillbirth

Along with birth defects, the risk for stillbirth in obese women increases with maternal weight and has been found to be a significant association in many different populations. A recent meta-analysis by Chu et al. [29]

Table 6.1 Summary of recent studies: obesity and risk of fetal anomalies

First author and reference	Year published	Years of study	Location of study	BMI 25–29.9 kg/m² OR	BMI 30–34.9 kg/m² OR	BMI ≥ 35 kg/m² OR
Neural tube defects						
Shaw [16]	2000	1999–2004	California	NS	NS	–
Watkins [15]	2003	1993–1997	Atlanta	NS	2.7	–
Waller [11]	2007	1997–2002	USA	NS	2.19	–
Rasmussen [10]	2008	Meta-analysis	USA	NS	1.7	3.11
Stothard [9]	2009	Meta-analysis	USA	1.2	1.87	–
Oddy [28]	2009	1997–2000	Australia	NS	NS	–
Congenital heart defects						
Watkins [24]	2001	1968–2000	Atlanta	NS	NS	–
Cedergren [21]	2003	1998–2001	Sweden	NS	1.18	1.41
Watkins [15]	2003	1993–1997	Atlanta	2.0	2.0	–
Martinez [23]	2005	1996–2004	Spain	NS	3.47	–
Waller [11]	2007	1997–2002	USA	NS	1.33	–
Stothard [9]	2009	Meta-analysis	USA	1.17	1.30	–
Oddy [28]	2009	1997–2000	Australia	NS	NS	–

Table 6.1 (*Continued*)

First author and reference	Year published	Years of study	Location of study	BMI 25–29.9 kg/m² OR	BMI 30–34.9 kg/m² OR	BMI ≥35 kg/m² OR
Orofacial clefts						
Watkins [15]	2003	1993–1997	Atlanta	NS	NS	–
Cedergren [25]	2005	1992–2001	Sweden	NS	1.3	–
Waller [11]	2007	1997–2002	USA	NS	NS	–
Stothard [9]	2009	Meta-analysis	USA	NS	1.20–1.23	–
Oddy [28]	2009	1997–2000	Australia	NS	NS	–
Hypospadias						
Watkins [15]	2003	1993–1997	Atlanta	NS	NS	–
Waller [11]	2007	1997–2002	USA	1.24	NS	–
Akre [26]	2008	2000–2005	Scandinavia	1.7	2.6	–
Stothard [9]	2009	Meta-analysis	USA	NS	NS	–
Limb reduction defects						
Waller [11]	2007	1997–2002	USA	NS	NS	–
Stothard [9]	2009	Meta-analysis	USA	NS	1.34	–
Oddy [28]	2009	1997–2000	Australia	NS	NS	–

BMI, body mass index; NS, not significant; OR, odds ratio.

highlights these associations. In their study, these authors found that women who were overweight had an adjusted OR for stillbirth of 1.47 (95% CI 1.08–1.94), and women who were obese had an adjusted OR of 2.07 (95% CI 1.59–2.74). Given an overall risk for stillbirth of 7 per 1,000 births [30], an OR that doubles the risk would lead to an overall risk for 14 per 1,000 births, or 1.4% of all births in this at-risk population.

One of the largest studies to show this association was that of Cnattingius et al. [31]. In their study of over 167,000 Swedish women from 1992 to 1993, the risk for stillbirth increased with maternal weight and was highest among obese women, with an overall OR of 4.3 (95% CI 2.0–9.3). The risk was lower in multiparous women (OR 2.0) but still statistically significant. In adjusting for nulliparous women with hypertensive disease, the risk for stillbirth did not change in this population. Kristensen et al. [32] found a similar overall risk for stillbirth in obese Danish women and reported that the stillbirth risk was greatest at term or post-term. This finding was confirmed in a separate study from Denmark [33] in an analysis of the Danish National Birth Cohort. The risk for fetal death in women with a BMI of $30 \, kg/m^2$ or more was directly related to gestational age when compared to normal-weight women. The overall OR at 37–39 weeks was 3.5 (95% CI 1.9–6.4), and that for greater than 40 weeks was 4.6 (95% CI 1.6–13.4). However, in a Chinese population of over 29,000 from 1995 to 2005, Leung et al. [34] found no association of obesity with stillbirth.

Another compounding risk factor for stillbirth in obese women is maternal race and ethnicity. Salihu et al. [35] evaluated stillbirth in a Missouri, USA, cohort and found that morbidly obese African-American women had the highest risk for stillbirth in this population, with a hazard ratio of 2.3 (compared to a hazard ratio of 1.8 in morbidly obese white women). One potential risk factor that appears to have to impact on the risk for stillbirth in obese women is total pregnancy weight gain [36]. In this case-control study of Swedish nulliparous women, only the lowest weight gain group (≤0.24 kg [0.5 lb] per week) had an increased risk for early and late pregnancy stillbirths (OR 1.7 and 1.8, respectively). No other weight gain increment was associated with stillbirth in obese women.

One important issue to consider is whether obesity is an independent risk factor for stillbirth or is in some way causative of stillbirth. This issue was addressed in a population-based study by Villamor and Cnattingius [37]. In this national study of Swedish women who delivered between 1992 and 2001, the change in pre-pregnancy BMI from the first to the second pregnancy was studied, and the risk for adverse pregnancy outcomes, including stillbirth, was then assessed. When comparing women with no significant change in BMI (change of −1.0 to 0.9 units) to women who gained 3 or more units during a 2-year average period, these investigators found an adjusted OR for stillbirth of 1.63 (95% CI 1.20–2.21) in the women who gained weight. Moreover, the OR for stillbirth was higher for late-pregnancy stillbirth, consistent with other epidemiological studies. These data indicate that being overweight or obese is potentially causative for stillbirth. The pathophysiological mechanisms to explain this finding are not clear, although the abnormal inflammatory or endocrine milieu that characterizes obesity has been speculated to contribute to a patho-physiological sequence leading to stillbirth.

Table 6.2 summarizes recent studies that have addressed the association of maternal obesity with stillbirth. Several studies have been included in this table that were not described above [38–42]. There is a clear consensus from these studies that obesity (BMI $\geq$ 30 kg/m^2) is strongly associated with stillbirth. Given the increase in obesity in the last 20 years, one wonders whether or not this may contribute to the lack of progress in decreasing perinatal mortality rates in the USA.

Clinical implications

Although the data implicating obesity as being an independent risk factor for stillbirth are compelling, and may even be causative, there are no clear therapeutic or management options that have been shown to decrease the stillbirth risk. Since about a third of pregnant women are obese, and about a half are overweight or obese, performing fetal surveillance merely because of maternal weight seems unreasonably costly and labor-intensive, given that there are no data to show that such an approach will improve perinatal mortality. Prudence dictates, however, that women who are obese and have other co-morbidities such as diabetes or hypertension should undergo some form of fetal surveillance.

Elective early delivery also seems excessive and, like so many treatment options, is not supported by currently available data. Until new data show that a specific intervention improves outcome, current recommendations for fetal surveillance should be followed regardless of maternal weight. However, a higher index of suspicion in obese women with liberal indications for fetal surveillance seems a wise measure.

Pre-eclampsia

An increased risk for pre-eclampsia in pregnant obese women is a clear and consistent finding. As early as 2003, enough studies had been completed for a systematic overview [43]. This study included 13 cohort studies with 1.4 million women, and the authors found that the risk for pre-eclampsia doubled with each 5–7 BMI units (kg/m^2), or 0.54% for each 1 kg/m^2 increase in BMI. For example, women with a normal weight (BMI

Table 6.2 Summary of recent studies: obesity and risk of stillbirth

First author and reference	Year published	Years of study	Location of study	Descriptors	BMI 25–29.9 OR	BMI 30–34.9 OR	BMI ≥ 35 OR
Cnattingius [31]	1998	1992–1993	Sweden	Nullipara	3.2	4.3	–
				Multipara	NS	2.0	–
Stephansson [36]	2001	1987–1996	Sweden		1.9	2.1	–
Sebire [38]	2001	1989–1997	England		NS	1.4	–
				Black	–	1.3	1.4–1.8
Cedergren [39]	2004	1992–2001	Sweden	>28 weeks	–	1.79	1.99–2.79
Kristensen [32]	2005	1989–1996	Denmark		NS	3.1	–
Nohr [33]	2005	1998–2001	Denmark		2.0	3.2	–
Salihu [35]	2007	1978–1997	Missouri	White	–	1.6	1.9–2.3
Chu [29]	2007	Meta-analysis	USA		1.47	2.07	–
Bhattacharya [40]	2007	1976–2005	Scotland		NS	1.8	NS
Leung [34]	2008	1995–2005	China		NS	NS	–
Denison [41]	2008	1998–2002	Sweden		1.7	2.87	3.90
Khashan [42]	2009	2004–2006	UK		NS	NS	NS

BMI, body mass index; NS, not significant; OR, odds ratio.

20–24.9 kg/m^2) had an approximately 2–4% incidence of pre-eclampsia, whereas women with a BMI greater than 30 kg/m^2 had an 8–12% risk for developing pre-eclampsia.

Since this review, several studies have confirmed this risk and provided new insights into the presumed causation and pathophysiological events leading to disease. Rosenberg et al. [44] studied the influence of race and ethnicity on the risk for pre-eclampsia of over 213,000 women in New York City. Women who weighed greater than 300 lb had an OR of 5.0 for pre-eclampsia (95% CI 3.5–7.1), and black women accounted for a disproportionate share of obese women. Whereas black women constituted 27.6% of their sample population, they accounted for 64% of women weighing greater than 300 lb. Ramos and Caughey [45], in a study of 22,658 Californian women, found that pre-eclampsia was increased in obese Latina women (OR 1.93; 95% CI 1.24–3.01). However, African-American women in this population did not have an increased risk for pre-eclampsia (OR 0.95; 95% CI 0.61–1.48).

Bodnar et al. [46] evaluated data from 38,000 women enrolled in the Collaborative Perinatal Project from 1958 to 1964 and found that there was a dose–response relationship between BMI and risk for both mild and severe hypertensive diseases of pregnancy. Furthermore, the risk for severe pre-eclampsia increased with BMI, such that white women with a BMI of 25 kg/m^2 had an OR of 1.7 (95% CI 1.1–2.5) and a BMI of 30 had an OR of 3.4 (95% CI 2.1–5.6). Moreover, the risk in black women with a BMI of 25 was 2.1 (95% CI 1.4–3.2) and with a BMI of 30 was 3.2 (95% CI 2.1–5.0). Similar to the study by Rosenberg, these investigators found that almost 22% of black women had a BMI of over 25 kg/m^2, compared to about 15% of white women. Of note, black women with a BMI of greater than 35 had a slightly lower risk for pre-eclampsia than did white women with the same BMI.

The effect of gestational weight gain on pregnancy outcomes was studied in obese women by Kiel et al. [47]. Obese women who had little or no weight gain had a significantly lower risk for developing pre-eclampsia. Obese women who gained 15 lb or less had an OR of 0.5–1.0, while women who gained greater than 15 lb had an OR of about 1.2–1.7 for pre-eclampsia. Based on these results, these investigators recommended that weight gain be limited to less than 15 lb in women with BMI of greater than 30.

The pathophysiology of pre-eclampsia in obese women appears to be the same as in lean or normal-weight women, but the precise mechanisms remain unclear. Walsh [48] noted that obesity and pre-eclampsia share many common pathophysiological abnormalities. For example, both obesity and pre-eclampsia are characterized by increases in circulating proinflammatory mediators such as interleukin-1 and tumor necrosis factor-α. In addition, both conditions are associated with increased oxidative stress, dyslipidemia, hyperinsulinemia, and altered endothelial cell function. However, how these common features result in an increased risk for pre-eclampsia in obese women is not clear.

Table 6.3 summarizes recent studies that have evaluated the association of maternal obesity with pre-eclampsia. Several studies not described above are included for illustration [49–54]. There is a strong consensus that maternal obesity is associated with a much higher risk for pre-eclampsia, and that this risk is weight dependent, with heavier women having a greater risk. Moreover, this risk remains elevated for mild and severe disease and regardless of race and ethnicity or parity.

Clinical implications

No specific intervention has been shown that decreases the incidence of pre-eclampsia. Clearly, increased vigilance on the part of the obstetrician to identify women who develop pre-eclampsia is prudent. However, no therapy to date, including low-dose aspirin, calcium supplementation, salt restriction, or activity restrictions, has been shown to decrease the incidence of pre-eclampsia. If weight loss cannot be accomplished prior to pregnancy, maintaining a weight gain of less than 15 lb throughout the pregnancy appears to be one way to decrease the risk for developing pre-eclampsia.

In addition, care must be taken to obtain accurate blood pressure readings. Since 1967 [55], physicians have known the importance of appropriate cuff size in order to obtain accurate blood pressure readings. A recent review by Pickering [56], as well as a report by Umana et al. [57], highlights the importance of accurate measurements of blood pressure. In this last report, the investigators found that, if the appropriate cuff size was used correctly, usual oscillometric techniques were as accurate an intra-arterial techniques. These findings highlight the important of using appropriate cuff size as per standard recommendations [58]. This issue is more thoroughly addressed in Chapter 8.

Preterm labor and birth

For any association of a factor with an adverse pregnancy outcome, there needs to be a plausible pathophysiological process to prove causality. Obesity is associated with increased proinflammatory processes [59], as adipose tissue is characterized by the active production of inflammatory cytokines. Inflammation and proinflammatory cytokines characterize many, if not most, instances of spontaneous preterm birth [60]. Hence, one could rationally postulate the obesity could be causative for an increased risk for preterm birth.

Table 6.3 Summary of recent studies: obesity and risk of pre-eclampsia

First author and reference	Year published	Years of study	Location of study	Descriptors	BMI 25–29.9 OR	BMI 30–34.9 OR	BMI ≥ 35 OR
Baeten [49]	2001	1992–1996	Washington	Pre-eclampsia	2.0	3.3	–
				Eclampsia	2.0	3.0	–
Sebire [38]	2001	1989–1997	England		1.44	2.14	–
Stephansson [36]	2001	1987–1996	Sweden		NS	1.8	–
Jensen [50]	2003	1992–1996	Denmark		NS	3.8	–
Weiss [51]	2004	1999–2002	USA		NS	1.6	3.3
Cedergren [39]	2004	1992–2001	Sweden		–	2.62	3.9–4.82
Bodnar [52]	2005	1997–2001	Pennsylvania		2.1–2.6	2.9	2.3–2.8
Ramos [45]	2005	1981–2001	California	White	–	2.54	–
				Black	–	1.58	–
				Latina	–	2.56	–
				Asian	–	3.46	–

Study	Year	Country				
Doherty [53]	2006	Australia	Pre-eclampsia	NS	3.74	–
			Hypertension	2.6	2.93	–
Smith [54]	2007	Scotland	Nullipara	1.68	2.57	3.60
			Multipara	1.72	2.89	4.57
Bhattacharya [40]	2007	Scotland		1.6	3.1	7.2
Bodnar [46]	2007	USA	Mild/white	1.8	3.0	4.9
			Mild/black	2.2	3.1	4.2
			Severe/white	1.7	3.4	7.6
			Severe/black	2.1	3.2	5.3
Denison [41]	2008	Sweden		1.8	2.9	4.24
Leung [34]	2008	China		1.6–3.25	3.97	–

BMI, body mass index; NS, not significant; OR, odds ratio.

However, studies regarding the potential association of maternal obesity and preterm birth provide conflicting results. One difficulty in interpreting the available evidence is determining if obesity is an independent risk factor for gestational length. Many confounding factors determine the length of gestation, including co-morbidities that may require delivery prior to 37 weeks, physician factors, and difficulties in assigning specific gestational age determinations in obese women. Given these confounders, the evidence must be carefully reviewed with careful consideration of these variables.

For example, Nohr et al. [61], in their evaluation of preterm birth in the context of maternal obesity using the Danish National Birth Cohort, found that obese women had an adjusted hazard ratio for preterm premature rupture of the membranes (PPROM) of 1.5 (95% CI 1.2–1.9), as well as induced preterm birth (hazards ratio 1.2). After they made adjustments for the many confounders in the data, the risk for induced preterm birth was not increased over that for normal-weight women, while the risk for PPROM remained elevated. Notably, they found that the risk for all types of preterm birth was greater in women with a low weight gain, as defined by a weight gain of less than 275 g per week. Also, Bhattacharya et al. [40] found that obese women in Aberdeen, UK, had an increased risk for preterm delivery at less than 33 weeks (OR 2.0; 95% CI 1.3–2.9). After adjusting for confounders, they confirmed that the morbidly obese women had an increased risk for spontaneous preterm birth with an OR of 1.2 (95% CI 1.1–2.8). Weiss et al. [51], in a secondary analysis of the FASTER trial, found a similar OR for preterm delivery in morbidly obese women (OR 1.5; 95% CI 1.1–2.1).

Conversely, the Maternal Fetal Medicine Units Network evaluated the impact of maternal weight on preterm birth in a subanalysis of their preterm prediction study [62]. They found that obese women had a significantly lower risk for preterm birth (OR 0.57; 95% CI 0.39–0.83). Notably, the lower risk for preterm birth was weight-dependent, such that women with a BMI of 35 kg/m² or more had a 5.2% incidence of spontaneous preterm birth compared to women with a BMI of less than 19 kg/m², who had a preterm birth rate of 16.6%. Similarly, Denison et al. [41] found that Swedish women with a higher BMI had an increased risk for post-term pregnancies. In addition, Sebire et al. [38], in an analysis of the impact of obesity on pregnancy outcomes in English women, found that obesity was protective against preterm delivery at less than 37 weeks (OR 0.82; 95% CI 0.78–0.86) and 32 weeks (OR 0.73; 95% CI 0.65–0.82). Kumari [63] found a much lower risk for preterm birth in obese Arab women (0.5% in obese women versus 5.3% in non-obese women), but this study was marked by a relatively small sample size. Bianco et al. [64], in their study of morbidly obese women in New York City also found no increased risk for preterm delivery.

There are many potential reasons for these conflicting data. The published reports use different methods in their analyses, have different sample sizes, and evaluate markedly different populations. Perhaps the strongest confounder is that many epidemiological studies cannot distinguish between indicated and spontaneous preterm births. In order to address this issue, Smith et al. [54] carefully evaluated a large database of over 187,000 Scottish women to determine the relative contributions of spontaneous and "elective" (indicated) preterm births in obese women. These investigators determined that morbidly obese nulliparous women overall had an increased risk for preterm birth (OR 1.34; 95% CI 1.15–1.56). However, spontaneous preterm delivery was not associated with maternal weight (OR for morbidly obese women 0.81; 95% CI 0.64–1.03) while the risk for elective preterm delivery was significantly elevated (OR 2.13; 95% CI 1.75–2.58). In this study, a common reason for "elective" delivery was pre-eclampsia, so the delineation "elective" delivery likely represents the fact that a clinical indication for preterm delivery was evident. In overweight women (BMI 25–29.9 kg/m^2), nulliparas actually had a decreased risk for preterm delivery (OR 0.89; 95% CI 0.82–0.98). Obese multiparous women overall were not an increased risk for preterm delivery but, as with nulliparas, these women had an increased OR for elective preterm delivery (1.45; 95% CI 1.21–1.75). As with nulliparas, the multiparous women had a decreased OR for spontaneous preterm birth. They concluded from this study that morbid obesity was associated with preterm delivery in nulliparas, but that the increased risk was entirely accounted for by elective, or indicated, preterm deliveries.

Table 6.4 summarizes recent studies evaluating potential associations between maternal obesity and preterm birth. There is no clear consensus regarding the effect of obesity on the occurrence of preterm birth. Clearly, more study is needed to ascertain the precise role of maternal weight and maternal weight gain on the incidence and causes of preterm birth. Even if the relative risk for preterm birth is modest, the overall numbers of obese women who deliver preterm may be substantial. For example, if approximately 4 million women deliver in the USA every year and one-third are obese, about 1.3 million obese women will deliver per year. Given an overall risk for preterm birth of 13% [64], even a 0.5% increase would be 8,450 women. On a population basis, even modest increases in the preterm birth risk would result in substantial morbidity, mortality, and costs.

Clinical implications

No specific interventions to prevent preterm birth in obese women, outside of standard of care, is indicated unless new evidence comes forth to show that any specific intervention improves outcome. Given this, standard care with a high index of suspicion seems prudent.

Table 6.4 Summary of recent studies: obesity and risk of preterm birth (PTB)

First author and reference	Year published	Years of study	Location of study	Descriptors	BMI 25–29.9 OR	BMI 30–34.9 OR	BMI ≥35 OR
Cnattingius [31]	1998	1992–1993	Sweden	Nullipara <32 weeks	NS	1.6	–
Sebire [38]	2001	1989–1997	England		0.82	0.93	–
Baeten [49]	2001	1992–1997	Washington	<37 weeks	1.2	1.3	–
				<32 weeks	1.3	1.6	–
Jensen [50]	2003	1992–1996	Denmark		NS	NS	–
Weiss [51]	2004	1999–2002	USA		–	NS	1.5
Cedergren [39]	2004	1992–2001	Sweden	<37 weeks	–	1.22	1.48–1.85
				<32 weeks	–	1.45	1.95–2.32
Hendler [62]	2005	1992–1994	USA	<37 weeks	–	0.5	–
				<34 weeks	–	0.4	–
				<32 weeks	–	0.5	–

Author	Year	Period	Country	Category			
Smith [54]	2007	1991–2001	Scotland	Nullipara: total	NS	1.12	1.34
				Nullipara: spontaneous	NS	NS	NS
				Nullipara: elective	1.15	1.52	2.13
Bhattacharyra [40]	2007	1976–2005	Scotland	All	NS	1.2	1.6
				Spontaneous	NS	NS	1.2
Nohr [61]	2007	1996–2002	Denmark	All PTB (22–36 weeks)	NS	1.5	–
				Late PTB (33–36 weeks)	1.2	1.5	–
				Early PTB (22–33 weeks)	NS	1.6	–
Leung [34]	2008	1995–2005	China	All	NS	1.55	–
				Spontaneous	NS	NS	–
				Induced	1.4	2.04	–
Khashan [42]	2009	2004–2006	UK		0.89	0.90	NS

BMI, body mass index; NS, not significant; OR, odds ratio.

Neonatal mortality

Given these adverse pregnancy outcomes, maternal obesity, not surprisingly, is associated with increased neonatal mortality (death of a liveborn infant within the first 28 days of life). Given this, obstetricians need to intervene appropriately for maternal and fetal complications on behalf of the fetus regardless of maternal weight.

Cedergren [39] reported a prospective population-based cohort study of 3,480 women and found that morbidly obese women with a BMI of greater than $40\,kg/m^2$ had an increased risk for early neonatal death (death within the first 7 days after birth), with an OR of 3.4 (95% CI 2.07–5.63). Moreover, women who were overweight and obese had an increased risk for early neonatal death (overweight OR 1.59, 95% CI 1.25–2.01; and obese OR 2.09, 95% CI 1.50–2.91). Smith et al. [54] similarly found an increased risk for neonatal death in their study of Scottish women. They found that nulliparous women with a BMI of $35\,kg/m^2$ or over had an increased risk for neonatal death (OR 2.77; 95% CI 1.54–4.99), but that there was no increased risk for multiparas. However, this association was not significant after adjusting for gestational age at delivery, indicating that the increased risk for neonatal death was accounted for by prematurity.

In reviewing the data from the Danish National Birth Cohort, Nohr et al. [65] found that overweight and obese women had increased risk for neonatal mortality with an OR of 1.7 (95% CI 1.2–2.5) for overweight women and 1.6 (95% CI 1.0–2.4) for obese women. This risk was independent of parity or fetal birth defects. The main association of neonatal death and obesity was found in the PPROM population of women, where the risk for death more than tripled for overweight women and showed a sixfold increase for obese women. Salihu et al. [66] evaluated the role of race in neonatal mortality of infants of obese women and found that neonatal mortality was increased in all women with morbid obesity (hazard ratio 1.3; 95% CI 1.1–1.5). Furthermore, they found that the risk for neonatal mortality was increased with increasing increments of BMI in black women (adjusted hazard ratio 1.5–2.0 for all neonatal deaths across all obesity classifications).

Table 6.5 summarizes recent studies evaluating the association of maternal obesity with neonatal mortality. Only one study is included that was not discussed above [67]. Whereas most studies show an association of maternal obesity with neonatal mortality, other confounding factors often account for the increased risk for neonatal death, so proving that obesity is an independent risk factor for neonatal mortality is difficult. Regardless of this, these studies underscore the high-risk nature of pregnancy in obese women.

Table 6.5 Summary of recent studies: obesity and risk of neonatal death

First author and reference	Year published	Years of study	Location of study	Descriptors	BMI 25–29.9 OR	BMI 30–34.9 OR	BMI ≥ 35 OR
Chattingius [31]	1998	1992–1993	Sweden		NS	NS	–
Baeten [49]	2001	1992–1997	Washington	Infant death	NS	1.9	–
Cedergren [39]	2004	1992–2001	Sweden		–	1.59	2.09–3.41
Kristensen [32]	2005	1989–1996	Denmark		NS	2.7	–
Nohr [65]	2007	1996–2002	Denmark		1.8	NS	–
Smith [54]	2007	1991–2001	Scotland	Nullipara	NS	NS	2.77
				Multipara	NS	NS	NS
Salihu [66]	2008	1978–1997	Missouri		–	1.1	1.2–1.3
Gardosi [67]	2009	1992–1995	Sweden		1.34	1.62	–
Khashan [42]	2009	2004–2006	UK		0.57	NS	NS

BMI, body mass index; NS, not significant; OR, odds ratio.

Clinical implications

Decreasing neonatal mortality requires vigilance on the part of the obstetrician to identify and manage co-morbid conditions. Even then, a key consideration must be that obese women should be managed the same as normal-weight women. Fetal surveillance may be more difficult in obese women because of the technical difficulties posed by these patients. The obstetrician may be reluctant to intervene because of these technical considerations, but they should not be dissuaded from acting on behalf of the fetus when indicated.

Preventing adverse pregnancy outcomes

The prevention of adverse pregnancy outcomes in obese women often requires a multidisciplinary team approach, including obstetricians, perinatologists, internists, nutritionists, and perinatal nursing. However, to date, there are no specific recommendations for obese women except to attempt weight reduction when not pregnant [68,69]. Unfortunately, this effort is often not realized, and obese women commonly present in the early stages of pregnancy. Management of pregnancy in these women should focus on vigilance for common medical and obstetric complications that may occur throughout the course of the pregnancy [70]. The following measures may improve outcome but have not been tested in randomized controlled trials focused on improving perinatal outcomes in obese women:

- When women present with pregnancy in the first trimester, vaginal sonography should be encouraged to establish firm dating criteria.
- A thorough physical examination should be performed to diagnose or confirm medical complications, such as hypertension and diabetes.
- If diabetes has not previously been diagnosed, obese women should have screening for diabetes with a 1-hour glucose challenge. If negative, this should be repeated at 24–28 weeks and then again at 32 weeks. Indications for confirmatory 3-hour glucose tolerance testing should be liberal.
- Serum screening for fetal anomalies should be encouraged, and, if positive, a genetic sonogram performed. Given the technical limitations of sonography, this should be considered later than usual, at 20–22 weeks' gestation.
- If the patient declines serum screening, a detailed genetic sonogram can be a useful test independent of the serum screen.
- Vigilant prenatal care, with specific questioning for preterm labor and PPROM, may help to identify women with early symptomatology.

Cervical length measurements and fetal fibronectin testing may be useful in diagnosing women at risk, but should not be performed unless there are specific indications for such testing.

• Careful assessment of blood pressure according to standard guidelines [58] should occur at each visit, and consideration should be made to seeing obese women more frequently throughout their pregnancies in order to make a timely diagnosis of hypertensive complications.

• Fetal surveillance, including non-stress testing and biophysical profile assessment, should occur as indicated by the maternal and fetal conditions, but not solely for the presence of maternal obesity.

• Indications for delivery should be the same for obese women as for women of normal weight. Maternal weight should only enter consideration for delivery with the recognition that pregnancy outcomes are typically worse for these women than for women of normal weight.

A more detailed analysis of clinical management during labor and delivery is included in Chapter 12.

Conclusions

Maternal obesity is clearly a significant risk factor for adverse pregnancy outcomes, with a higher overall perinatal mortality rate noted for these pregnancies. While the relative risk for a specific condition often seems small and perhaps clinically insignificant, the sheer volume of women who are overweight and obese who become pregnant over the course of the year indicates that, although the individual risk may seem low, the overall population risk is much higher, given that at least one-third of women who achieve pregnancy are obese, with a BMI of greater than 30kg/m^2. In this regard, even small increases in relative risk have broad implications in a general population.

Therefore, specific interventions to attempt to improve perinatal outcome in obese women are warranted. Unfortunately, there are few such interventions that have been shown to definitively improve these generally worse perinatal outcomes. Much more research, with specific interventions designed for overweight and obese women, must be performed so that obstetricians can have timely, relevant, and efficacious interventions proven in appropriately designed trials with sufficient power to address the myriad of problems that obese women face during pregnancy. While one is tempted to merely recommend losing weight, obstetricians often do not have that luxury when obese women present for initial prenatal care. Identifying effective interventions specifically designed to improve pregnancy outcomes in obese women is imperative.

Summary

- Maternal obesity is associated with adverse pregnancy outcomes, including an increased risk for fetal anomalies, spontaneous abortion, stillbirth, pre-eclampsia, and preterm birth.
- The most common fetal anomalies found in infants of obese mothers include neural tube defects, cardiac defects, and abdominal wall defects.
- Approximately 20–25% of obese women suffer a first trimester pregnancy loss, compared to an overall population risk for approximately 15%.
- While the overall stillbirth rate is 7 per 1,000 pregnancies, the risk for obese women ranges from 12 to 16 per 1,000 pregnancies.
- The risk for pre-eclampsia and preterm birth is increased in obese women, accounting for an overall increased risk for prematurity of about 15–20%.
- Improved perinatal outcomes could be achieved if the rate of obesity declined.

References

1. Edwards LE, Dickes WF, Alton IR, et al. Pregnancy in the massively obese: course, outcome, and obesity prognosis of the infant. Am J Obstet Gynecol 1978;131:479–83.
2. Johnson SR, Kolberg BH, Varner MW, et al. Maternal obesity and pregnancy. Surg Obstet Gynecol 1987;164:431–7.
3. Lashen H, Fear K, Sturdee DW. Obesity is associated with increased risk of first trimester and recurrent miscarriage: matched case-control study. Hum Reprod 2004;19:1644–6.
4. Fedorcsak P, Storeng R, Dale PO, et al. Obesity is a risk factor for early pregnancy loss after IVF or ICSI. Acta Obstet Gynecol Scand 2000;79:43–8.
5. Metwally M, Saravelos SH, Ledger WL, et al. Body mass index and risk of miscarriage in women with recurrent miscarriage. Fertil Steril 2009 May 11. [Epub ahead of print]
6. Metwally M, Ong KJ, Ledger WL, et al. Does high body mass index increase the risk of miscarriage after spontaneous and assisted conception? A metaanalysis of the evidence. Fertil Steril 2008;90:714–26.
7. Porter TF, Scott JR. Evidence-based care of recurrent miscarriage. Best Pract Res Clin Obstet Gynecol 2005;19:85–101.
8. Scialli AR. Public Affairs Committee position paper. Maternal obesity and pregnancy. Birth Defects Res A Clin Mol Teratol 2006;76:73–7.
9. Stothard KJ, Tennant PWG, Bell R, et al. Maternal overweight and obesity and the risk of congenital anomalies: a systematic review and metaanalysis. JAMA 2009;301: 636–50.
10. Rasmussen Sa, Chu SY, Kim SY, et al. Maternal obesity and risk of neural tube defects: a metaanalysis. Am J Obstet Gynecol 2008;198:611–19.
11. Waller DK, Shaw GM, Rasmussen SA, et al., for the National Birth Defects Prevention Study. Prepregnancy obesity as a risk factor for structural birth defects. Arch Pediatr Adolesc Med 2007;161:745–50.

12. Anderson JL, Waller DK, Canfield MA, et al. Maternal obesity, gestational defects, and central nervous system birth defects. Epidemiology 2005;16:87–92.

13. Hendricks KA, Nuno OM, Suarez L, et al. Effects of hyperinsulinemia and obesity on risk of neural tube defects among Mexican Americans. Epidemiology 2001;12: 630–5.

14. Ray JG, Wyatt PR, Vermeulen MJ, et al. Greater maternal weight and the ongoing risk of neural tube defects after folic acid flour fortification. Obstet Gynecol 2005; 105:261–5.

15. Watkins ML, Rasmussen SA, Honein MA, et al. Maternal obesity and risk for birth defects. Pediatrics 2003;111:1152–8.

16. Shaw GM, Todoroff K, Finnell RH, et al. Spina bifida phenotypes in infants or fetuses of obese mothers. Teratology 2000;61:376–81.

17. Shaw GM, Carmichael SL. Prepregnancy obesity and risks of selected birth defects in offspring. Epidemiology 2008;19:616–20.

18. Garcia-Patterson A, Erdozain L, Ginovart G, et al. In gestational diabetes mellitus congenital malformations are related to prepregnancy body mass index and to severity of diabetes. Diabetologia 2004;47:509–14.

19. Werler MM, Louik C, Shapiro S, et al. Prepregnant weight in relation to risk of neural tube defects. JAMA 1996;275:1089–92.

20. Carmichael SL, Shaw GM, Schaffer DM, et al. Dieting behaviors and risk of neural tube defects. Am J Epidemiol 2003;158:1127–31.

21. Cedergren MI, Kallen B. Maternal obesity and infant heart defects. Obes Res 2003; 11:1065–71.

22. Khalil HS, Saleh AM, Subhani SN. Maternal obesity and neonatal congenital cardiovascular defects. Int J Gynecol Obstet 2008;102:232–6.

23. Martinez-Frias ML, Frias JP, Bermejo E, et al. Pre-gestational maternal body mass index predicts an increased risk of congenital malformations in infants of mothers with gestational diabetes. Diabet Med 2005;22:775–81.

24. Watkins Ml, Botto LD. Maternal prepregnancy weight and congenital heart defects in the offspring. Epidemiology 2001;11:439–46.

25. Cedergren MI, Kallen B. Maternal obesity and the risk for orofacial clefts in the offspring. Cleft Palate Craniofac J 2005;42:367–71.

26. Akre O, Boyd H, Ahlgren M, et al. Maternal and gestational risk factors for hypospadias. Environ Health Perspect 2008;116:1071–6.

27. Siega-Riz AM, Herring AH, Olshan AF, et al. The joint effects of maternal pre-pregnancy body mass index and age on the risk of gastroschisis. Paediatr Perinat Epidemiol 2008;23:51–7.

28. Oddy WH, De Klerck NH, Miller M, et al. Association of maternal pre-pregnancy weight with birth defects: evidence from a case-control study in Western Australia. Aust NZ J Obstet Gynecol 2009;49:11–15.

29. Chu SY, Kim SY, Lau J, et al. Maternal obesity and risk of stillbirth: a metaanalysis. Am J Obstet Gynecol 2007;197:223–8.

30. MacDorman MF, Kirmeyer S. Fetal and perinatal mortality, United States, 2005. National Vital Statistics Reports. Vol. 57, No. 8. Hyattsville, MD: National Center for Health Statistics, 2009.

31. Cnattingius S, Bergstrom R, Lipworth L, et al. Prepregnancy weight and the risk of adverse pregnancy outcomes. N Eng J Med 1998;338:147–52.

32. Kristensen J, Vestergaard M, Wisborg K, et al. Prepregnancy weight and the risk of stillbirth and neonatal death. Br J Obstet Gynecol 2005;112:403–8.

33. Nohr EA, Bech BH, Davies MJ, et al. Prepregnancy obesity and fetal death: a study within the Danish National Birth Cohort. Obstet Gynecol 2005:106:250–9.

34. Leung TY, Leung TN, Sahota DS, et al. Trends in maternal obesity and associated risks of adverse pregnancy outcomes in a population of Chinese women. Br J Obstet Gynecol 2008;115:1529–37.

35. Salihu HM, Dunlop AL, Hedayatzadeh M, et al. Extreme obesity and risk of stillbirth among black and white gravidas. Obstet Gynecol 2007;110:552–7.

36. Stephansson O, Dickman PW, Johansson A, et al. Maternal weight, pregnancy weight gain, and the risk of antepartum stillbirth. Am J Obstet Gynecol 2001;184: 463–9.

37. Villamor E, Cnattingius S. Interpregnancy weight change and risk of adverse pregnancy outcomes: a population-based study. Lancet 2006;368:1164–70.

38. Sebire NJ, Jolly M, Harris JP, et al. Maternal obesity and pregnancy outcome: a study of 287213 pregnancies in London. In J Obes 2001;25:1175–82.

39. Cedergren MI. Maternal morbid obesity and the risk of adverse pregnancy outcomes. Obstet Gynecol 2004;103:219–24.

40. Bhattacharya S, Campbell DM, Liston WA, et al. Effect of body mass index on pregnancy outcomes in nulliparous women delivering singleton babies. BMC Public Health 2007;7:168–76.

41. Denison FC, Price J, Graham C, et al. Maternal obesity, length of gestation, risk of postdates pregnancy and spontaneous onset of labor at term. Br J Obstet Gynecol 2008;115:720–5.

42. Khashan AS, Kenny LC. The effects of maternal body mass index on pregnancy outcome. Eur J Epidemiol 2009;24:697–705.

43. O'Brien TE, Ray JG, Chan WS. Maternal body mass index and the risk of preeclampsia: a systematic overview. Epidemiology 2003;14:368–74.

44. Rosenberg TJ, Garbers S, Chavkin W, et al. Prepregnancy weight and adverse perinatal outcomes in an ethnically diverse population. Obstet Gynecol 2003;102:1022–7.

45. Ramos GA, Caughey AB. The interrelationship between ethnicity and obesity on obstetric outcomes. Am J Obstet Gynecol 2005;193:1089–93.

46. Bodnar LM, Catov JM, Klebanoff MA, et al. Prepregnancy body mass index and the occurrence of severe hypertensive disorders of pregnancy. Epidemiology 2007;18: 234–9.

47. Kiel DW, Dodson EA, Artal R, et al. Gestational weight gain and pregnancy outcomes in obese women: how much is enough? Obstet Gynecol 2007;110:752–8.

48. Walsh SW. Obesity: a risk factor for preeclampsia. Trends Endocrinol Metabol 2007; 18:365–70.

49. Baeten JM, Bukusi EA, Lambe M. Pregnancy complications and outcomes among overweight and obese nulliparous women. Am J Public Health 2001;91:436–40.

50. Jensen DM, Damm P, Sorensen B, et al. Pregnancy outcome and prepregnancy body mass index in 2459 glucose-tolerant Danish women. Am J Obstet Gynecol 2003:189: 239–44.

51. Weiss JL, Malone FD, Emig D, et al., for the FASTER Research Consortium. Obesity, obstetric complications and cesarean delivery rate – a population-based screening study. Am J Obstet Gynecol 2004;190:1091–7.

52. Bodnar LM, Ness RB, Markovic N, et al. The risk of preeclampsia rises with increasing prepregnancy body mass index. Ann Epidemiol 2005;15:475–82.

53. Doherty DA, Magaan EF, Francis J, et al. Prepregnancy body mass index and pregnancy outcomes. Int J Obstet Gynecol 2006;95:242–7.

54. Smith GC, Shah I, Pell JP, Crossley JA, et al. Maternal obesity in early pregnancy and risk of spontaneous and elective preterm deliveries: a retrospective cohort study. Am J Public Health 2007;97:157–62.

55. King GE. Errors in clinical measurement of blood pressure in obesity. Clin Sci 1967;32:223–37.
56. Pickering TG. Principles and techniques of blood pressure measurement. Cardiol Clin 2002;20:207–23.
57. Umana E, Ahmed W, Fraley MA, et al. Comparison of oscillometric and intraarterial systolic and diastolic blood pressures in lean, overweight, and obese patients. Angiology 2006;57:41–5.
58. Pickering TG, Hall JE, Appel LJ, et al.; Subcommitee of Professional and Public Education of the American Heart Association Council on High Blood Pressure Research. Recommendations for blood pressure measurement in humans and experimental animals. Part 1: Blood pressure measurement in humans. Hypertension 2005:45:142–61.
59. Ramsay JE, Ferrell WR, Crawford L, et al. Maternal obesity is associated with dys-regulation of metabolic, vascular, and inflammatory pathways. J Clin Endocrinol Metab 2002;87:4231–7.
60. Dudley DJ. The role of cytokines in normal and abnormal parturition. In Hill J (ed.), Cytokines in human reproduction. Wiley-Liss, 2000, pp. 171–202.
61. Nohr EA, Bech BH, Vaeth M, et al. Obesity, gestational weight gain and preterm birth: a study within the Danish National Birth Cohort. Paediatr Perinat Epidemiol 2007;21:5–14.
62. Hendler I, Goldenberg RL, Mercer BM, et al. The preterm prediction study: associa-tion between maternal body mass index and spontaneous and indicated preterm birth. Am J Obstet Gynecol 2005;192:882–6.
63. Kumari AS. Pregnancy outcome in women with morbid obesity. Int J Gynecol Obstet 2001;73:101–7.
64. Bianco AT, Smilen SW, Davis Y, et al. Pregnancy outcome and weight gain recom-mendations for the morbidly obese woman. Obstet Gynecol 1998;91:97–102.
65. Nohr EA, Vaeth M, Bech BH, et al. Maternal obesity and neonatal mortality accord-ing to subtypes of preterm birth. Obstet Gynecol 2007;110:1083–90.
66. Salihu HM, Alio AP, Wilson RE, et al. Obesity and extreme obesity: new insights into the black–white disparity in neonatal mortality. Obstet Gynecol 2008;1410–16.
67. Gardosi J, Clausson B, Francis A. The value of customized centiles in assessing perinatal mortality risk associated with parity and maternal size. Br J Obstet Gynecol, in press; doi:10.1111/j.1471-0528.2009.02245.x.
68. Yu CKH, Teoh TG, Robinson S. Obesity in pregnancy. Br J Obstet Gynecol 2006; 113:1117–25.
69. Castro LC, Avina RL. Maternal obesity and pregnancy outcomes. Curr Opin Obstet Gynecol 2002;14:601–6.
70. Catalano PM. Management of obesity in pregnancy. Obstet Gynecol 2007;109: 419–33.

CHAPTER 7

Abnormal Fetal Growth Related to Maternal Obesity

Hugh M. Ehrenberg

Ohio State University Medical Center, Columbus, Ohio, USA

The number of adults burdened with obesity in the USA continues to increase, with recent data suggesting that up to 30–35% of US adults are obese (body mass index [BMI] > 30 kg/m^2), with as many as 65% at least overweight (BMI > 25 kg/m^2) [1,2]. The multitude of adverse health consequences associated with increasing adult weight, including diabetes, hypertension, hyperlipidemia, and cardiovascular disease, joint disease, risk for venous thromboembolic events, and some malignancies, has far-reaching implications for public health. The effects of obesity in pregnancy, including complications encountered along the course of prenatal care, at the time of delivery, and in the postpartum period, have been thoroughly described, and are discussed in detail elsewhere in this volume. In light of these healthcare concerns, public health officials regard obesity as the second most prevalent cause of preventable death in the USA, behind only tobacco abuse [3].

Identifying the roots of the epidemic of obesity is complicated, with proposed mechanisms that include genetics, the increase in sedentary lifestyles and urban living, dietary changes, and ultimately the increase in newborn size. Attention has increasingly been paid to the consequences of abnormal body habitus in pregnancy for future generations: the increasing frequency of fetal overgrowth and excessive adipose deposition, and in turn the higher rate of infant, childhood, and adolescent obesity. Along with the striking increase in childhood obesity and overweight body habitus comes early lipid irregularities, and eventually obesity in pregnancy as the cycle repeats itself. This chapter will focus on the implications of maternal obesity for the developing fetus, newborn, and adolescent, with reference to growth and body composition.

Macrosomia is increasing in prevalence worldwide. Recent studies from both North America and Europe have reported an increase in mean

Pregnancy in the Obese Woman, 1st edition. Edited by Deborah L. Conway.
© 2011 Blackwell Publishing Ltd.

birthweights, as well as in infants classified as large for gestational age (greater than the 90th percentile for gestational age) or macrosomic (birth-weight greater than 4 kg [approximately 9 lb]) [4,5]. In Denmark, the percentage of macrosomic newborns increased from 16.7% in 1990 to 20.0% in 1999 [6]. Factors such as decreased maternal smoking, an increased incidence of diabetes, and increasing maternal BMI have all been implicated. In work completed in Cleveland, USA, Catalano et al. observed a mean 116 g increase in term singleton birthweight over the last 30 years. The increase in maternal weight at delivery was the factor most strongly correlated with the increase in birthweight [7].

Factors Associated with Fetal Growth

If we are to better understand the relationship between maternal obesity and fetal overgrowth, a review of factors related to fetal growth is in order (Table 7.1). There are multiple factors that influence the rate of fetal growth and fetal body composition, including maternal nutrition and anthropometrics, pregnancy weight gain, age, parity, and glucose intolerance. There is also limited influence from paternal factors.

Nutrition

Maternal nutrition is obviously an important factor in the determination of growth velocity and body composition of the fetus. Data collected from

Table 7.1 Factors associated with fetal growth

Factor	Influence on growth
Maternal weight	↑↑↑
Maternal weight gain*	Nulliparous (↑↑), parous (↑)
Maternal nutritional deficit	Early (↑), late (↑)
Maternal height†	↑
Maternal age‡	↑
Parity§	↑
Glucose intolerance	Weight (↑↓), fat content (↑)
Paternal influence	↑

* Influence falls as pregravid weight rises.
† No longer significant when controlled for weight.
‡ No longer significant after controlling for parity.
§ Decreasing influence as parity rises.

the Dutch famine of 1944–45 illustrated that the period of gestation at which nutritional deprivation occurs is important [8,9]. If the famine peaked in early pregnancy followed by increased access to food in later pregnancy, the result was heavier babies at birth when compared to those born either before or after the famine. In contrast, if the famine occurred during late gestation, the babies weighed less and were thinner at birth, with no change in length. [10]. These findings imply that the placenta can be "programmed" by environmental factors, and that this in turn can have immediate and lifelong consequences. The mechanisms and implications of placental programming are the subject of much ongoing work.

The role of the mother

Maternal anthropometric variables are also important factors relating to fetal growth. Pregravid weight has a very strong correlation with birthweight [11]. Increasing maternal height is also associated with an increase in birthweight; however, when maternal height is adjusted for weight, there is no longer a significant correlation between maternal height and birthweight [12]. Gestational weight gain is positively correlated with birthweight, [13], although the correlation is stronger in nulliparous women ($r = 0.26$) than in parous women ($r = 0.16$).

The interaction of maternal pregravid weight and weight gain was examined by Abrams and Laros [14]. There was a progressively stronger correlation between maternal weight gain and birthweight as maternal pregravid weight dropped. Among women conceiving at a weight closer to normal or underweight, excessive maternal weight gain played a larger role in the increased risk for macrosomia than it did among women who began pregnancy with an overweight or obese BMI. Conversely, in women beyond 135% of ideal weight for height at conception, there was no correlation between gestational weight gain and birthweight. These findings are likely due in part to the glucose intolerance, which is an effect of excessive weight. That is, in women who are already overweight or obese, glucose intolerance plays a role in overgrowth at baseline, without a need for bolstering by excessive weight gain. In the normal or underweight patient, excessive weight gain is required to create the glucose intolerance involved with fetal overgrowth.

Maternal age and parity also show a positive correlation with birthweight, although McKeown and Gibson reported that when maternal age was adjusted for parity, there was no consistent correlation between maternal age and birthweight [15]. Thompson et al. found a mean 100–150 g increase in birthweight in a subsequent pregnancy [16], although the additional effect of parity on birthweight was noted to diminish with increasing parity.

The role of the father

In clinical practice, there is often a concern related to large babies when viewing the size of the father. In reality, however, when compared to maternal factors, paternal anthropometric factors have a limited impact on fetal growth. Morton reported that among half-siblings who shared the mother as the common parent, the correlation between birthweight in each half-sibling was significantly higher ($r = 0.58$) than when half-siblings shared the father as the common parent ($r = 0.10$) [17]. Klebanoff et al., using a Danish population-based registry, reported that paternal birthweight, adult height, and adult weight collectively explained approximately 3% of the variance in birthweight, compared to 9% for the corresponding maternal factors [18].

The contribution of adipose tissue

As early as 1923, research by Moulton found that the variability in weight in mammals was explained by the amount of adipose tissue, while the amount of lean body mass was relatively constant, changing predictably over time [19]. Sparks used autopsy data and chemical analysis in 169 human stillborn infants to describe body composition across the spectrum of fetal growth. The rate of accretion of lean body mass was noted to be relatively constant in small-for-gestational age (SGA), average-for-gestational age (AGA), and large-for-gestational age (LGA) fetuses, while there was considerable variation in the accretion of fetal fat. Fat accretion in the SGA fetus was considerably less than in the AGA fetus, which in turn was less than that of the LGA fetus [20]. The term human newborn has the greatest percentage of body fat (approximately 12%) compared to other mammals [21]. In light of all these factors, it follows that variation in weight at birth would primarily be due to change in body composition, and specifically the degree to which fat is deposited during gestation.

Body composition

In some of the most detailed studies of fetal overgrowth and macrosomia, Catalano et al. concentrated on measures of neonatal body composition: fat content and fat-free (lean) body mass. A small group of newborns was studied for the influence of maternal glycemia on fetal growth. In the group as a whole, the mean birthweight was 3,553 g (range $\pm$ 462 g), with a mean percentage body fat of 13.7% (range $\pm$ 4.2%). Fat-free mass, which accounted for approximately 86% of mean birthweight, was responsible for 83% of the variance in that weight. In contrast, body fat, which accounted for only around 14% of birthweight, explained 46% of its variance [22]. These findings indicated that adipose tissue, which makes up a relatively smaller fraction of the newborn's body composition, is responsible for a relatively greater impact on newborn weight than lean body mass.

Dividing the cohort by maternal glucose tolerance into women with normal glucose tolerance (NGT) and subjects with gestational diabetes mellitus (GDM), the body composition of these babies was determined within 48 hours of birth, and the variation in body fat content between these two groups was described [23]. Although there was no significant difference in birthweight or fat-free mass between the groups, there was a significant increase in fat mass and percentage body fat in the infants of the mothers with GDM. After data were adjusted for potential confounding variables such as parity and gestational age, there was no significant change in results. These women were not evaluated for the influence of maternal weight or weight gained in pregnancy. These findings suggested that maternal glucose intolerance plays a role in fetal growth through an impact on body composition, specifically an increase in fat mass.

This same group of infants was then divided along lines of newborn size into AGA ($n = 37$) and LGA ($n = 38$) groups. Among the AGA infants, there were no differences in birthweight between the GDM and NGT groups, but there was again a significant increase in fat mass, percentage body fat, and skinfold measures in the infants of the GDM mothers compared to the NGT mothers. Interestingly, the fat-free mass in the infants of the GDM mothers was significantly less than that of infants in the NGT group. Similar results were obtained when the analysis was limited to LGA neonates alone [24]. The relative increase in fat mass but not body weight may have obstetric implications, such as the increased incidence of shoulder dystocia in GDM when compared to NGT neonates in similar birthweight categories [25,26].

These results illustrate the complicated role that adipose accretion during fetal life plays in the body composition differences seen in newborns, such that birthweight alone may not be a sensitive enough measure to recognize subtle but important characteristics in fetal growth among certain populations, such as the infants of mothers with diabetes. Furthermore, maternal control over fetal growth via a control of blood glucose levels through pregnancy remains an important area of study.

Maternal obesity versus diabetes

Both obesity and diabetes have a significant impact on fetal growth. Poorly controlled blood glucose levels and maternal weight gain each contribute to abnormal fetal growth, as well as to differences in fetal adipose deposition leading to perturbations in neonatal body composition. Abnormal glucose tolerance is commonly seen among obese women, so it is difficult to establish the independent influence of one or the other on fetal growth.

To examine the contribution of each factor, Catalano et al. performed a stepwise logistic regression analysis on the 220 infants of NGT and 195 term infants of GDM mothers previously described (Table 7.2) [24].

Table 7.2 Stepwise aggression analysis of factors relating to fetal growth and body composition in infants of women with gestational diabetes ($n = 195$) and normal glucose tolerance ($n = 220$)

Birthweight	r^2	Δr^2	
EGA	0.114	–	
Pregravid weight	0.162	0.048	
Weight gain	0.210	0.048	
Smoking (–)	0.227	0.017	
Parity	0.239	0.012	$p = 0.0001$
Lean body mass			
EGA	0.122	–	
Smoking (–)	0.153	0.031	
Pregravid weight	0.179	0.026	
Weight gain	0.212	0.033	
Parity	0.225	0.013	
Maternal height	0.241	0.016	
Paternal weight	0.250	0.009	$p = 0.0001$
Fat mass	r^2	Δr^2	
Pregravid body mass index	0.066	–	
EGA	0.136	0.070	
Weight gain	0.171	0.035	
Group (gestational diabetes mellitus)	0.187	0.016	$p = 0.0001$
% Body fat			
Pregravid body mass index	0.072	–	
EGA	0.116	0.044	
Weight gain	0.147	0.031	
Group (gestational diabetes mellitus)	0.166	0.019	$p = 0.0001$

EGA, estimated gestational age.

Pregravid BMI had the strongest correlation with neonatal fat mass and percentage body fat, explaining approximately 7% of the variance in both fat mass and percentage body fat. Although approximately 50% of the subjects had GDM, only 2% of the variance in fat mass in this population was explained by abnormal maternal glucose tolerance. Not surprisingly, gestational age at delivery was the independent variable with the strongest correlation with both birthweight and lean body mass. In keeping with previous investigations, maternal smoking was found to have a negative correlation with both birthweight and lean body mass, and paternal weight had a weak correlation with only lean body mass.

In work completed among an urban population of mixed racial backgrounds [27], we reported that the odds of having an LGA neonate were greater for women with a history of pre-existing diabetes (odds ratio [OR] 4.4) compared to maternal obesity (OR 1.6). On the other hand, the absolute number of LGA infants was fourfold greater in obese women compared to diabetic women, because the prevalence of overweight/obesity was 47% compared to a 5% prevalence of diabetes. Therefore, at least in our population, it is maternal obesity and not diabetes that is the more crucial factor for increase in birthweight.

Effects on the offspring

It is increasingly clear that maternal obesity increases the risk for excessive fetal growth. The most immediate risk to the newborn resulting from this excess growth is encountered during birth, as the risk for shoulder dystocia and associated injuries is increased in this population. The obstetric implications of maternal obesity are discussed in detail in Chapter 12. More far-reaching risks for LGA and macrosomic infants include metabolic syndrome (obesity, hypertension, insulin resistance, dyslipidemia), similar to the risk seen in infants born SGA [28].

There is abundant evidence linking higher birthweights to increased obesity in adolescents as well as adults [29,30]. Large cohort studies, such as the Nurses Health Study [31] and the Health Professional Follow-up Study [32], report an increase in BMI among the population overall, but a far greater increase in BMI among those who were born large [33]. The increased prevalence of adolescent obesity is related to an increased risk for the metabolic syndrome, and accounts for much of the 33% increase in type 2 diabetes seen in recent years, particularly among the young. Between 50% and 90% of adolescents with type 2 diabetes have a BMI of over 27kg/m^2 [34] and 25% of obese children 4–10 years of age have impaired glucose tolerance [35]. It is becoming clear that the epidemic of obesity, the subsequent risk for diabetes, and components of the metabolic syndrome may begin *in utero* with fetal overgrowth and changes in body composition.

A retrospective cohort study by Whitaker looked at over 8,400 children in the USA from the early 1990s. Children who were born to obese mothers were twice as likely to be obese by 2 years of age compared to those who were not [36]. If a women had a BMI of over 30kg/m^2 in the first trimester, the prevalence of childhood obesity (BMI > 95th percentile based on Center for Disease Control criteria) at ages 2, 3, and 4 years was 15.1%, 20.6%, and 24.1%, respectively. This was 2.4–2.7 times the prevalence of obesity observed in children of mothers whose BMI was in the normal range ($18.5–24.9 \text{kg/m}^2$). Of note, birthweight had only a modest effect on the relationship between maternal obesity in early pregnancy and childhood obesity.

There is an independent effect of maternal pregravid weight and diabetes not only on birthweight, but also on the adolescent risk for obesity. In a cohort of women with GDM who were in good glycemic control on diet treatment alone, Langer and colleagues reported that obese women had a higher risk for fetal macrosomia (OR 2.12) compared to lean women (BMI $18.5–24.9 \text{kg/m}^2$) [37]. Similar results were reported in women with GDM who were poorly controlled on diet or insulin. Only in those women with GDM whose glucose was well controlled with insulin was there no increased risk for macrosomia, regardless of the pregravid BMI. Dabelea et al. also reported that the mean BMI was 2.6kg/m^2 greater in the offspring of diabetic pregnancies than in siblings born prior to the diagnosis of glucose intolerance in the mother [38]. Hence, both maternal pregravid weight and the presence of maternal diabetes may independently affect the risk for adolescent obesity in the offspring.

The risk for developing the metabolic syndrome in adolescence was addressed by Boney et al. in a prospective longitudinal cohort study of AGA and LGA infants of women with NGT and GDM [39]. They defined the metabolic syndrome as two or more of the following components: obesity, hypertension, glucose intolerance, and dyslipidemia. They defined maternal obesity as a pregravid BMI of over 27.3kg/m^2. Children who were LGA at birth had an increased hazard ratio for the metabolic syndrome of 2.19 (95% confidence interval [CI] 1.25–3.82, $p = 0.01$) by 11 years of age. Children who were the offspring of obese women also had an increased hazard ratio of 1.81 (95% CI 1.03–3.19, $p = 0.04$) for the metabolic syndrome. An independent influence of maternal GDM on the development of metabolic syndrome in adolescent offspring could not be established. However, the risk for developing metabolic syndrome was significantly higher in LGA offspring than in AGA offspring of women with GDM, showing a 3.6-fold greater risk by age 11.

The role of maternal behavior

The *in utero* environment to which the growing fetus is exposed clearly has both short- and long-term implications for the offspring of a pregnancy affected by abnormal maternal body habitus. Questions remain regarding whether interventions on behalf of the fetus have any effect on postnatal development. Ongoing work is attempting to establish the time periods during gestation at which weight control (or lack thereof) or glucose control (or lack thereof) have the greatest effect on the size or body composition of the newborn.

Weight gain

Ideally, the time to approach more appropriate weight for a healthy pregnancy and avoid complications attendant to abnormal body habitus is prior to pregnancy. In this way, potential risks of ketosis, which may be associated with rapid weight loss due to starvation, can be avoided, and the metabolic needs of pregnancy are not a concern while aggressive diet and exercise plans are pursued. As many as half of all pregnancies are unplanned in the USA, making pre-pregnancy counseling or planning in this regard difficult, and leaving weight control in pregnancy as the only option.

Increasing attention has been paid to recommendations for pregnancy weight gain, stratified by pregravid BMI. Recommendations by the Institute of Medicine, modified in May 2009, have varied only slightly over time (Table 7.3). Data on which these recommendations are based come principally from large population-based cohorts studied by Keil [40] and Cedergren et al. [41]. These studies looked at the critical risks of obesity in pregnancy, such as fetal overgrowth, pre-eclampsia, and cesarean delivery, balanced against the risks of poor maternal weight gain, including SGA. As pregravid BMI increased, the risk for untoward pregnancy outcomes was limited in women who gained a decreasing amount of weight. This occurred without an appreciable increase in SGA risk.

Table 7.3 Institute of Medicine weight gain recommendations: then and now

Recommended weight gain (lb)	1990	2009	Late pregnancy weight gain (lb/week (range))
Underweight	28–40	28–40	1 (1–1.3)
Normal	25–35	25–35	1 (0.8–1)
Overweight	15–25	15–20	0.6 (0.5–0.7)
Obese	>15	11–20	0.5 (0.4–0.6)

Surely the gravida who is not gaining weight in pregnancy is modifying her own body composition through gestation. The developing fetus, amniotic fluid, placenta, and plasma volume expansion would result in an increase in body weight that would be compensated by loss of maternal adipose tissue. The effect of this maternal modification is difficult to study due to the limited number of subjects available. Clausen et al. failed to see a difference in birthweight among women who successfully limited their weight gained in pregnancy [42,43]. However, these women and their offspring were not evaluated for changes in body composition.

Blood glucose control

Hyperglycemia during pregnancy is associated with a host of complications that are similar to those of obesity. These include fetal overgrowth [44] and death [45], anomaly, and cesarean delivery [46] Hillier et al. assessed the risk for macrosomia associated with gestational weight gain and increasing blood glucose levels. Among women with both normal and abnormal GDM screening tests, increasing level of maternal glucose on GDM screening was closely related to macrosomia risk ($p < 0.001$ for trend in all groups). Women who gained more than 40 lb during pregnancy had nearly double the risk for fetal macrosomia for each level of maternal glucose compared to those with a gestational weight gain of 40 lb or less. Among women with normal GDM screening results and excessive weight gain, 16.5% had macrosomic newborns, compared to 9.3% of women who gained appropriate weight. A total of 29.3% of women with GDM who gained more than 40 lb had a macrosomic newborn, compared to only 13.5% of women with GDM who gained 40 lb or less during pregnancy ($p = 0.018$). The risk for macrosomia due to glucose intolerance is modified by a control of blood sugar, but may be more heavily influenced by maternal weight gain [47]. Hyperglycemia may have more of an effect on body composition than total weight of the newborn.

Conclusions

The origins of fetal macrosomia and excessive adiposity in the newborn appear to be related to maternal weight at conception, gestational weight gain, and blood glucose levels, and it is difficult to separate the attributable risk for each. Furthermore, study of the modification of macrosomia risk with blood glucose control or limited weight gain is only beginning. This limits our ability to make safe and effective clinical recommendations regarding these factors in order to optimize fetal growth. As efforts to find a break in the cycle of obesity continue, the consistent point of intervention is weight loss and optimization of blood glucose control prior to conception. Data concerning the impact of control of weight gain during gestation on the rate of fetal overgrowth, as well as the impact of glycemic control, are encouraging, but long-term results are yet to be studied. There is an urgent need to do this, however, because the implications of fetal overgrowth on global health are far reaching.

References

1. Ogden CL, Carroll MD, Curtin LR, et al. Prevalence of overweight and obesity in the United States, 1999–2004. JAMA 2006;295:1549–55.
2. Hedley AA, Ogden CL, Johnson CL, et al. Prevalence of overweight and obesity among US children, adolescents, and adults, 1999–2002. JAMA 2004;291:2847–50.
3. Catalano PM, Ehrenberg HM. The short- and long-term implications of maternal obesity on the mother and her offspring. Br J Obstet Gynaecol 2006;113:1126–33.
4. Surkan PJ, Hsieh C-C, Johansson AL, et al. Reasons for increasing trends in large for gestational age births. Obstet Gynecol 2004;104:720–6.
5. Anath CV, Wen SW. Trends in fetal growth among singleton gestations in the United States and Canada, 1985 through 1998. Semin Perinatol 2002;26:260–7.
6. Orskou J, Kesmodel U, Henrikson TB, et al. An increasing proportion of infants weigh more than 4000 grams at birth. Acta Obstet Gynecol Scand 2001;80:931–6.
7. Catalano P, Ashmead GG, Huston-Presley L, et al. The obesity cycle comes full circle: increasing trends in birth weight. Diabetes in Pregnancy Study Group 37th Annual Meeting, Mykonos, Greece, September 15–18, 2005.
8. Ozanne SE, Fernandez-Twinn D, Hales CN. Fetal growth and adult disease. Semin Perinatol 2004;28:81–7.
9. Khan IY, Lakasing L, Poston L, et al. Fetal programming for adult disease: where next? J Matern Fetal Neonatal Med 2003;13:292–99.
10. Lechtig A, Habracht J-P, Delgado H, et al. Effect of food supplementation during pregnancy on birthweight. Pediatrics 1975;56:508–20.
11. Eastman NJ, Jackson E. Weight relationships in pregnancy. Obstet Gynecol Surv 1968;23:1003–25.
12. Whitaker RC. Predicting preschooler obesity at birth: the role of maternal obesity in early pregnancy. Pediatrics 2004;114:29–35.
13. Humphreys RC. An analysis of the maternal and foetal weight factors in normal pregnancy. J Obstet Gynecol Br Emp 1954;61:764–71.
14. Abrams BF, Laros RK. Prepregnancy weight, weight gain and birth weight. Am J Obstet Gynecol 1986;154:503–9.
15. McKeown T, Gibson JR. Observations on all births (23,970) in Birmingham, 1947. Part II: Birth weight. Br J Soc Med 1951;5:98–112.
16. Thompson AM, Billewicz WZ, Hytten FE. The assessment of fetal growth. J Obstet Gynecol 1968;75:903–16.
17. Whitaker RC. Predicting preschooler obesity at birth: the role of maternal obesity in early pregnancy. Pediatrics 2004;114:29–35.
18. Klebanoff MA, Mednick BR, Schulsinger C, et al. Father's effect on infant birth weight. Am J Obstet Gynecol 1998;178:122–6.
19. Moulton CR. Age and chemical development in mammals. J Biol Chem 1923;57:79–97.
20. Sparks JW. Human intrauterine growth and nutrient accretion. Semin Perinatol 1984;8:74–93.

21. Girard J, Ferre P. Metabolic and hormonal changes around birth. In Jones CT (ed.), Biochemical development of the fetus and neonate. New York: Elsevier Biomedical Press, 1982, pp. 517–551.

22. Catalano PM, Tyzbir ED, Allen SR, et al. Evaluation of fetal growth by estimation of body composition. Obstet Gynecol 1992;79:46–50.

23. Catalano PM, Thomas A, Huston-Presley L, et al. Increased fetal adiposity: a very sensitive marker of abnormal in utero development. Am J Obstet Gynecol 2003; 189:1698–704.

24. Durnwald C, Huston-Presley L, Amini S, et al. Evaluation of body composition of large-for-gestational-age infants of women with gestational diabetes mellitus compared with women with normal glucose tolerance levels. Am J Obstet Gynecol 2004; 191:804–8.

25. Langer O, Berkus MD, Huff RW, et al. Shoulder dystocia: should the fetus weighing greater than or equal to 4,000 grams be delivered by cesarean section? Am J Obstet Gynecol 1991;165:831–7.

26. Ecker JL, Greenberg JA, Norwitz ER, et al. Birth weight as a predictor of brachial plexus injury. Obstet Gynecol 1997;89:643–7.

27. Ehrenberg HM, Mercer BM, Catalano PM. The influence of obesity and diabetes on the prevalence of macrosomia. Am J Obstet Gynecol 2004;191:964–8.

28. Oken E, Gillman MW. Fetal origins of obesity. Obes Res 2003;11:496–506.

29. Garn SM, Clark DC. Trends in fatness and the origins of obesity. Pediatrics 1976; 57:443–56.

30. Garn SM, Cole PE, Bailey SM. Living together as a factor in family line resemblances. Hum Biol 1979;51:565–87.

31. Curhan GC, Cherton GM, Willet WC, et al. Birth weight and adult hypertension and obesity in women. Circulation 1996;94:1310–15.

32. Curhan GC, Willett WC, Rimm EB, et al. Birth weight and adult hypertension, diabetes mellitus and obesity in U.S. men. Circulation 1996;94:3246–50.

33. Martorell R, Stein AD, Schroeder DG. Early nutrition and adiposity. J Nutr 2001;131:8745–805.

34. Mokdad AH, Ford ES, Bowman BA, et al. Diabetes trends in the U.S. 1990–1998. Diabetes Care 2000;23:1278–83.

35. Sinha R, Fisch G, Teague B, et al. Prevalence of impaired glucose tolerance among children and adolescents with marked obesity. N Engl J Med 2002;346:802–10.

36. Whitaker RC. Predicting preschooler obesity at birth: the role of maternal obesity in early pregnancy. Pediatrics 2004;114:29–36.

37. Langer O, Yogev Y, Xenakis EMJ, et al. Overweight and obese in gestational diabetes: the impact on pregnancy outcome. Am J Obstet Gynecol 2005;192:1368–76.

38. Dabelea D, Hanson RL, Lindsay RS, et al. Intrauterine exposure to diabetes conveys risks for type 2 diabetes and obesity: a study of discordant sibships. Diabetes 2000; 49:2208–11.

39. Boney CM, Verma A, Tucker R, et al. Metabolic syndrome in childhood: association with birth weight, maternal obesity and gestational diabetes mellitus. Pediatrics 2005;115:290–6.

40. Kiel DW, Dodson EA, Artal R, et al. Gestational weight gain and pregnancy outcomes in obese women: how much is enough? Obstet Gynecol 2007;110:752–8.

41. Cedergren MI. Optimal gestational weight gain for body mass index categories. Obstet Gynecol 2007;110:759–64.

42. Claesson IM, Brynhildsen J, Cedergren M, et al. Weight gain restriction during pregnancy is safe for both the mother and neonate. Acta Obstet Gynecol Scand 2009;88:1158–62.

43. Claesson IM, Sydsjo G, Brynhildsen J, et al. Weight gain restriction for obese pregnant women: a case-control intervention study. Br J Obstet Gynaecol 2008;115:44–50.

44. Biri A, Korucuoglu U, Ozcan P, et al. Effect of different degrees of glucose intolerance on maternal and perinatal outcomes. J Matern Fetal Neonatal Med 2009;22:473–8.

45. Rackham O, Paize F, Weindling AM. Cause of death in infants of women with pregestational diabetes mellitus and the relationship with glycemic control. Postgrad Med 2009;121:26–32.

46. Ehrenberg HM, Durnwald CP, Catalano P, et al. The influence of obesity and diabetes on the risk of cesarean delivery. Am J Obstet Gynecol 2004;191:969–74.

47. Hillier TA, Pedula KL, Vesco KK, et al. Excess gestational weight gain: modifying fetal macrosomia risk associated with maternal glucose. Obstet Gynecol 2008;112: 1007–14.

CHAPTER 8

Special Considerations in Prenatal Care

Hugh M. Ehrenberg

Division of Maternal Fetal Medicine, Ohio State University Medical Center Columbus, Ohio, USA

As obesity increases in prevalence in the USA and abroad, the number of women of childbearing age affected by the disease has mirrored the epidemic, with as many as one in three pregnant women classified as obese [1,2]. Management of the pregnancy in the obese woman is a challenge that will face most obstetricians, necessitating alterations in practice that range from the subtle to the severe, and sometimes requiring referral for specialized care, consultations, or co-management. Awareness of the potential pitfalls in the care of the obese gravida is vital in order to avoid complications and minimize the effect of abnormal maternal body habitus on both mother and child.

Numerous high-risk conditions associated with obesity may impact pregnancy: hypertension and heart disease, hypercholesterolemia and hyperlipidemia, joint disease [3,4], sleep apnea [5], diabetes, venous thromboembolic disease, and biliary tract disease. Obesity at conception and excessive weight gained during gestation can increase the risk to the fetus such as perturbations in fetal growth [6], malformation [7–10], and miscarriage [11]. Obstetric risks include increased rates of labor dystocia [12,13], cesarean delivery [14], and postoperative complications, such as maternal infectious morbidity, and wound infection and breakdown (Box 8.1) [15]. With these risks in mind, this chapter addresses the impact of obesity on the delivery of prenatal care, with suggested modifications that may help maintain healthy outcomes for both mother and child.

Preconceptual counseling

The woman seeking preconceptual counseling represents a unique opportunity for an introduction to healthy living. Motivations for healthy change include the interests of an expectant mother's pregnancy, if not

---

Pregnancy in the Obese Woman, 1st edition. Edited by Deborah L. Conway.
© 2011 Blackwell Publishing Ltd.

> **Box 8.1 Conditions significantly associated with obesity in pregnancy**
>
> Hypertension and pre-eclampsia
>
> Diabetes
>
> Macrosomia
>
> Shoulder dystocia
>
> Venous thromboembolism
>
> Miscarriage
>
> Fetal malformation
>
> Labor arrest and cesarean delivery
>
> Failed attempt at vaginal birth after cesarean
>
> Postoperative wound complications

her longer term health. Whenever possible, the most optimal time to introduce lifestyle changes such as diet and exercise, and to lose excessive weight, is prior to conception. Many of the adverse effects of maternal obesity can be offset by a loss of weight prior to pregnancy to approach ideal body weight, and advice on optimal weight gain in pregnancy can be provided. Attention can be paid to limitations on first-trimester weight gain, which in excess has been associated with an increased risk for gestational diabetes [16]. Ideally, the changes in behavior are best attempted prior to conception. More aggressive programs for weight loss should be avoided after conception, as loss of weight due to starvation may be associated with ketosis in pregnancy, which may have an untoward effect on neonatal neurodevelopment [17]. By initiating weight loss prior to pregnancy, nutritional concerns for pregnancy can be avoided. In the event of pregnancy, the relationship with healthcare professionals begun early can be continued though prenatal care, allowing for the reinforcement of positive behaviors with continuous feedback. Modifications of diet and physical activity are first-line therapy for obesity and are central to any extended management scheme. Chapter 3 provides recommendations in this regard.

Sadly, preconceptual counseling regarding the steps an obese woman can take to prepare for pregnancy is infrequently employed, due in part to the high proportion of unplanned pregnancies in the USA. Furthermore, when preconceptual counseling does occur, providers often focus on the morbidities associated with obesity rather than on the root cause. It is therefore essential that physicians and other healthcare workers who see women of childbearing age familiarize themselves with basic advice on lifestyle modification and weight loss, and become comfortable discussing these issues with their obese and overweight patients.

Other preconceptual evaluations to be considered depending on clinical scenario include screening for diabetes, thyroid dysfunction, and cardiac disease. Properly motivated patients may benefit from consultations with nutritionists and exercise advisors. The introduction of well-defined exercise programs is rarely successful when done during pregnancy, but many obese women are so severely out of condition that even seemingly insignificant exertion like walking a short distance, walking up steps, or walking in a swimming pool are enough to raise the heart rate to target levels. For the woman willing to put pregnancy off for a year, referral to bariatric surgery professionals for evaluation and management may offer protection from complications due to obesity in pregnancy. Goals of preconceptual care in the obese woman considering pregnancy are summarized in Box 8.2.

First-trimester interventions

Early pregnancy care must be focused on the identification of complications associated with obesity, as well as minimizing weight gained during pregnancy as a way to reduce the exacerbation of such risk (Box 8.3) [18]. Women with abnormal body habitus are known to be affected by irregular menstruation [19] due to anovulatory cycles [20,21], which may adversely affect the accuracy of menstrual pregnancy dating. Early sonographic confirmation of pregnancy dates is therefore integral to the appropriate

---

Box 8.2 Preconceptual goals in the care of pregnancies in obese women

Approach ideal body weight (BMI < 25 kg/m^2)

Diabetes screening

Thyroid function testing

Nutrition consultation

Exercise program planning

Bariatric surgery referral

Box 8.3 Management points for early pregnancy

Limitation of maternal weight gain

Early ultrasound dating of pregnancy

Early screening for gestational diabetes

Reinforce exercise and weight gain plan

Ongoing nutrition consultation

management of the later pregnancy complications common in obese and overweight gravidas, such as pertubations in fetal growth, pre-eclampsia, diabetes, and post-datism. Early testing for carbohydrate intolerance using standard testing algorithms may uncover undiagnosed pregestational diabetes. Particularly in cases accompanied by abnormal levels of glycated hemoglobin, such women should be managed in a manner similar to those with known pre-existing diabetes (see Chapter 11).

Obesity can interfere with sonographic imaging conducted as a matter of routine prenatal care [7], affecting both the utility of anomaly screening and the assessment of aneuploidy risk. With the advent of first-trimester genetic risk assessment utilizing ultrasound measurements of nuchal translucency or detection of a nasal bone, the impact of obesity on these modalities is of significant importance in counseling patients. Although body mass index (BMI) is not known to affect the utility of the analytes included in the first- or second-trimester maternal serum screening for aneuploidy risk, the quality of ultrasound images is certainly affected, and in turn the accuracy of a nuchal translucency measurement or nasal bone detection. The rates of successfully completed targeted ultrasounds are significantly lower in those who are overweight or obese, with an uncertain impact on the rate of anomaly detection in this population [22]. Obesity appears to affect the utility of second-trimester sonographic assessment of genetic risk, with an impact on the detection of "soft" sonographic markers for aneuploidy [23]. Caution should be used when counseling women affected by obesity in terms of the accuracy of such screening tools in their case.

Unfortunately, many of these same women are difficult candidates for invasive testing, such as amniocentesis. Careful consideration should be paid to site selection, and should include a judgment of needle placement where tissue depth is minimized. Beyond the concern that a short needle may not reach the amniotic fluid, uncompressed target depth from the skin surface of greater than about 3 inches (8.3 cm) will make manipulation of the needle during the procedure more difficult, and requires that a 5-inch-long needle be used. This longer needle requires particular attention to fine movements translated through its extended length. Although there has been no report of any increased rate of procedure-related complications in this population undergoing amniocentesis, circumspection is warranted.

The prevalence of sleep apnea in pregnancy is poorly described [24,25] but is significant, with implications for fetal well-being, pregnancy outcome, and maternal health postpartum. The risk for hypertensive disorders of pregnancy and diabetes is increased in those who are obese when sleep apnea has been diagnosed. Early intervention with continuous positive-pressure ventilation may hold promise in averting some of these risks [26].

Screening early in prenatal care, with provider inquiry as to snoring behavior, may identify patients who require further evaluation with sleep studies to establish the diagnosis and guide therapy.

Accurate determination of maternal blood pressure in the setting of obesity has long been a difficult topic. For most women, the use of the large adult cuff is adequate. However, particularly in the woman affected by a high peripheral adipose content, even these fit poorly, and their use will lead to inaccurate, falsely elevated values. Alternative placement of blood pressure cuffs on the ankle or forearm in some cases offers an improvement in the ability to obtain measurements. Although formulae have been proposed for the translation of values obtained using the forearm [27], blood pressures obtained more distally from the trunk are subject to exponentially more variation due to position relative to the maternal heart [28]. Whatever monitoring technique is employed, change from the "normal" can be assessed when baseline values are followed with consistency through pregnancy, and this can be useful in raising any initial suspicion of pre-eclampsia. Care should be taken in the interpretation of these results in isolation. Similar statements can be made of the use of thigh cuffs on the upper arm for blood pressure monitoring. Monitoring that utilizes the patient's digits is notoriously unreliable, and should be avoided, despite ease of use.

With the elevated risk for hypertensive complications in pregnancy that is present in these patients, high blood pressure should be assumed to be correctly assessed until proven otherwise, prompting further evaluation and treatment as necessary.

Mid-trimester testing (Box 8.4)

The adequacy of a mid-trimester sonographic survey for fetal anomalies, commonly performed between 18 and 20 weeks' gestational age, is known to be adversely affected by maternal size [7,29,30]. The ability to adequately capture images for detailed anatomical evaluation has been shown to be impaired [22,31], while at the same time obese women have been

---

Box 8.4 Mid-trimester management concerns

Limitations of ultrasound in anomaly detection

Difficult invasive testing

Interval assessment of fetal growth

Reinforce exercise and weight gain plan

Ongoing nutrition consultation

seen to be at increased risk for fetal anomalies [8–10]. Whether this is a bona fide increase in risk, or the result of a decreased sensitivity of ultrasound in the detection of defects, remains to be determined. The increase in maternal girth may be related to troubling trends in sonographer health. Between 54% and 80% of sonographers report work-related injuries in survey data [32–34], requiring limitations in the studies performed and modifications in the office such as motorized tables and ergonomic seating to reduce such injury [35].

Some have proposed a 2-week delay of initial imaging in those who are obese [36] until 20–22 weeks of gestational age, or repeated studies for completion of poorly visualized anatomy on earlier scans [37], although results are mixed. Transumbilical placement of the transvaginal probe has been attempted, which has improved the ability to image more extremely obese subjects, but this is impractical for most overweight and obese patients [38]. Unfortunately, while delayed imaging may provide larger structures to be interrogated, the additional interference from calcified bony skeleton may add an artifact that outweighs this benefit. Additional studies *may* be more effective in increasing study completion rates, but are of questionable utility in view of time, expense, and sonographer exposure to additional injury risk. Most crucially, when it has been shown to be useful in improving visualization, delayed imaging was performed at approximately 22 weeks' gestation. Should an anomaly be discovered this late in pregnancy, there is an extremely limited amount of time to adequately counsel the patient on the findings, perform additional diagnostic testing (e.g. amniocentesis) and obtain the results, and allow the patient and her family to make difficult decisions before the option to terminate pregnancy becomes limited by state laws.

Pregnancies affected by maternal obesity and overweight body habitus are at risk for fetal overgrowth [6]. This risk is independent of the influence of gestational diabetes [39]. Interestingly, diabetic pregnancies tend to show asymmetric growth acceleration, commonly seen as large abdominal circumference relative to the head circumference, whereas pregnancies in those who are obese but not diabetic may result in more symmetrically overgrown fetuses. This is important, since asymmetric growth acceleration should prompt a consideration of repeated testing for glucose intolerance after routine testing for gestational diabetes has been conducted between 24 and 28 weeks' gestational age. Assessment of fetal growth requires serial ultrasounds, particularly near term, when fetal overgrowth in a diabetic pregnancy imparts a risk for shoulder dystocia with attempted vaginal delivery. Sonographic measurements of fetal soft tissue, particularly in the abdominal circumference view, may provide an insight into the increased risk for fetal overgrowth [42,41] and dystocia, particularly in the fetus of a diabetic mother [40,42].

Macrosomia may be the result of poor compliance with care and poor glucose control, and correlates with an increased risk for fetal demise. Management schemes in this regard vary, with sonography for interval assessment of fetal growth and amniotic fluid performed monthly by many providers. Fundal height assessment in those who are overweight and obese may initially seem to be impossible, and of limited utility. Contrary to this belief, according to unpublished data, fundal heights measured near term remain sensitive in the detection of fetal under- and overgrowth when compared to previously obtained measurements in the same patient. As such, this simple, easy, and inexpensive screening tool retains value in the overweight and obese gravida.

Late pregnancy and early labor

As pregnancy nears term, the obese gravida may benefit from some additional planning and counseling regarding delivery. Late pregnancy and delivery are unique experiences for these women, and anticipation of some of the difficulties imposed by increased maternal girth will aid in the normalization of the process. Most patients will appreciate and welcome a frank discussion of the anticipated course of labor and delivery, as well as the potential risks. A detailed discussion of labor and delivery risks and processes is found in Chapters 12 and 13. A brief overview, for the purposes of antenatal counseling and preparation, is provided here.

The issues and risks of providing safe and effective anesthesia to obese women are well documented [43–45]. Landmarks used in the placement of regional anesthesia can be obscured by soft tissue, and intubation in the event of emergency can be extremely difficult. In this light, early consultation with obstetric anesthesia providers may be helpful in planning treatment of the obese parturient in labor. Providers proficient in the placement of difficult regional anesthesia or fiber optic intubations may be most helpful in this regard.

Fetal overgrowth must be considered when planning for delivery. Given the morbidity associated with cesarean delivery in this population, a trial of labor is preferred. However beyond the 90th percentile for gestational age-adjusted fetal weight, the risk for failure with a labor dystocia or shoulder dystocia begins to increase. Management late in pregnancy should include an estimation of fetal weight by ultrasound, although these measurements are known to be subject to error [46]. The American College of Obstetricians and Gynecologists currently supports offering unlabored cesarean delivery for estimated fetal weights beyond 5,000 g in the nondiabetic pregnancy and 4,200–4,500 g in the diabetic mother [47,48]. The threshold for diabetic women is lower due to the increased risk for shoulder dystocia in these asymmetrically grown infants, particularly in fetuses with a ratio of head circumference to abdominal circumference lower than 0.90 [49,50]. Again, an assessment of fetal soft tissue depth may be of use in further characterizing this risk.

Other difficulties in late pregnancy and delivery for women affected by abnormal body habitus include the increased risk for fetal death [11,51], as well as post-term pregnancy [52,53]. While there are currently no recommendations in place for testing fetal well-being in these patients, non-stress testing represents a non-invasive means of weekly reassurance in women who may be at increased risk for an adverse event. In light of this increase in risk for late pregnancy demise, allowing post-datism may be ill advised even though the induction of labor presents a particular challenge in the obese. Once in labor, labor curves may be flattened [12,54], with prolongation of both active and second-stage progress [12,54]. In the absence of other fetal or maternal indications for expedited delivery, this prolongation of labor can be allowed. The obstetrician must consider the competing risks of postoperative complications after cesarean section in the obese woman and the increased risk for a cesarean with the induction due to obesity.

Management of breech presentation

The management of fetal malpresentation can present similar difficulty in this at-risk group. While abnormal body habitus does not necessarily increase the risk for breech presentation [55], obstetric caregivers presented with this combination of factors near term face a management dilemma. Allowing a breech fetus at term to labor is no longer considered standard management [56], so the risks for operative complications after a cesarean should be weighed against the possible failure of an attempt at external cephalic version. Several reports based on small numbers of patients have been unable to show an increased risk for failure of attempting external cephalic version in those who are obese, particularly when regional anesthesia is used [57–60]. In light of these data, an attempt at version of the breech near term in the obese and overweight population is a reasonable alternative to a planned cesarean in an effort to avoid maternal morbidity [61].

Route of delivery

A significant debate surrounds the issue of trial of labor in obese women [62], particularly regarding attempted vaginal birth after cesarean [3,63]. Although data show an increased risk for failed trial of labor with increasing pregravid BMI and gestational weight gain [64], the chances of successful vaginal delivery remain above 50% in most studies. Furthermore, although some have suggested the avoidance of labor due to the high failure rate and morbidity of a labored cesarean, it appears that the morbidity of cesarean delivery attributed to obesity is independent of whether or not that cesarean was performed in labor [65]. In light of this, we suggest that the obese and overweight gravida deserves a concerted effort to avoid abdominal delivery, in keeping with the standard of care for normal-weight women [66]. Should a cesarean be required in this population, the direction of the incision should be dictated by attention to the shallowest depth of adipose, which can be accomplished through horizontal incisions [67]. Similar consideration should be paid to the cosmetic result in obese women as it would to women of normal body habitus. Although vertical incisions may be performed with slightly greater speed, there is no benefit conferred upon the neonate, and these more dramatic scars may in fact infer a risk for complications on the mother [68].

Conclusions

The prenatal management of the obese pregnant woman will be an increasingly prevalent challenge as the population increases in weight. These at-risk women require heightened vigilance and honest, forthright counseling regarding the complications discussed. Early awareness of such risks, with consultations and coordination of specialized care where indicated, is critical to insure the best chances of a healthy outcome for both mother and baby. Early referral for consultation with maternal–fetal medicine subspecialists may help delineate patients who might benefit from ongoing tertiary care. Ongoing research continues to evaluate opportunities for intervention to avoid such complications in future generations, but the results are few and inconsistent. In the meantime, multidisciplinary care, with input from maternal–fetal medicine specialists, dietitians, diabetologists, exercise trainers, and anesthesiologists regarding obstetrical management, and active participation on the part of the patient in her care, remain pivotal for a healthy pregnancy outcome.

References

1. Ogden CL, Carroll MD, Curtin LR, et al. Prevalence of overweight and obesity in the United States, 1999–2004. JAMA 2006;295:1549–55.
2. Ehrenberg HM, Dierker L, Milluzzi C, et al. Prevalence of maternal obesity in an urban center. Am J Obstet Gynecol 2002;187:1189–93.
3. Anandacoomarasamy A, Smith G, Leibman S, et al. Cartilage defects are associated with physical disability in obese adults. Rheumatology (Oxford) 2009;48:1290–3.

4. Nunez M, Lozano L, Nunez E, et al. Total knee replacement and health-related quality of life: factors influencing long-term outcomes. Arthritis Rheum 2009;61:1062–9.

5. Idris I, Hall AP, O'Reilly J, et al. Obstructive sleep apnoea in patients with type 2 diabetes: aetiology and implications for clinical care. Diabetes Obes Metab 2009;11: 733–41.

6. Ehrenberg HM, Mercer BM, Catalano PM. The influence of obesity and diabetes on the prevalence of macrosomia. Am J Obstet Gynecol 2004;191:964–8.

7. Hendler I, Blackwell SC, Bujold E, et al. The impact of maternal obesity on midtrimester sonographic visualization of fetal cardiac and craniospinal structures. Int J Obes Relat Metab Disord 2004;28:1607–11.

8. Cedergren M, Kallen B. Maternal obesity and the risk for orofacial clefts in the offspring. Cleft Palate Craniofac J 2005;42:367–71.

9. Cedergren MI, Kallen BA. Maternal obesity and infant heart defects. Obes Res 2003;11:1065–71.

10. Watkins ML, Rasmussen SA, Honein MA, et al. Maternal obesity and risk for birth defects. Pediatrics 2003;111:1152–8.

11. Kristensen J, Vestergaard M, Wisborg K, et al. Pre-pregnancy weight and the risk of stillbirth and neonatal death. Br J Obstet Gynaecol 2005;112:403–8.

12. Nuthalapaty FS, Rouse DJ, Owen J. The association of maternal weight with cesarean risk, labor duration, and cervical dilation rate during labor induction. Obstet Gynecol 2004;103:452–6.

13. Buhimschi CS, Buhimschi IA, Malinow AM, et al. Intrauterine pressure during the second stage of labor in obese women. Obstet Gynecol 2004;103:225–30.

14. Sheiner E, Levy A, Menes TS, et al. Maternal obesity as an independent risk factor for caesarean delivery. Paediatr Perinat Epidemiol 2004;18:196–201.

15. Chelmow D, Rodriguez EJ, Sabatini MM. Suture closure of subcutaneous fat and wound disruption after cesarean delivery: a meta-analysis. Obstet Gynecol 2004;103: 974–80.

16. Hedderson MM, Gunderson EP, Ferrara A. Gestational weight gain and risk of gestational diabetes mellitus. Obstet Gynecol;115:597–604.

17. Rizzo T, Metzger BE, Burns WJ, et al. Correlations between antepartum maternal metabolism and child intelligence. N Engl J Med 1991;325:911–16.

18. Kiel DW, Dodson EA, Artal R, et al. Gestational weight gain and pregnancy outcomes in obese women: how much is enough? Obstet Gynecol 2007;110:752–8.

19. Wei S, Schmidt MD, Dwyer T, et al. Obesity and menstrual irregularity: associations with SHBG, testosterone, and insulin. Obesity (Silver Spring) 2009;17:1070–6.

20. Loret de Mola JR. Obesity and its relationship to infertility in men and women. Obstet Gynecol Clin North Am 2009;36:333–46, ix.

21. Wilkes S, Murdoch A. Obesity and female fertility: a primary care perspective. J Fam Plann Reprod Health Care 2009;35:181–5.

22. Khoury FR, Ehrenberg HM, Mercer BM. The impact of maternal obesity on satisfactory detailed anatomic ultrasound image acquisition. J Matern Fetal Neonatal Med 2009;22:337–41.

23. Ehrenberg HM, Fischer RL, Hediger ML, et al. Are maternal and sonographic factors associated with the detection of a fetal echogenic cardiac focus? J Ultrasound Med 2001;20:1047–52.

24. Richman RM, Elliott LM, Burns CM, et al. The prevalence of obstructive sleep apnea in an obese female population. Int J Obes Relat Metab Disord 1994;18:173–7.

25. Maasilta P, Bachour A, Teramo K, et al. Sleep-related disorder breathing during pregnancy in obese women. Chest 2001;120:1448–54.

26. Chebonneau M, Falcone T, Cosio M, et al. Obstructive sleep apnea during pregnancy. Therapy and implications for fetal health. Am Rev Respir Dis 1991;144:461–3.

27. Pierin AM, Alavarce DC, Gusmao JL, et al. Blood pressure measurement in obese patients: comparison between upper arm and forearm measurements. Blood Press Monit 2004;9:101–5.

28. Pickering TG. Principles and techniques of blood pressure measurement. Cardiol Clin 2002;20:207–23.

29. Catanzarite V, Quirk JG. Second-trimester ultrasonography: determinants of visualization of fetal anatomic structures. Am J Obstet Gynecol 1990;163:1191–5.

30. Wolfe HM, Sokol RJ, Martier SM, et al. Maternal obesity: a potential source of error in sonographic prenatal diagnosis. Obstet Gynecol 1990;76:339–42.

31. Dashe JS, McIntire DD, Twickler DM. Maternal obesity limits the ultrasound evaluation of fetal anatomy. J Ultrasound Med 2009;28:1025–30.

32. Friesen MN, Friesen R, Quanbury A, et al. Musculoskeletal injuries among ultrasound sonographers in rural Manitoba: a study of workplace ergonomics. AAOHN J 2006;54:32–7.

33. Russo A, Murphy C, Lessoway V, et al. The prevalence of musculoskeletal symptoms among British Columbia sonographers. Appl Ergon 2002;33:385–93.

34. Schoenfeld A, Goverman J, Weiss DM, et al. Transducer user syndrome: an occupational hazard of the ultrasonographer. Eur J Ultrasound 1999;10:41–5.

35. Nelson TR, Fowlkes JB, Abramowicz JS, et al. Ultrasound biosafety considerations for the practicing sonographer and sonologist. J Ultrasound Med 2009;28:139–50.

36. Lantz ME, Chisholm CA. The preferred timing of second-trimester obstetric sonography based on maternal body mass index. J Ultrasound Med 2004;23:1019–22.

37. Hendler I, Blackwell SC, Bujold E, et al. Suboptimal second-trimester ultrasonographic visualization of the fetal heart in obese women: should we repeat the examination? J Ultrasound Med 2005;24:1205–9; quiz 1210–11.

38. Rosenberg JC, Guzman ER, Vintzileos AM, et al. Transumbilical placement of the vaginal probe in obese pregnant women. Obstet Gynecol 1995;85:132–4.

39. Sacks DA. Fetal macrosomia and gestational diabetes: what's the problem? Obstet Gynecol 1993;81:775–81.

40. Mintz MC, Landon MB, Gabbe SG, et al. Shoulder soft tissue width as a predictor of macrosomia in diabetic pregnancies. Am J Perinatol 1989;6:240–3.

41. Petrikovsky BM, Oleschuk C, Lesser M, et al. Prediction of fetal macrosomia using sonographically measured abdominal subcutaneous tissue thickness. J Clin Ultrasound 1997;25:378–82.

42. Bochner CJ, Medearis AL, Williams J, 3rd, et al. Early third-trimester ultrasound screening in gestational diabetes to determine the risk of macrosomia and labor dystocia at term. Am J Obstet Gynecol 1987;157:703–8.

43. Roofthooft E. Anesthesia for the morbidly obese parturient. Curr Opin Anaesthesiol 2009;22:341–6.

44. Vallejo MC. Anesthetic management of the morbidly obese parturient. Curr Opin Anaesthesiol 2007;20:175–80.

45. Saravanakumar K, Rao SG, Cooper GM. The challenges of obesity and obstetric anaesthesia. Curr Opin Obstet Gynecol 2006;18:631–5.

46. Rovetto B, Palai N, Zatti S, et al. OC26.02: Fetal weight estimation in pregnancy complicated by obesity: comparison between conventional and a new 3D ultrasound method. Ultrasound Obstet Gynecol 2009;34:51.

47. Fetal macrosomia. ACOG Technical Bulletin Number 159 – September 1991. Int J Gynaecol Obstet 1992;39:341–5.

48. ACOG practice bulletin clinical management guidelines for obstetrician-gynecologists. Number 40, November 2002. Obstet Gynecol 2002;100:1045–50.

49. Chauhan SP, Gherman R, Hendrix NW, et al. Shoulder dystocia: comparison of the ACOG Practice Bulletin with another national guideline. Am J Perinatol 2010;27:129–36.

50. Rose VL. ACOG releases practice pattern on shoulder dystocia. Am Fam Physician 1998;57:2546, 2548.

51. Chibber R. Unexplained antepartum fetal deaths: what are the determinants? Arch Gynecol Obstet 2005;271:286–91.

52. Caughey AB, Stotland NE, Washington AE, et al. Who is at risk for prolonged and postterm pregnancy? Am J Obstet Gynecol 2009;200:683 e1–5.

53. Stotland NE, Washington AE, Caughey AB. Prepregnancy body mass index and the length of gestation at term. Am J Obstet Gynecol 2007;197:378 e1–5.

54. Vahratian A, Zhang J, Troendle JF, et al. Maternal prepregnancy overweight and obesity and the pattern of labor progression in term nulliparous women. Obstet Gynecol 2004;104:943–51.

55. Tilton Z, Hodgson MI, Donoso E, et al. Complications and outcome of pregnancy in obese women. Nutrition 1989;5:95–9.

56. Hodnett E, Hannah M. Term breech trial. Birth 2002;29:217–19; author reply 219–20.

57. Fortunato SJ, Mercer LJ, Guzick DS. External cephalic version with tocolysis: factors associated with success. Obstet Gynecol 1988;72:59–62.

58. Predanic M. External cephalic version for breech presentation with or without spinal analgesia in nulliparous women at term: a randomized controlled trial. Obstet Gynecol 2008;111:776; author reply 776–7.

59. Shalev E, Battino S, Giladi Y, et al. External cephalic version at term – using tocolysis. Acta Obstet Gynecol Scand 1993;72:455–7.

60. Weiniger CF, Ginosar Y, Elchalal U, et al. External cephalic version for breech presentation with or without spinal analgesia in nulliparous women at term: a randomized controlled trial. Obstet Gynecol 2007;110:1343–50.

61. Chervenak FA, Berkowitz RL. Successful external cephalic version in a massively obese patient. Obstet Gynecol 1983;62:8s–9s.

62. Edwards RK, Harnsberger DS, Johnson IM, et al. Deciding on route of delivery for obese women with a prior cesarean delivery. Am J Obstet Gynecol 2003;189:385–9; discussion 389–90.

63. Carroll CS, Sr., Magann EF, Chauhan SP, et al. Vaginal birth after cesarean section versus elective repeat cesarean delivery: weight-based outcomes. Am J Obstet Gynecol 2003;188:1516–20; discussion 1520–2.

64. Jensen H, Agger AO, Rasmussen KL. The influence of prepregnancy body mass index on labor complications. Acta Obstet Gynecol Scand 1999;78:799–802.

65. Myles TD, Gooch J, Santolaya J. Obesity as an independent risk factor for infectious morbidity in patients who undergo cesarean delivery. Obstet Gynecol 2002;100:959–64.

66. Brill Y, Windrim R. Vaginal birth after Caesarean section: review of antenatal predictors of success. J Obstet Gynaecol Can 2003;25:275–86.

67. Tixier H, Thouvenot S, Coulange L, et al. Cesarean section in morbidly obese women: supra or subumbilical transverse incision? Acta Obstet Gynecol Scand 2009;88:1049–52.

68. Alderdice F, McKenna D, Dornan J. Techniques and materials for skin closure in caesarean section. Cochrane Database Syst Rev 2003:CD003577.

CHAPTER 9

Nutrition and Weight Gain in the Obese Gravida

Naomi E. Stotland[1], Janet King[2], and Barbara Abrams[3]

[1]University of California, San Francisco, California, USA
[2]Children's Hospital Oakland Research Institute and University of California at Berkeley & Davis, Oakland, California, USA
[3]School of Public Health, University of California, Berkeley, California, USA

It is physiologically normal and healthy for women to gain weight during pregnancy. Weight gained during a normal pregnancy is a combination of weight from the fetus, placenta, and amniotic fluid, increased maternal blood volume, and maternal lean and fat mass. Although the optimal weight gain for women who begin pregnancy obese remains controversial, it is clear that excessive weight gain exacerbates the perinatal risks associated with obesity. Avoidance of excessive gestational weight gain may reduce the risk for adverse health outcomes during pregnancy, delivery, and the postpartum period.

While there is an abundance of epidemiological data supporting an association between weight gain and health outcomes in obese pregnant women, few studies exist that examine the optimal energy intake and dietary composition for obese pregnant women. There is also a lack of studies comparing strategies for counseling obese pregnant women to make healthful behavior changes. This chapter will examine the existing literature, make recommendations based on the evidence, and, where adequate evidence is lacking, provide expert opinion.

Recommended weight gain – the Institute of Medicine Guidelines

In 1990, the Institute of Medicine (IOM) issued recommendations for gestational weight gain that have been widely accepted and endorsed by healthcare authorities, including the American College of Obstetricians and Gynecologists [1]. These guidelines provided recommended weight gain ranges based on a woman's pre-pregnancy body mass index (BMI), with lower gains recommended for women with a higher BMI. The report recommended a lower limit of 15 lb for obese women (pre-pregnancy

Pregnancy in the Obese Woman, 1st edition. Edited by Deborah L. Conway.
© 2011 Blackwell Publishing Ltd.

Table 9.1 Institute of Medicine weight gain in pregnancy – guidelines by pre-pregnancy body mass index (BMI)

Prepregnancy BMI	Total Weight Gain		Rates of Weight Gain* 2nd and 3nd Trimester	
	Range in kg	Rang in lbs	Mean (range) in kg/week	Mean (range) in lbs/week
Underweight (<18.5 kg/m²)	12.5–18	28–40	0.51 (0.44–0.58)	1 (1–13)
Normal weight (18.5–24.9 kg/m²)	11.5–16	25–35	0.42 (0.35–0.50)	1 (0.8–1)
Overweight (2.50–29.9 kg/m²)	7–11.5	15–25	0.28 (0.23–0.33)	0.6 (0.5–0.7)
Obese (≥30.0 kg/m²)	5–9	11–20	0.22 (0.17–0.27)	0.5 (0.4–0.6)

* Calculations assume a 0.5–2 kg (1.1–4.4 lbs) weight gain in the first trimester (based on Siega et al., 1994; Abrams et al., 1995; Carmichael et al., 1997)

For references in table, see Institute of Medicine (US) Subcommittee on Nutritional Status and Weight Gain during Pregnancy [2]; reprinted with permission from the National Academies Press, Copyright 2009, National Academy of Sciences.

BMI ≥ 29 kg/m²) but concluded that data were too limited to suggest an upper limit of weight gain. In May 2009, the IOM issued a new report on pregnancy weight gain (Table 9.1) with guidelines similar to those put forth in 1990; however, the 2009 report now advises obese women (BMI ≥ 30 kg/m²) to gain between 11 and 20 lb [2].

The IOM based its 2009 recommendations on a large body of epidemiological studies, several of which were commissioned specifically for the report. Using these data, the committee identified the range of weight gain in which the lowest rates of maternal and child adverse outcomes were observed, balancing the risks of low gestational weight gain against the risks of excessive weight gain (Box 9.1).

Optimal weight gain in class 2 and 3 obesity

The IOM committee noted a dramatic increase in the prevalence of class 2 and 3 obesity among women of childbearing age in the USA during the last decade. However, they identified only one study with adequate numbers of women of class 2 and 3 obesity to study these groups separately [3]. Kiel et al. analyzed birth certificate data including self-reported weight for more than 120,000 obese (approximately 30,000 class 2 and 20,000 class 3) women who delivered in Missouri. They reported that, for

---

Box 9.1 Outcomes included by the Institute of Medicine in establishing gestational weight gain guidelines

Outcomes primarily associated with inadequate weight gain

Small-for-gestational-age infant

Preterm birth

Outcomes primarily associated with excessive weight gain

Large-for-gestational-age infant

Cesarean delivery

Postpartum weight retention

Childhood obesity

---

women of class 2 and 3 obesity, the lowest risk for pre-eclampsia, cesarean delivery, and large-for-gestational-age (LGA) infants was seen at a weight gain of 0–9 lb. For women with class 1 obesity, the lowest risk for these outcomes was seen at a gain of 10–25 lb. Of note, the committee was concerned that the observed association between pre-eclampsia and weight gain might be confounded by edema associated with pre-eclampsia. The committee called for further studies examining the association between weight gain in the first two trimesters (before fluid retention occurs) and pre-eclampsia.

Although the Kiel study suggests that low or even no gestational weight gain may be beneficial for these outcomes among women with higher classes of obesity, the committee considered the data from only one observational study insufficient to provide separate guidelines for women of class 1, 2, and 3 obesity. The committee was particularly concerned with potential harm relating to lower gestational weight gain for these mothers, including small-for-gestational-age (SGA) infants and the neurological effects of ketonemia associated with dietary restriction. It therefore made only one recommendation for obese women of all classes and called for future studies to explicitly determine the benefits and risks of gestational weight gain for class 2 and 3 obesity.

Gestational weight gain among obese women

From a population perspective, obese women gain less weight on average than non-obese women during the course of their pregnancies. However, there is great variation among women in the amount of weight gained, and a large percentage of obese women gain above the IOM guidelines. Bianco et al. found that the mean weight gain for 613 obese (BMI > 35 kg/m^2) women averaged 9.1 kg (20 lb; standard deviation 7.4 kg) [4]. Thirteen per cent of the women, however, gained more than 16 kg (35 lb), and 9% either lost or failed to gain weight. In Kiel and colleagues' large birth certificate cohort of obese women in Missouri discussed earlier, 23% gained less than 15 lb, 31% gained 15–25 lb, and 46% gained more than 25 lb [3]. Among women of class 3 obesity (BMI ≥ 40 kg/m^2), 15% gained less than 2 lb. A prospective study of a cohort of 245,526 Swedish women confirmed that gestational weight gain among obese women (BMI = 30–34.9) and very obese women (BMI ≥ 35) was lower (11.1 kg [24.5 lb] and 8.7 kg [19.2 lb], respectively) than among non-obese women [5]. Low weight gain, defined as less than 8 kg (17.6 lb) occurred in 30.2% and 44.6% of the obese and very obese women, respectively. In summary, the higher the BMI, the lower the observed weight gain, and it is not a rare event for obese women to gain no weight or lose weight during pregnancy.

Ongoing controversy over optimal weight gain range for obese women: studies supporting restricted weight gain (less than IOM guidelines) for obese women

As noted above, Kiel found that obese women who gained less than 7 kg [15.4 lb] had reduced rates of pre-eclampsia, cesarean birth, and LGA infants compared to women gaining over 7 kg [3]. Cedergren et al. studied 298,648 births from the Swedish Medical Birth Registry, and calculated the risk for selected pregnancy outcomes categorized by pre-pregnancy BMI [6]. This study included several maternal and infant outcomes that may or may not be related to maternal weight gain, including pre-eclampsia, and did not weight the outcomes for frequency or severity. Cedergren found the optimal weight gain for obese women (pre-pregnancy BMI ≥ 30 kg/m^2) to be less than 13 lb. Obese women gaining less than this amount had the lowest frequency of adverse perinatal outcomes. Inclusion of SGA births in the analysis did not substantially affect the results.

Possible risks associated with restricted weight gain among obese women

Low birthweight/small-for-gestational-age infants

Schieve et al. examined the relationship between weight gain and birthweight among 173,066 full-term births in a Centers for Disease Control dataset, stratifying by maternal BMI and race/ethnicity [7]. Among obese women who gained less than 5 lb, there was a statistically significant increased odds of low birthweight (<2500 g) compared to women gaining within the lower half of the guidelines. However, the degree of risk was different for different racial and ethnic groups. For non-Hispanic white women, the adjusted odds ratio (OR) was 1.6 (95% confidence interval [CI] 1.04–2.4), for non-Hispanic black women it was 2.6 (95% CI 1.5–4.5), and for Hispanic women it was 1.0 (95% CI 0.4–2.5). There was no increased risk for obese women in any racial/ethnic group gaining 6–14 lb. In the Kiel study, the odds of SGA at birth were higher among those gaining less than 7 kg, but other neonatal outcomes were not reported (due to lack of validity in birth certificate variables) [3]. In a cohort study of 2,946 births at the University of California, San Francisco, weight gain had a negligible effect on mean birthweight among obese women [8]. Overall, it appears that very low weight gain carries a small but statistically significant increased risk for term low birthweight among obese women.

In a study of 104,980 singleton births from the Pregnancy Risk Assessment Monitoring System (PRAMS) database in the USA, Dietz et al. reported that the association between low gestational weight gain and SGA was weak and was *not* modified by maternal pre-pregnancy BMI [9]. The authors estimated that only 1.2% of SGA was attributable to low weight gain. It is important to note that as term low birthweight is relatively rare among obese women, this increased odds still represents a low absolute risk, whereas the absolute risk for macrosomia among obese women is much higher, and increases with higher weight gain.

Preterm birth

Data are conflicting in terms of the role of gestational weight gain in spontaneous preterm birth among obese women. Multiple studies have shown that the risk associated with very low weight gain diminishes as pre-pregnancy BMI increases. However, even among obese women, there appears to be some elevation of risk associated with low weight gain. In a study of 113,019 births from PRAMS in 21 US states, Dietz et al. categorized women as obese (BMI 29–34.9 kg/m^2) or very obese (BMI ≥ 35 kg/m^2) [10]. In both groups, very low weight gain (<0.12 kg [0.3 lb] per week) was associated with an increased risk for very preterm birth (20–31 weeks) among obese (OR 3.6; 95% CI 2.9–4.6) and very obese (OR 2.6; 95% CI 2.0–3.2) women. Of note, excessive weight gain (>0.79 kg [1.7 lb] per week) was also associated with an increased risk for preterm birth in all BMI categories. Low weight gain was not associated with moderately preterm birth (32–36 weeks) among obese women.

Schieve et al. studied 3511 mother–infant pairs from the National Maternal and Infant Health Survey in 1988. They excluded pregnancies with medical complications, including diabetes and hypertension, as well as medically indicated preterm births. They also found that the risk for preterm birth associated with low weight gain decreased as maternal BMI increased. In addition, they found no increased risk for spontaneous preterm birth among overweight and obese women. Schieve also studied 266,172 births among low-income US women, and again found no increased risk for preterm birth among the subgroup of obese women [11].

Ketonemia and fetal neurological development

Pregnant women are especially susceptible to the development of ketonemia during periods of fasting. This is presumably a protective mechanism to provide fuel for the fetal brain when maternal intake is insufficient. Studies have associated maternal ketonemia with reduced IQ and other measures of neurological development in the child [12,13]. However, these studies have focused on women with diabetes, and it is unknown whether ketonemia is harmful to fetal development in non-diabetic obese women, or whether the association seen between ketonemia and adverse development is related to caloric restriction, or the ketonemia is a marker for poor glycemic control or some other factor. The IOM committee was concerned that a recommendation of severely restricted weight gain for obese women would lead to caloric restriction and resultant ketonemia, with possible adverse fetal effects.

It is critical to make the distinction between epidemiological studies, which associate lower weight gain with good birth outcomes, and intervention studies, which intentionally restrict caloric intake to produce lower weight gain. It is unknown to what degree the women who did not gain weight in the epidemiological studies were actually restricting caloric intake, or whether they had ketonemia or other metabolic effects of starvation/fasting. Resting energy expenditure increases during pregnancy, and adipose tissue increases energy expenditure during pregnancy [14]. This increased metabolic rate seen among overweight and obese women during pregnancy may be an adaptive mechanism to prevent the adverse effects of weight gain on the fetus. If this is the case, it may not be advantageous to try to compensate for low weight gain with added caloric intake.

At the time of this writing, a study is underway at the University of Adelaide, Australia, randomizing 2,500 overweight and obese pregnant women to an intervention that attempts to limit weight gain to 0–5 kg (0–11 lb). This study hopes to answer the above questions regarding the safety of restricted gestational weight gain for the infant, and will include detailed metabolic and anthropometric measures of both mother and child.

The role of prenatal counseling

More research is needed about how information is given to pregnant women regarding diet, nutrition, and maternal weight gain in various systems of healthcare, whether they follow it, and how this information influences their behavior. Two surveys of pregnant women have shown that approximately a third of women report receiving no advice about how much weight to gain during pregnancy [15,16]. Women who reported that they received no advice were more likely to gain an amount outside the IOM guidelines, compared to women who recalled receiving advice consistent with the guidelines. Therefore, the role of effective counseling by prenatal care providers has been emphasized as a key strategy in the prevention of excessive gestational weight gain among obese women. Studies suggest that although prenatal care providers recognize that obesity and weight gain are important factors in pregnancy outcome, they are not always comfortable giving such counseling [17–19]. In one qualitative study, providers reported several barriers to weight gain counseling, including concern over shaming or stigmatizing patients, a lack of knowledge about nutrition, and doubt about the effectiveness of such counseling.

As noted above, it is quite common for obese women to gain no weight or even lose weight during pregnancy. If dietary intake is adequate and fetal growth is normal by physical examination and/or ultrasound, these women may be reassured that their weight gain is appropriate (Box 9.2). More research is needed to determine the optimal pregnancy weight gain recommendations for obese women, particularly for those with a pre-pregnancy BMI of over $40\,kg/m^2$.

Because the optimal gestational weight gain for obese women remains controversial, it is particularly important for the clinician to be vigilant for

---

Box 9.2 Practical recommendations for implementing the Institute of Medicine weight gain guidelines

1. Whenever possible, measure and record a preconception height and weight in the medical record

2. Calculate and record the woman's pre-pregnancy body mass index in the prenatal record

3. At the first prenatal visit, set a weight gain goal together with the patient based on her pre-pregnancy body mass index and other considerations, and explain to her the association between pregnancy weight gain and health outcomes

4. Monitor weight gain at each prenatal visit, plot the weight gain on a chart, and discuss the results with the patient. When an abnormal weight gain is apparent, try to identify the causes and develop and implement corrective actions together with the patient

5. Encourage moderate exercise, such as water aerobics (see Chapter 10)

6. Eliminate "empty" calories (e.g. soda, sweetened beverages, sweets, refined flours) from the diet

7. Encourage the consumption of foods naturally high in fiber and nutrients: fruits, vegetables, legumes, and whole grains

> **Box 9.3 What to do if weight gain is below guidelines for the obese patient**
>
> 1. Assess energy (calorie) and nutrient intake using a 24-hour diet recall. Consult a dietitian if possible
> 2. Rule out identifiable causes (below)
> 3. Assess fetal growth using ultrasound
> 4. If the diet is inadequate, advise the patient to take corrective action with her diet to meet intake recommendations. (Again, consult a dietitian if possible)
> 5. If diet and fetal growth are adequate, continue to monitor fetal growth using fundal height and/or ultrasound. *Reassure the patient that a low weight gain does not require dietary alteration in this setting, and may indeed be beneficial.*
> 6. If fetal growth is less than expected, consult maternal–fetal medicine professional and look for non-dietary causes (hypertension, infection, etc.)
>
> **Questions to ask when weight gain is slow or weight loss occurs**
>
> 1. Is there a measurement or recording error?
> 2. Is the overall pattern acceptable? Was a lack of gain preceded by a higher than expected gain?
> 3. Was there evidence of edema at the last visit, and has it resolved?
> 4. Is nausea, vomiting, or diarrhea a problem?
> 5. Is there a problem with access to food?
> 6. Have psychosocial problems led to poor appetite?
> 7. Does the woman have an eating disorder? Is she excessively restricting her caloric intake?
> 8. Is the patient smoking? How much?
> 9. Is she using drugs or alcohol (especially cocaine or methamphetamines)?
> 10. Does her energy expenditure exceed her intake?
> 11. Does she have an illness or infection that requires treatment?
>
> *In the majority of cases, there will be no evidence of the above etiologies when an obese patient fails to gain weight, but these must be excluded.*

conflicting messages the patient may be receiving. Dietitians may be required to advise patients to meet the IOM guidelines, and may advise obese women who are gaining below the guidelines to increase caloric intake despite evidence of adequate diet and fetal growth (Box 9.3). Therefore it is imperative that the provider, dietitian, and other members of the care team work together to present consistent advice to patients. Patients may also receive conflicting advice from family members and friends about weight gain. Asking the patient to bring her partner or other close family members along to a prenatal visit can be helpful to reduce conflicting advice.

Studies of interventions to prevent excessive gestational weight gain among obese women

Few studies have tested interventions to reduce excessive gestational weight gain among non-diabetic obese women. In Denmark, Wolff and colleagues randomized 50 non-diabetic obese pregnant women to either a weight gain restriction program or usual care [20]. The intervention group underwent 10 1-hour dietary consultations beginning at 15 weeks' gestation, and were instructed to eat according to the official Danish dietary recommendations (≤30% fat, 15–20% protein, 50–55% carbohydrate). The energy intake was restricted based on individually estimated energy requirements and estimated energetic cost of fetal growth. The women in the intervention group consumed fewer calories and gained less weight than the control group: 6.6 kg [14.6 lb] versus a gain of 13.3 kg [29.3 lb] ($p = 0.002$; 95% CI 2.6–10.8 kg). This study demonstrated that weight gain can be successfully restricted among obese pregnant women using intensive dietary counseling.

In a non-randomized Swedish study by Claesson et al., 155 obese women (BMI = 30–40 kg/m^2) participating in a prenatal intervention gained less weight (adjusted weight gain = 7.52 kg [16.6 lb]) than matched obese controls (adjusted weight gain = 9.78 kg [21.6 lb]) [21]. The intervention consisted of weekly motivational talks and aqua-aerobics classes. There were no statistically significant differences between the groups in length of gestation, mode of delivery, or infant birthweight, but the study was not powered to detect such differences.

Artal and colleagues studied 96 overweight and obese women (BMI > 25 kg/m^2) with gestational diabetes who self-selected into either a diet (D) or diet plus exercise (ED) group in the early third trimester [22]. Women in the D group were prescribed a eucaloric (energy-balanced) diet and counseled by a registered dietitian. Women were instructed to consume a daily meal plan based on BMI: 25 kcal/kg for overweight, 20 kcal/kg for obese, and 15 kcal/kg for morbidly obese (BMI ≥ 40 kg/m^2) women. The meal plan included 40–45% carbohydrates. The ED group received the same dietary counseling as the D group, plus additional education in reducing fat intake and advice to engage in moderate exercise. The ED group was encouraged to use a treadmill and a recumbent bike available in the study's laboratory, as well as to exercise at home.

The addition of exercise to a calorie-restricted diet lowered the weekly weight gain from 0.3 to 0.1 kg [0.7 to 0.2 lb] ($p < 0.05$). The incidence of

LGA tended to be higher among the women who gained weight versus those who lost weight or had no weight change (10 versus one macrosomic baby), but the difference did not reach significance ($p = 0.12$). No adverse pregnancy outcomes were observed with weight maintenance or loss, but the study was not powered to detect differences in SGA or other infant outcomes. However, the study suggests that a prevention of excessive weight gain or, possibly, weight maintenance among obese pregnant women with gestational diabetes may reduce the risk for fetal overgrowth. It is unclear, however, to what degree the findings of this study apply to obese pregnant women without gestational diabetes.

Five groups have studied behavioral interventions, consisting of dietary counseling and weight gain monitoring, to prevent excessive weight gain in pregnancy, but *not* exclusively in obese women [23–27]. One of the four studies, a community-based intervention [24], failed to find an effect of the intervention on gestational weight gain. In Polley and colleagues' study [27], normal-weight women in the intervention group had lower percentages that exceeded the IOM recommendation; however, the intervention did not work for overweight/obese women. In Olson et al.'s study [26], a significant effect was seen only among the low-income women (adjusted OR 0.41 and 95% CI 0.20–0.81) for excessive gestational weight gain associated with the intervention. The fourth study, carried in Finland, found that women increased their intakes of fruit, vegetables, and high-fiber bread, but the prevalence of excessive weight gain was not reduced [25]. Asbee et al. randomized 100 women and found a decreased mean weight gain in the intervention group, but no difference in the percentage that met the IOM weight gain guidelines [23].

In summary, there is moderately strong evidence that gestational weight gain can be reduced in obese women through prenatal counseling and modification of diet and physical activity during pregnancy.

Nutrition for obese pregnant women (Table 9.2)

Although one might assume that obese pregnant women have an adequate nutritional intake, there is evidence that the obese gravida has a poorer *quality* diet compared to that of leaner women. Oken and colleagues examined the diets of a cohort of 1,777 women in Project Viva [28]. They used the Alternative Healthy Eating Index (AHEI), slightly modified for pregnancy. The AHEI calculates a score based on a balance between healthful foods such as fruits and vegetables versus unhealthful foods such as trans fats. Women in the highest BMI category had the lowest AHEI scores (the poorest diet). Siega-Riz studied the diets of a cohort of 2,247 women in North Carolina, USA, and found that high-calorie, nutrient-poor foods such as sodas, juices, and refined flours were

Table 9.2 Macronutrient needs during pregnancy

Macronutrient	Range (% of energy)	
	4–18 years	Adults
Fat	25–35	20–35
Omega-6 fats	5–10	5–10
Omega-3 fats	0.6–1.2	0.6–1.2
Carbohydrate	46–65	46–65
Protein	10–30	10–35
Cholesterol	As low as possible while consuming a nutritionally adequate diet	
Trans fats		
Saturated fats		
Added sugars	Limit to no more than 25% of total energy	

major contributors to the overall caloric intake [29]. The diets were also high in saturated fats.

The additional caloric needs of pregnancy are small relative to the needs for many other nutrients. Although an extra 340–450 kcal could be consumed by simply adding a glass of 2% milk and a small sandwich, this would not meet increased micronutrient requirements of pregnancy. The fact that the relative increase required for many other nutrients is more dramatic than for energy indicates the importance of emphasizing *nutrient-dense* foods during pregnancy. Following the dictum of "eating for two" may result in excessive maternal weight gain.

Vitamin and mineral supplementation
The consumption of a daily prenatal multivitamin should ensure that women are meeting their micronutrient requirements. However, supplements should not be considered to be an equivalent substitute for a diet rich in fruits, vegetables, and whole grains, which contain a myriad of beneficial substances, such as antioxidants, that are not present in supplements.

Folic acid
Obese women have higher rates of neural tube defects (NTDs) compared to women of lower BMI [30]. It is not known to what degree this higher rate is related to folic acid intake. It has also been theorized that relative hyperglycemia, even among women without a diagnosis of diabetes, contributes to the higher rates of NTD among obese women. In a retrospective, population-based Canadian study of NTDs pre- and post-universal

folic acid fortification of flour, there was less reduction of risk among obese women [31]. The current recommendation for periconception folic acid intake – 400 μg per day – is the same for women of all BMIs.

Caloric intake

The Dietary Reference Intakes of the IOM recommend that pregnant women should, on average, consume an extra 340 kcal per day in the second trimester and 452 kcal per day in the third trimester [32]. Whether this energy prescription is suitable for overweight and obese women is unknown. Research is needed in this area to support dietary recommendations that result in appropriate weight gain for overweight and obese pregnant women. Women can get an individualized diet plan, based on height, weight, gestational age, and activity level, at http://www.mypyramid. gov/mypyramidmoms/index.html.

The association between caloric intake and gestational weight gain is very weak. This may reflect the fact that gestational weight gain is driven largely by hormonal changes in pregnancy, and that weight gain is a combination of blood volume, edema, fetal and placental weight, amniotic fluid, and tissue hypertrophy, as well as maternal fat stores.

Small studies of obese women with gestational diabetes show that caloric restriction (to around 1800 kcal per day) will limit weight gain without significant ketosis and improve maternal glycemia [33]. These studies did not show any adverse effect on infant birthweight, but the numbers of subjects were too small to rule out such adverse effects. Again, it is unknown whether these findings can be generalized to obese women without diabetes.

Special diets

Unfortunately, there is a lack of data regarding the optimal diet for obese women during pregnancy. Therefore, current nutritional recommendations are the same for obese pregnant women as for all pregnant women. Whether or not specific diets, such as a low-glycemic diet, can improve pregnancy outcomes specifically among obese pregnant women is an active area of research. See Table 9.3 for a comparison of diets that may be beneficial for obese pregnant women.

Low-glycemic diet

The postprandial blood glucose response is primarily determined by the rate of intestinal carbohydrate absorption, with the most rapidly absorbed refined sugars causing the highest response, and the more complex, slowly absorbed carbohydrates causing the lowest response. Thus, shifting the *source* carbohydrates to a higher proportion of complex, low-glycemic foods may play a role in the prevention of gestational diabetes among obese women.

Table 9.3 Comparison of diets that may be beneficial for obese pregnant women

Name of diet	Description	Supporting evidence	Disadvantages/risks	Online reference
MyPyramid Diet	Same diet composition as recommended for non-pregnant adults Emphasizes vegetables, fruits, and whole grains	Based on epidemiological data on diet and chronic disease in non-pregnant adults	May not provide adequate potassium, vitamin E, and iron for pregnancy, but would be adequate with supplementation (prenatal vitamin)	http://www.mypyramid. gov/mypyramidmoms/
Sweet Success Diet	Diet designed for pregnant women with gestational diabetes to prevent hyperglycemia. Emphasizes small, frequent meals/snacks and avoidance of concentrated sweets. Caloric restriction of 30% for obese women	Has been used for many years in pregnant diabetic women without evidence of harm May decrease the risk for excessive weight gain	Has never been studied in normoglycemic obese women Caloric restriction may be associated with increased risk for small-for-gestational-age infants	http://www.cdph.ca.gov/ programs/cdapp
Low-glycemic Diet	Diet modifying the type of carbohydrate – the goal is to lower the insulin and glycemic response to meals	Epidemiological data support a reduced risk for gestational diabetes [34]	Limited data in pregnancy Associated with small-for-gestational age infant in an observational study [38]. Adherence may be especially difficult	http://www.glycemicindex. com/

A prospective, epidemiological cohort study confirmed that the source of dietary carbohydrate influences the risk for gestational diabetes. Among 13,110 women in the Nurses' Health Study, high dietary fiber intake was strongly associated with a reduced risk for gestational diabetes. Each 10 g per day increment in total fiber intake was associated with a 26% reduction in the risk for gestational diabetes. Conversely, a low cereal fiber/high-glycemic load diet was associated with a 2.15-fold increased risk for gestational diabetes compared to the reciprocal diet [34]. In 2008, a Cochrane review assessed the efficacy of either a high-fiber or a low-glycemic index diet for preventing gestational diabetes. Three trials (107 women) were included in the review [35–37], but the data were insufficient for determining whether a diet rich in complex carbohydrates reduced the risk for gestational diabetes. In an observational study of 1,082 low-income women in New Jersey, USA, a lower glycemic diet was associated with a twofold increased risk for having an SGA infant [38].

Postpartum weight concerns in obese women

In a cohort study from the USA, overweight and obese women who gained excessive weight during pregnancy were more likely to retain this weight postpartum compared to women with a normal pre-pregnancy BMI [39]. This is yet another reason to avoid excessive pregnancy weight gain. Pregnancy weight gain above the IOM guidelines is the strongest predictor of postpartum weight retention at 1 year [40]. However, there is also evidence that diet and exercise interventions during the postpartum period can help women return to their pre-pregnancy weight. Breastfeeding for at least 6 months has been associated with lower postpartum weight [41]. Obese women may have more difficulty breastfeeding (see Chapter 14) so lactation support may also help with postpartum weight loss [42].

Summary

Both excessive and inadequate weight gain carry risks for the obese pregnant woman, but there appear to be greater risks associated with excessive gain. There is evidence that excessive weight gain can be reduced or prevented by prenatal counseling and behavior modification (nutrition and exercise). The optimal diet for obese pregnant women is unknown, but it is prudent to consider recommending that women make dietary improvements during pregnancy and beyond, including replacing refined carbohydrates, saturated and trans fats with fruits, vegetables, legumes, and whole grains. Obese women should be advised to target a total weight gain within the IOM recommendations; however, many will gain less, and if weight gain is below the recommended range despite adequate dietary intake, we do not recommend adding further calories to increase weight gain. Women who gain weight during pregnancy should be given support during the postpartum period to implement healthful behavior changes to lose the added weight. Future research will address the safety of dietary and weight gain restriction during pregnancy among obese women.

References

1. Institute of Medicine (US) Subcommittee on Nutritional Status and Weight Gain during Pregnancy, Institute of Medicine (US) Subcommittee on Dietary Intake and Nutrient Supplements during Pregnancy. Nutrition during pregnancy. Part I: Weight gain. Part II: Nutrient supplements. Washington, DC: National Academy Press, 1990.
2. Institute of Medicine (US) Subcommittee on Nutritional Status and Weight Gain during Pregnancy. Weight gain during pregnancy: reexamining the guidelines. Washington, DC: National Academy Press, 2009.
3. Kiel DW, Dodson EA, Artal R, et al. Gestational weight gain and pregnancy outcomes in obese women: how much is enough? Obstet Gynecol 2007;110:752–8.
4. Bianco AT, Smilen SW, Davis Y, et al. Pregnancy outcome and weight gain recommendations for the morbidly obese woman. Obstet Gynecol 1998;91:97–102.
5. Cedergren M. Effects of gestational weight gain and body mass index on obstetric outcome in Sweden. Int J Gynaecol Obstet 2006;93:269–74.
6. Cedergren MI. Optimal gestational weight gain for body mass index categories. Obstet Gynecol 2007;110:759–64.
7. Schieve LA, Cogswell ME, Scanlon KS. An empiric evaluation of the Institute of Medicine's pregnancy weight gain guidelines by race. Obstet Gynecol 1998;91:878–84.
8. Abrams BF, Laros RK, Jr. Prepregnancy weight, weight gain, and birth weight. Am J Obstet Gynecol 1986;154:503–9.
9. Dietz PM, Callaghan WM, Smith R, et al. Low pregnancy weight gain and small for gestational age: a comparison of the association using 3 different measures of small for gestational age. Am J Obstet Gynecol 2009;201:53 e51–7.
10. Dietz PM, Callaghan WM, Cogswell ME, et al. Combined effects of prepregnancy body mass index and weight gain during pregnancy on the risk of preterm delivery. Epidemiology 2006;17:170–7.
11. Schieve LA, Cogswell ME, Scanlon KS. Maternal weight gain and preterm delivery: differential effects by body mass index. Epidemiology 1999;10:141–7.
12. Rizzo T, Metzger BE, Burns WJ, et al. Correlations between antepartum maternal metabolism and child intelligence. N Engl J Med 1991;325:911–16.
13. Silverman BL, Rizzo T, Green OC, et al. Long-term prospective evaluation of offspring of diabetic mothers. Diabetes 1991;40(Suppl. 2):121–5.
14. Bronstein MN, Mak RP, King JC. Unexpected relationship between fat mass and basal metabolic rate in pregnant women. Br J Nutr 1996;75:659–68.
15. Cogswell ME, Scanlon KS, Fein SB, et al. Medically advised, mother's personal target, and actual weight gain during pregnancy. Obstet Gynecol 1999;94:616–22.
16. Stotland NE, Haas JS, Brawarsky P, et al. Body mass index, provider advice, and target gestational weight gain. Obstet Gynecol 2005;105:633–8.
17. Power ML, Cogswell ME, Schulkin J. Obesity prevention and treatment practices of U.S. obstetrician-gynecologists. Obstet Gynecol 2006;108:961–8.

18. Power ML, Cogswell ME, Schulkin J. US obstetrician-gynaecologist's prevention and management of obesity in pregnancy. J Obstet Gynaecol 2009;29:373–7.
19. Stotland NE, Gilbert P, Bogetz A, et al. Preventing excessive weight gain in pregnancy: how do prenatal care providers approach counseling? J Womens Health (Larchmt) 2010;19:807–14.
20. Wolff S, Legarth J, Vangsgaard K, et al. A randomized trial of the effects of dietary counseling on gestational weight gain and glucose metabolism in obese pregnant women. Int J Obes (Lond) 2008;32:495–501.
21. Claesson IM, Sydsjo G, Brynhildsen J, et al. Weight gain restriction for obese pregnant women: a case-control intervention study. Br J Obstet Gynaecol 2008;115:44–50.
22. Artal R, Catanzaro RB, Gavard JA, et al. A lifestyle intervention of weight-gain restriction: diet and exercise in obese women with gestational diabetes mellitus. Appl Physiol Nutr Metab 2007;32:596–601.
23. Asbee SM, Jenkins TR, Butler JR, et al. Preventing excessive weight gain during pregnancy through dietary and lifestyle counseling: a randomized controlled trial. Obstet Gynecol 2009;113:305–12.
24. Gray-Donald K, Robinson E, Collier A, et al. Intervening to reduce weight gain in pregnancy and gestational diabetes mellitus in Cree communities: an evaluation. CMAJ 2000;163:1247–51.
25. Kinnunen TI, Pasanen M, Aittasalo M, et al. Preventing excessive weight gain during pregnancy – a controlled trial in primary health care. Eur J Clin Nutr 2007;61:884–91.
26. Olson CM, Strawderman MS, Reed RG. Efficacy of an intervention to prevent excessive gestational weight gain. Am J Obstet Gynecol 2004;191:530–6.
27. Polley BA, Wing RR, Sims CJ. Randomized controlled trial to prevent excessive weight gain in pregnant women. Int J Obes Relat Metab Disord 2002;26:1494–502.
28. Rifas-Shiman SL, Rich-Edwards JW, Kleinman KP, et al. Dietary quality during pregnancy varies by maternal characteristics in Project Viva: a US cohort. J Am Diet Assoc 2009;109:1004–11.
29. Siega-Riz AM, Bodnar LM, Savitz DA. What are pregnant women eating? Nutrient and food group differences by race. Am J Obstet Gynecol 2002;186:480–6.
30. Stothard KJ, Tennant PW, Bell R, et al. Maternal overweight and obesity and the risk of congenital anomalies: a systematic review and meta-analysis. JAMA 2009;301:636–50.
31. Ray JG, Wyatt PR, Vermeulen MJ, et al. Greater maternal weight and the ongoing risk of neural tube defects after folic acid flour fortification. Obstet Gynecol 2005;105:261–5.
32. Institute of Medicine. Dietary reference intakes for energy, carbohydrate, fiber, fat, fatty acids, cholesterol, protein, and amino acids. Part 1. Washington, DC: National Academies Press, 2002.
33. Gunderson EP. Gestational diabetes and nutritional recommendations. Curr Diab Rep 2004;4:377–86.
34. Zhang C, Liu S, Solomon CG, et al. Dietary fiber intake, dietary glycemic load, and the risk for gestational diabetes mellitus. Diabetes Care 2006;29:2223–30.
35. Clapp JF, 3rd. Maternal carbohydrate intake and pregnancy outcome. Proc Nutr Soc 2002;61:45–50.
36. Fraser RB, Ford FA, Milner RD. A controlled trial of a high dietary fibre intake in pregnancy – effects on plasma glucose and insulin levels. Diabetologia 1983;25:238–41.
37. Moses RG, Luebcke M, Davis WS, et al. Effect of a low-glycemic-index diet during pregnancy on obstetric outcomes. Am J Clin Nutr 2006;84:807–12.

38. Scholl TO, Chen X, Khoo CS, et al. The dietary glycemic index during pregnancy: influence on infant birth weight, fetal growth, and biomarkers of carbohydrate metabolism. Am J Epidemiol 2004;159:467–74.
39. Gunderson EP, Abrams B, Selvin S. Does the pattern of postpartum weight change differ according to pregravid body size? Int J Obes Relat Metab Disord 2001;25: 853–62.
40. Phelan S. Pregnancy: a "teachable moment" for weight control and obesity prevention. Am J Obstet Gynecol 2010;202:135 e1–8.
41. Baker JL, Gamborg M, Heitmann BL, et al. Breastfeeding reduces postpartum weight retention. Am J Clin Nutr 2008;88:1543–51.
42. Oddy WH, Li J, Landsborough L, et al. The association of maternal overweight and obesity with breastfeeding duration. J Pediatr 2006;149:185–91.

Other useful online resources

- American College of Obstetricians and Gynecologists. Webtreats: Diet, Weight Management and Obesity: http://www.acog.org/departments/dept_notice.cfm?recno=20& bulletin=4531
- Royal College of Obstetricians and Gynaecologists. Obesity and Reproductive Health, Study Group Statement: http://www.rcog.org.uk/womens-health/clinical-guidance/ obesity-and-reproductive-health-study-group-statement
- US Department of Agriculture. MyPyramid for Pregnancy and Breastfeeding: http:// www.mypyramid.gov/mypyramidmoms/index.html

CHAPTER 10

Exercise Recommendations for the Obese Gravida

Krista L. Rompolski and John M. Jakicic
University of Pittsburgh, Pittsburgh, Pennsylvania, US

Background

Obesity is related to a number of public health problems and presents a unique challenge for women. The prevalence of obesity is in women is higher than in men [1] and increases during the childbearing years [2]. Recent data from the National Health and Nutrition Examination Survey indicated that the prevalence of obesity among childbearing women aged 20–39 years reached 29% in 2004 [1].

Women who are overweight or obese in the prenatal period are heavier after pregnancy and may have a more difficult time losing weight given the new lifestyle of motherhood [3]. Weight gained during a woman's first pregnancy is often retained postpartum, and each subsequent pregnancy is likely to result in greater postpartum weight retention [2]. Having only one child doubles the 5- and 10-year incidence of obesity compared to women who never give birth [4]. Both excess weight before pregnancy and excess weight gain during pregnancy predispose women to adverse pregnancy-related outcomes [2,5–7].

Despite the complications associated with excess weight before, during, and after pregnancy, lifestyle strategies to manage gestational weight gain, particularly physical activity and exercise, are not always implemented. Without effective intervention, women are often left with excess weight postpartum. A considerable amount of evidence suggests that exercise not only helps to control adverse pregnancy outcomes in the obese woman, but may aid in the attenuation of pregnancy weight gain [8–11]. Women who are considering becoming pregnant are strongly advised to achieve a healthier body weight prior to pregnancy [2,12], but this is not always feasible. Losing excess body weight may take longer than a family would like to wait to have children, making safe and effective interventions during pregnancy

Pregnancy in the Obese Woman, 1st edition. Edited by Deborah L. Conway.
© 2011 Blackwell Publishing Ltd.

essential. Through careful dietary monitoring and appropriate physical activity, both lean and obese pregnant women may achieve optimal weight gain and prevent pregnancy-related complications [13–15].

Concern exists about the safety of exercise during pregnancy on maternal and fetal health, as well about as the appropriate type and dose of exercise that maximizes benefits and minimizes risk [16–18]. These concerns and challenges are magnified in the setting of obesity. The type and dose of exercise are influenced by weight status, prior history of exercise, and the special needs of women classified as having a high risk pregnancy for other reasons [17]. Exercise is not widely addressed among providers of maternal care, even in the postpartum period, when exercise can speed recovery, aid in the return to normal weight, and improve mood [19,20]. Obesity itself presents a challenge to professionals attempting to prescribe exercise. Obese people experience several barriers to exercise, including joint pain, gait abnormalities, temperature regulation, and low fitness levels. Obese women may become even less active during pregnancy due to the compounding effect on gait, balance, and thermoregulation. Clear recommendations on exercise for obese women are needed. This chapter will address the following:

- the benefits of exercise for the obese pregnant woman;
- the effect of exercise attenuation on gestational weight gain;
- the risks associated with exercise for the obese woman;
- the benefits of exercise for preventing and treating gestational diabetes;
- the effects of exercise during the postpartum period on future outcomes;
- recommendations for clinicians on appropriate exercise prescription

Safety of weight restriction in obese pregnant women

In obese women, weight gain restriction or weight loss during pregnancy is controversial but has been investigated to determine the safety of this goal as well as the influence on pregnancy outcomes. Across interventions, weight gain restriction of less than 7 kg (15.4 lb) was safe for both mother and neonate and did not adversely affect the delivery process or birthweight [9,21–23] (Table 10.1). Obese women with a low gestational weight gain have a lower risk for adverse outcomes than normal or overweight women with excessive pregnancy weight gain [24], indicating the potential value of weight restriction across all weight levels. This issue is discussed in greater detail in Chapter 9.

The effect of exercise on gestational weight gain

Lifestyle physical activity and structured exercise are important components of health and are considered predictive of long-term weight maintenance and prevention of weight gain [25]. When at a healthy body

Table 10.1 Summary of the Institute of Medicine 2009 guidelines for pregnancy weight gain

Prenatal body mass index (kg/m²)		Total weight gain (lb)	Rates (ranges) of weight gain* 2nd and 3rd trimesters (lb/week)
Underweight	<18.5	28–40	1 (1–1.3)
Normal	18.6–24.9	25–35	1 (0.8–1)
Overweight	25–29.9	15–25	0.6 (0.5–0.7)
Obese	≥30	11–20	0.5 (0.4–0.6)

*Calculations assume a 0.5–2 kg (1.1–4.4 lb) weight gain in the first trimester.

weight, the caloric deficit created through regular exercise may balance the occasional caloric surplus in those eating a eucaloric diet. Over time, women who continue to exercise during and after pregnancy gain less weight and deposit less fat than their non-exercising counterparts [26]. A sedentary lifestyle during pregnancy is more common in women who gain excessive weight [14]. During pregnancy, a woman's metabolic rate increases to support fetal growth, causing an increased caloric requirement [27]. Obese women may use this increase in metabolic rate in combination with the modest energy expenditure of exercise to help meet weight gain goals throughout pregnancy.

Few investigations have been conducted on the relationship between physical activity and gestational weight gain and postpartum weight retention, but those which exist yield promising results. An investigation that used aqua-aerobics classes and weekly motivational talks resulted in significantly lower weight gain during pregnancy compared to the group who received only talks. Participants also weighed less at their postnatal check-up compared to their weight during early pregnancy [9]. A behavioral intervention utilizing a stepped care behavioral approach (including education about weight gain, healthy eating, and exercise) significantly decreased the percentage of normal-weight women who exceeded the Institute of Medicine (IOM) recommendations compared to the control group (33% versus 58%) [15]. A cohort study of pregnant women across all body mass index (BMI) categories found that walking for 30 minutes per day or 30 minutes of vigorous physical activity per day decreased the risk for excessive gestational weight gain [14].

The recommended amount of physical activity for cardiovascular health alone may cause only modest weight loss in non-pregnant adults, yet it appears to be effective in balancing the calories women may consume above and beyond the increased requirement of pregnancy [25]. Since energy expenditure increases in exercising women during pregnancy, and increased energy expenditure leads to weight loss when the diet is maintained, obese pregnant women can use exercise in combination with healthy dietary practices to attenuate weight gain or maintain weight throughout gestation [28, 29].

Exercise in pregnant women

Exercise is widely recommended for all women with low-risk pregnancies [30]. Research continues to show that exercise in women of all weight categories carries multiple benefits for both mother and the child, both during pregnancy and in the postpartum period [17]. In addition to limiting weight gain and minimizing fat retention, maternal benefits include increased cardiovascular function, improved attitude and mental state, easier and less complicated labor, quick recovery, and greater fitness [17]. Women of all BMI categories who voluntarily continue to exercise during pregnancy are more likely to continue to exercise over time and to enter into menopause with a low cardiovascular risk profile [26]. The offspring of women who exercised throughout pregnancy are typically leaner at 5 years of age than children born to sedentary, overweight women [17]. This relationship may be due to both shared lifestyle factors between mother and offspring and to maternal habits during pregnancy. Women who are active throughout pregnancy also require less healthcare intervention during pregnancy and the postpartum period for both themselves and their infants [2,28]. Previously active women may be concerned that pregnancy will decrease their aerobic fitness levels. Research has shown that pregnant women who remain active throughout their pregnancy can maintain their fitness [16,28]. Pregnancy should not be viewed as a period of time to reach peak aerobic fitness or strength, but rather to maintain prior fitness levels throughout gestation [17,30].

Metabolic and mechanical adaptations

Several physiological adaptations that affect exercise performance occur during pregnancy. Heart rate, ventilation, skin blood flow, mass and dilation of the left ventricle, and total blood volume increase throughout pregnancy, while systemic vascular resistance decreases, all in order to optimize uterine blood flow and to increase heat dissipation for the maintenance of core temperature [2,31–33]. Due to the reliance of the fetus on maternal adaptations, women are advised to exercise at a lower intensity during pregnancy. However, previously active women exhibit a higher cardiac output, a lower rate of ventilation, and increased blood flow, oxygen and nutrient delivery to the uterus during exercise than previously sedentary women, allowing them to exercise safely at a higher intensity [28,34]. Adequate hydration and ventilation are essential for heat dissipation in exercising pregnant women, especially for obese women, who experience increased ventilation and decreased heat dissipation in response to exercise [8,35,36]. All exercising pregnant women are advised to use a fan to maximize heat dissipation and to exercise indoors or in the early morning or late evening if in a hot, humid environment [35,37].

Mechanical adaptations occur during pregnancy that may affect performance and mobility in pregnant women. As the fetus increases in size, a woman's center of gravity shifts forward, increasing the risk for falls. To compensate, lumbar lordosis occurs, causing or exacerbating back pain in some women. Obese women may experience greater pain and balance issues due to the increased stress of excess body weight. Exercises that are low impact and incorporate the major muscle groups are safe and decrease the risk for falls and abdominal trauma [35]. Pregnant women should avoid the supine position as well as standing in place for prolonged periods of time, as these positions will restrict uterine blood flow [2,35]. Pregnant women also experience greater ligament and joint laxity due to increases in estrogen and relaxin [8,31]. Although this might be expected to increase the risk for sprains or strains during pregnancy, increased rates of injury in pregnant women during exercise have not been reported [8,16,30,35,37].

Despite the benefits, there are risks associated with excessive exercise or lifestyle activity for fetal growth that receive attention. Our knowledge of the maternal physiological adaptations to pregnancy, including alterations in cardiac output, blood flow, and heat dissipation, has caused controversy over the safety of exercise during pregnancy. Focus has been on the possible competition between a pregnant woman's contracting skeletal muscle and the uteroplacental circulation for blood supply during exercise [36]. Hypothetical risks to the fetus include growth restriction, altered fetal development and the possibility of pre-term labor due to redistribution of blood flow during regular or prolonged exercise [8,36,38]. However, there are no reports to link adverse fetal outcomes with maternal exercise in women who exercise at recommended levels [8].

Barriers to exercise in pregnant women

In order to prescribe an appropriate exercise program to which women can adhere, it is important to understand the factors associated with inactivity during pregnancy, both in previously sedentary and in previously active women. Across studies that examine the barriers to leisure-time physical activity and exercise, the major barriers identified included fatigue, time constraints, and physical limitations such as obesity [3,20,39]. A low level of exercise self-efficacy, that is, how confident a person is in her ability to exercise when other lifestyle factors interfere, is related to inactivity during pregnancy, particularly among women of low income and less education [40,41]. Healthcare professionals should make efforts to understand each individual's beliefs about exercise and about her ability to perform exercise during pregnancy, in order to maximize health during the childbearing years [20]. These efforts will be more important in obese pregnant women who experience greater psychological and physical barriers to exercise, independent of pregnancy.

Exercise prescription for the obese pregnant woman

The American College of Sports Medicine and the Centers for Disease Control and Prevention have collaborated to establish exercise recommendations for both obese individuals as well as women during pregnancy and the postpartum period. In pregnancies of low risk and no complications, normal-weight pregnant women are encouraged to exercise at least three, but preferably all, days of the week at a moderate intensity (exercise intensity is described later in this chapter). Walking is highly encouraged in pregnant women, yet some women engaging in regular vigorous activity (e.g. running) before pregnancy are able to maintain this practice for most of the pregnancy until it becomes uncomfortable [42].

There are currently no standard recommendations for the obese pregnant woman. Guidelines recommend that obese women receive medical clearance from their physicians before the appropriate exercise prescription is determined in order to minimize potential risks [8,34,43]. The Canadian Society for Exercise Physiology's Physical Activity Readiness Medical Examination for Pregnancy (PARmed-X for Pregnancy) should be utilized for screening all pregnant women considering participating in an exercise program. The PARmed-X for Pregnancy is a checklist that can be used by healthcare providers to evaluate, prescribe, and monitor exercise in pregnant patients [44]. Once the low-risk nature of the pregnancy is established in the overweight or obese woman, exercise recommendations may follow a blend of those established for obese and pregnant women. In order to avoid fatigue and minimize risk, women who have been sedentary prior to pregnancy should gradually increase their activity over a few weeks until they meet the regular recommendations [2,34,37].

Aerobic exercise
Aerobic exercise for the obese woman during pregnancy is intended to increase energy expenditure, attenuate gestational weight gain, improve physical function, and decrease the risk for adverse pregnancy outcomes [16]. Even at low intensities, fitness will be increased among previously sedentary and obese women while increasing the likelihood of compliance with the program [2]. As with all exercise prescriptions, obese pregnant women should follow the FITT (Frequency, Intensity, Time, and Type)

Table 10.2 Aerobic exercise prescription for the obese gravida

Frequency	3–4 days/week
Intensity	Target heart rate* Ages 20–29: 110–131 bpm Ages 30–39: 108–127 bpm RPE 12–14†
Duration	30–50 minutes
Mode	Low-impact aerobic activity

bpm, beats per minute.
* Equivalent to 20–39% $VO_{2reserve}$[47].
† Utilize the "talk test"; based on Borg Rating of Perceived Exertion (RPE) scale 6–20.

principle for the initiation and progression of exercise (Table 10.2). The frequency, intensity, and duration of exercise should all begin at levels that do not result in pain, shortness of breath, or excess fatigue [35].

Frequency

Pregnant and obese women are advised to exercise most days of the week, yet the combination of obesity and pregnancy, especially in the second or third trimester, may lead to excess fatigue in previously sedentary women. Women are advised to exercise at least 3 or 4 days per week while maintaining leisure-time physical activity. As with all populations, pregnant women should minimize prolonged periods of sedentary time to maximize total daily energy expenditure. Exercising every other day versus on 3 or 4 consecutive days should minimize the fatigue that obese pregnant women may experience and allow for adequate recovery time [2].

Intensity

Perceived exertion may be higher at a given workload in obese women, who demonstrate increased ventilation responses to treadmill exercise, than in lean women. However, these responses do not appear until higher intensities, and obese women exhibit similar breathing patterns during submaximal workloads and activities of daily living [45]. The most common methods for monitoring intensity of exercise are the Rating of Perceived Exertion and target heart rate. The defined target heart rate zones based on age and the appropriate fitness levels can be used for exercise prescription in healthy pregnant women [46]. Since obese women are most compliant with exercise at a lower intensity and typically exhibit lower work capacities, Davenport et al. developed a target heart rate zone specifically for overweight and obese pregnant women [47]. A target heart rate of 110–131 or 108–127 beats per minute is appropriate for obese pregnant women ages 20–29 and 30–39, respectively. The Rating of Perceived Exertion scale may also be used alone or in combination with target heart rate during exercise.

The perceived exertion scale developed by Borg classifies intensity on a scale of 6–20, with 6 indicating no effort and 20 indicating maximal effort. A range of 12–14 on this scale is considered moderate intensity. Obese pregnant women should utilize the "talk test," indicating that the intensity of exercise results in a rate of breathing that is comfortable enough to simultaneously hold a conversation [36].

Duration

Obese women should perform 30–50 minutes of moderate-intensity aerobic exercise on 3 or 4 days per week, with a goal of achieving 150 minutes of recommended physical activity for health per week. The recommendations for non-pregnant obese adults are up to two times greater, at 300 minutes per week [34], but this prescription is to enhance weight loss or prevent weight regain when coupled with dietary restriction. Conversely, in obese pregnant women, exercise is intended to decrease the adverse health risks associated with obesity and to attenuate excessive gestational weight gain. Higher doses of exercise can be targeted in the postpartum period [2,35].

Type

Low-impact activities are most tolerable, especially during the third trimester when women have a decreased tolerance for weight-bearing exercise [35]. The type of exercise most recommended for both pregnant and overweight women is walking, but swimming, water aerobics, and stationary cycling can still provide a sufficient intensity and may be more appropriate for severely obese women with joint pain or other biomechanical constraints[2,34]. Non-weight-bearing activities do not cause any changes in oxygen uptake with pregnancy, whereas oxygen uptake increases during weight-bearing activities [34], making activities such as stationary cycling and water aerobics more feasible for previously sedentary obese women.

Progression

Obese women exhibit a lower capacity for intensity and duration during exercise testing, indicating the value of progressing slowly [45]. Women are advised to begin at 15 minutes a day, gradually building to 30–40 minutes, including 5-minute warm-up and cool-down periods [2]. As fitness improves, women may gradually increase the intensity to a target heart rate as reflected in Table 10.2, the range recommended for overweight pregnant women, thus maintaining the same levels of exertion. The second trimester is the optimal time for progression since physical discomfort and nausea are at their lowest and the increased discomforts of the third trimester have not yet begun [2]. Frequent self-assessments of fitness, mental and emotional well-being, quality of rest, and any muscle or joint pain are advised [35].

Strength and conditioning

Muscular conditioning and aerobic exercise are essential components of a well-rounded fitness program for obese pregnant women and can possibly decrease the need for insulin therapy in women with gestational diabetes [48]. Conditioning exercises that target the core may reduce the risk for injury, make for an easier birth process, and alleviate back and pelvic pain caused by the shift in the center of gravity [2]. In obese women, conditioning exercises may be more beneficial due to the compounding effects of obesity and pregnancy on physical discomfort. Muscular conditioning may also help keep previously sedentary women engaged in an exercise program by preventing boredom and providing an alternative to aerobic exercise if fatigued.

There is limited research on the effects or appropriate doses of muscular conditioning in pregnant women. Women are advised to avoid any type of strenuous lifting or straining during pregnancy, as they may temporarily reduce the uterine blood flow and oxygen supply to the fetus. However, light to moderate weight-conditioning exercises performed without any isometric or static components have been consistently proven safe and are not associated with adverse fetal outcomes [8,30,35,42,49]. The Valsalva maneuver – holding one's breathing while working against a resistance – can cause unsafe decreases in both maternal blood pressure and blood flow to the uterus and should be avoided during conditioning exercise [2,35,42]. The supine position should be avoided both during exercise and at rest as it decreases maternal cardiac output [42,44,50]. Weight machines or resistance bands may be used in place of free weights as they require less balance and a less extreme range of motion [35,42].

Cautions/risks

The American College of Obstetricians and Gynecologists (ACOG) has indentified relative and absolute contraindications for aerobic and muscular conditioning exercise for the pregnant woman [51]. Additional considerations may be necessary for the obese pregnant woman who is at an increased risk for pregnancy complications and risks associated with exercise (Table 10.3). Both relative and absolute contraindications are provided for pregnancy, some of which may be exacerbated by or a may be a direct result of obesity, including orthopedic limitations, chronic hypertension, and cardiovascular disease. Pregnant obese women with or without gestational diabetes or hypertension, both of which increase pregnancy risk in general, should consult with their physician before beginning any exer-

Table 10.3 Contraindications for exercise during pregnancy

Relative	Absolute
• Severe anemia	• Significant heart disease
• Unevaluated maternal cardiac arrhythmia	• Restrictive lung disease
• Chronic bronchitis	• Incompetent cervix or cerclage placement
• Poorly controlled type 1 diabetes	
• Extreme morbid obesity	• Multiple gestation at risk for premature labor
• Extreme underweight (body mass index <12 kg/m^2)	• Persistent second or third trimester bleeding
• History of an extremely sedentary lifestyle	• Placenta previa after 26 weeks gestation
• Intrauterine growth restriction in current pregnancy	• Premature labor during the current pregnancy
• Poorly controlled hypertension/pre-eclampsia	• Ruptured membranes
• Orthopedic limitations	• Pregnancy-induced hypertension
• Poorly controlled thyroid disease	
• Poorly controlled seizure disorder	
• Heavy smoker	

Adapted from the American College of Obstetricians and Gynecologists Committee Opinion 267 [51].

cise program [43]. Tables 10.2 and 10.3 can assist practitioners in recommending exercise to their patients based on their signs and symptoms. Additional warning signs to terminate exercise during pregnancy include vaginal bleeding, cramping, prolonged dizziness, nausea, shortness of breath before exercise, chest pain, and muscle weakness [8,30].

The ACOG recommends advising women that adverse pregnancy or neonatal outcomes are not increased for exercising women, and light to moderate exercise has been consistently proven safe and beneficial [30]. Research has demonstrated an inverse relationship between a high frequency of vigorous aerobic exercise and/or occupational activity and birthweight [52,53]. Furthermore, moderate exercise throughout pregnancy may prevent low birthweight, suggesting that energy expenditure in chronic vigorous exercisers may be exceeding the caloric consumption necessary to support fetal growth [33]. Birthweight appears to be normal in women who maintain an adequate energy intake [8]. Although normal-weight women are recommended to increase their caloric intake by 150–300 calories per day to ensure sufficient energy for fetal growth and support [8,14,35,50], caloric increases may not be necessary in the obese mother even when coupled with exercise due to her already excess energy stores. Obese active women would benefit from supervised nutrition sessions to determine a safe caloric intake that balances the increased needs

of pregnancy with weight loss goals and physical activity. Nutritional considerations are discussed in Chapter 9.

Exercise and gestational diabetes mellitus

Insulin resistance is an expected effect of pregnancy due to increases in
body weight and body fat, and to hormonal changes. By the third trimester, insulin resistance approximates the levels seen in individuals with type
2 diabetes, yet glucose tolerance remains normal in most gravidas [54].
The physiological changes that lead to insulin resistance during pregnancy
are similar to those which contribute to insulin resistance in the obese. If
a woman is already obese, insulin resistance is more likely to develop into
gestational diabetes mellitus. Indeed, rates of gestational diabetes are
higher among obese women than lean women [6,7,55]. In a meta-analysis
conducted on 21 studies of gestational diabetes risk between January 2000
and 2006, the unadjusted odds ratios of developing gestational diabetes
were 2.14, 3.56, and 8.56 among overweight, obese, and severely obese
women compared to normal-weight pregnant women. To decrease the
risk for complications both during and after pregnancy, aggressive prevention or management of gestational diabetes in all women, particularly
those who are overweight or obese, should be a priority in obstetric care.
Therefore, weight gain restriction during pregnancy may be of even greater
importance in women diagnosed with gestational diabetes. Exercise can
be a powerful tool in meeting this goal.

Habitual physical activity is directly related to insulin resistance, and
lack of physical activity is an independent risk factor for developing type
2 diabetes [56]. The relationship between obesity, a sedentary lifestyle,
and insulin resistance must be taken into consideration when examining
the combined effect of physical activity/inactivity and obesity on the risk
for developing gestational diabetes. Studies examining the effect of physical activity before and during pregnancy on the risk for developing gestational diabetes have returned with positive findings. Dye et al. found
that exercise during pregnancy significantly decreased the risk for gestational diabetes in women with BMIs classified as extremely obese [55].
An observational study found that women who participated in any physical activity during the year before conception experienced a 56% reduction in risk for gestational diabetes. When specific dose and intensity of
exercise were examined, women spending 4.2 or more hours per week
engaged in physical activity experienced a 76% reduction in risk, compared to inactive women. Women who engaged in any type of physical
activity both in the year before and during pregnancy experienced a 69%
reduced risk [57].

Despite their body weight, exercise can be a powerful tool for obese
women in the management of gestational diabetes. An intervention by

Davenport et al. that utilized a low-intensity walking program in combination with insulin therapy resulted in an additive effect on glucose control in women with gestational diabetes [10]. In order for exercise to be an effective treatment of gestational diabetes, proper exercise prescriptions must be established. Traditional management for women with gestational diabetes consists of medical and nutrition therapy with adjunctive exercise for at least 30 minutes per day, yet this may not be an adequate dose in obese women. Exercise recommendations to promote weight loss and weight management in non-pregnant obese adults advise at least 60 minutes of moderate-intensity aerobic exercise daily [25]. Houmard et al. conducted a prospective study in non-pregnant women to assess the relationship between differing intensities and volumes of weekly exercise and insulin action. They found that the total number of minutes of exercise per week was the only significant predictor of improved insulin action, likely related to total energy expenditure [58].

However, simply discussing exercise does not appear to be as effective as supervised interventions. Obese women diagnosed with gestational diabetes may benefit more from supervised interventions, versus simply being provided with information on physical activity, to prevent and treat both gestational diabetes and its associated excess pregnancy weight gain [9,10,59,60].

Exercise in the postpartum period

Women often retain excess weight during pregnancy and continue to gain in the postpartum years. Pre-pregnancy weight is strongly indicative of postpartum weight, which may be an indication of unhealthy lifestyle behaviors before pregnancy that are exacerbated by the demands of newborn care [27,61]. Women may maintain the caloric increase recommended during pregnancy into the postpartum period and may be less active during and after pregnancy [3]. In a 15 year follow-up study of women of childbearing age, the weight of women who had excessive gestational weight gain was significantly greater at the 1-year and 15-year follow-up than those who gained within or below IOM recommendations [62]. Women who have more than one child may experience even greater weight retention. Observational studies indicate a relationship between parity and obesity. Parous women have a higher incidence of obesity and have a 50% increased risk for weight retention compared to nulliparous women [4]. The relationship between parity and obesity appears to be stronger among minority women [4].

Several intervention and observational studies have focused on behavioral factors including physical activity and exercise related to postpartum weight retention and the subsequent development of obesity [3,19,63–68]. Across observational studies, a return to pre-pregnancy weight and normal gestational weight gain were significantly related to both structured exercise frequency and leisure-time physical activity 6 months to 1 year postpartum [3,67]. Women engaging in vigorous activity before, during, and after pregnancy retain even less weight postpartum [19]. Intervention studies that prescribed an exercise regimen or held guided exercise sessions had more favorable outcomes on postpartum weight retention than those which only provided counseling on diet and exercise and monitoring of weight gain [64,65,68]. However, educational materials alone and a continuous monitoring of weight gain significantly decreased postpartum weight retention and gestational weight gain among low-income women [68]. Low-income women also experience greater barriers to exercise, lower exercise self-efficacy, and less lifestyle physical activity, making this population a unique and important target for intervention.

In addition to aiding the loss of postpartum weight, exercise has been shown to speed recovery from delivery and improve mood. However, exercise interventions are less common in the postpartum period, and exercise advice is rarely a component of postpartum care [69]. In a survey of women, 90% of respondents were dissatisfied with their postpartum weight, and 71% were actively trying to prevent further weight gain [65], indicating that follow-up care related to weight retention is an area to target for improvement. New mothers experience several barriers to physical activity [20], yet research has shown that women who exercised prior to and during pregnancy were able to overcome these barriers and regain their previous levels of activity [19,42]. Beliefs about exercise among postpartum women do not necessarily influence their activity patterns. In general, women believe that exercise may control weight gain and improve mood, yet are consistently less active [20,70]. Women should be encouraged to exercise in shorter bouts of 10 minutes or more or incorporate their infants and children into their exercise routine. New mothers can utilize strollers to walk or jog, focusing on maintaining an upright posture and not leaning on the stroller throughout. Most health clubs offer free child care as well.

Exercise prescription for obese women in the postpartum period

A primary concern of women who would like to exercise after delivery is knowing when it is safe to resume exercise. The answer depends on several factors, including the method of delivery, intensity of labor, whether or not a cesarean section was performed, and whether perineal repair was required [42]. Some women have reported resuming normal activities within a few days, while others may require months to return to normal.

The ACOG guidelines recommend that "pregnancy exercise routines may be resumed gradually as soon as it is physically and medically safe" [8]. Exercise has not been shown to have a negative impact on the volume or the quality of breast milk, but it is advised that women nurse or pump before exercise to reduce discomfort [8,19,30,42]. Obese women already experience longer recovery periods and more complicated deliveries and may require a more extended recovery period before increasing their physical activity [13]. Gentle, non-weight-bearing exercise such as stationary cycling or swimming may be more feasible in the first few weeks postpartum until activities such as walking and low-impact aerobics can be resumed or initiated. It should be noted, with obese women as well as non-obese women attempting to lose weight postpartum, that physical activity alone appears to have little impact on the magnitude of weight loss compared to reductions in energy intake [43]. However, the combination maximizes weight loss in the overweight and obese and appears to be a crucial factor in sustaining significant weight loss throughout life [25].

Once exercise is deemed safe, obese women should begin to progress to the minimum recommended level of physical activity and gradually reach the dose of exercise recommended for overweight and obese adults (Table 10.4). Postpartum women who are cleared for exercise should begin at the minimal volume (i.e. frequency and time) of exercise to improve health, and gradually progress to the dose of exercise recommended for weight loss and long-term weight maintenance [25,43]. A frequency of 5 days per week is recommended, with the goal of reaching 7 days to maximize caloric expenditure. Exercise intensity should begin at the moderate level and eventual progress to vigorous intensity, whether combined with bouts of moderate exercise or used alone on various days. Intensity may be determined using the target heart rate method previously mentioned. Sessions should begin at 30 minutes per day with a goal of 150 minutes

Table 10.4 Exercise recommendations for overweight and obese adults

Frequency	5–7 days/week
Intensity	Moderate to vigorous (40–60% to 50–75% $HR_{reserve}$)
Duration	30–60 minutes/day Gradual increase to 300 minutes moderate or 150 minutes vigorous per week, or an equivalent combination
Type	Low-impact aerobic activity

$HR_{reserve}$, [(maximal heart rate – resting heart rate) × % exercise intensity desired] + resting heart rate.

Adapted from the American College of Sports Medicine's Guidelines for Exercise Testing and Prescription [43].

per week, gradually increasing to a total of 300 minutes per week of moderate activity or 150 minutes of vigorous or a combination of both intensities. As with exercise during pregnancy, the mode of exercise should be comfortable given excess body weight but involve the major muscle groups in order to achieve cardiovascular benefits. For obese women, walking, cycling, and water activities are widely recommended. As weight loss progresses and fitness increases, intensity levels should be re-evaluated to continue to experience benefits.

Finally, structured exercise should not be considered a substitute for leisure-time or lifestyle physical activity such as house cleaning, walking instead of driving when possible, and using the stairs, all of which further promote caloric expenditure throughout the day. Obese women may experience added benefits from technologies such as accelerometers, which estimate caloric expenditure, or pedometers to receive daily feedback on their physical activity levels [29]. The promotion of a healthy body weight and the benefits associated with increased physical activity should not be missed in obese postpartum women, particularly in those planning to have additional children.

Conclusions

Women who are overweight or obese prior to pregnancy would benefit by achieving a healthy body weight prior to pregnancy, before the stressors of pregnancy and the postpartum period begin. The prevalence of obesity continues to rise in the USA and developed countries worldwide, making the time before pregnancy an important target for intervention. Exercise has been proven both safe and effective for obese women. In addition to controlling weight gain during pregnancy, exercise can offset some of the complications associated with pregnancy and provide a more comfortable, functional experience during the pregnancy and postpartum period. Regardless of weight status, all women can experience benefits from exercise and lifestyle physical activity both during and following pregnancy.

References

1. Ogden CL, Carroll MD, Curtin LR, et al. Prevalence of overweight and obesity in the United States, 1999–2004. JAMA 2006;295(13):1549–55.
2. Mottola MF. Exercise prescription for overweight and obese women: pregnancy and postpartum. Obstet Gynecol Clin North Am 2009;36(2):301–16, viii.
3. Pereira MA, Rifas-Shiman SL, Kleinman KP, et al. Predictors of change in physical activity during and after pregnancy: Project Viva. Am J Prev Med 2007;32(4): 312–19.

4. Davis EM, Zyzanski SJ, Olson CM, et al. Racial, ethnic, and socioeconomic differences in the incidence of obesity related to childbirth. Am J Public Health 2009; 99(2):294–9.

5. Baeten JM, Bukusi EA, Lambe M. Pregnancy complications and outcomes among overweight and obese nulliparous women. Am J Public Health 2001;91(3):436–40.

6. Chu SY, Callaghan WM, Kim SY, et al. Maternal obesity and risk of gestational diabetes mellitus. Diabetes Care 2007;30(8):2070–6.

7. Doherty DA, Magann EF, Francis J, et al. Pre-pregnancy body mass index and pregnancy outcomes. Int J Gynaecol Obstet 2006;95(3):242–7.

8. Artal R, O'Toole M. Guidelines of the American College of Obstetricians and Gynecologists for exercise during pregnancy and the postpartum period. Br J Sports Med 2003;37(1):6–12; discussion.

9. Claesson IM, Sydsjo G, Brynhildsen J, et al. Weight gain restriction for obese pregnant women: a case-control intervention study. BJOG 2008;115(1):44–50.

10. Davenport MH, Mottola MF, McManus R, et al. A walking intervention improves capillary glucose control in women with gestational diabetes mellitus: a pilot study. Appl Physiol Nutr Metab 2008;33(3):511–17.

11. Oken E, Ning Y, Rifas-Shiman SL, et al. Associations of physical activity and inactivity before and during pregnancy with glucose tolerance. Obstet Gynecol 2006; 108(5):1200–7.

12. Olafsdottir AS, Skuladottir GV, Thorsdottir I, et al. Maternal diet in early and late pregnancy in relation to weight gain. Int J Obes (Lond) 2006;30(3):492–9.

13. Robinson HE, O'Connell CM, Joseph KS, et al. Maternal outcomes in pregnancies complicated by obesity. Obstet Gynecol 2005;106(6):1357–64.

14. Stuebe AM, Oken E, Gillman MW. Associations of diet and physical activity during pregnancy with risk for excessive gestational weight gain. Am J Obstet Gynecol 2009;201(1):58 e1–8.

15. Polley BA, Wing RR, Sims CJ. Randomized controlled trial to prevent excessive weight gain in pregnant women. Int J Obes Relat Metab Disord 2002;26(11):1494–502.

16. Kramer MS, McDonald SW. Aerobic exercise for women during pregnancy. Cochrane Database Syst Rev 2006;(3):CD000180.

17. Clapp JF, 3rd. Exercise during pregnancy. A clinical update. Clin Sports Med 2000; 19(2):273–86.

18. Dye TD, Oldenettel D. Physical activity and the risk of preterm labor: an epidemiological review and synthesis of recent literature. Semin Perinatol 1996;20(4):334–9.

19. Sampselle CM, Seng J, Yeo S, et al. Physical activity and postpartum well-being. J Obstet Gynecol Neonatal Nurs 1999;28(1):41–9.

20. Symons Downs D, Hausenblas HA. Women's exercise beliefs and behaviors during their pregnancy and postpartum. J Midwifery Womens Health 2004;49(2):138–44.

21. Claesson IM, Brynhildsen J, Cedergren M, et al. Weight gain restriction during pregnancy is safe for both the mother and neonate. Acta Obstet Gynecol Scand 2009;26:1–5.

22. Kiel DW, Dodson EA, Artal R, et al. Gestational weight gain and pregnancy outcomes in obese women: how much is enough? Obstet Gynecol 2007;110(4):752–8.

23. Olson CM. Achieving a healthy weight gain during pregnancy. Annu Rev Nutr 2008;28:411–23.

24. Cedergren M. Effects of gestational weight gain and body mass index on obstetric outcome in Sweden. Int J Gynaecol Obstet 2006;93(3):269–74.

25. Donnelly JE, Blair SN, Jakicic JM, et al. American College of Sports Medicine Position Stand. Appropriate physical activity intervention strategies for weight loss and prevention of weight regain for adults. Med Sci Sports Exerc 2009;41(2):459–71.

26. Clapp JF, 3rd. Long-term outcome after exercising throughout pregnancy: fitness and cardiovascular risk. Am J Obstet Gynecol 2008;199(5):489 e1–6.

27. Giroux I, Inglis SD, Lander S, et al. Dietary intake, weight gain, and birth outcomes of physically active pregnant women: a pilot study. Appl Physiol Nutr Metab 2006; 31(5):483–9.

28. Pivarnik JM, Ayres NA, Mauer MB, et al. Effects of maternal aerobic fitness on cardiorespiratory responses to exercise. Med Sci Sports Exerc 1993;25(9):993–8.

29. Stein AD, Rivera JM, Pivarnik JM. Measuring energy expenditure in habitually active and sedentary pregnant women. Med Sci Sports Exerc 2003;35(8):1441–6.

30. Davies GA, Wolfe LA, Mottola MF, et al. Exercise in pregnancy and the postpartum period. J Obstet Gynaecol Can 2003;25(6):516–29.

31. Davis E, Olson C. Obesity in pregnancy. Prim Care 2009;36(2):341–56.

32. Pivarnik JM. Cardiovascular responses to aerobic exercise during pregnancy and postpartum. Semin Perinatol 1996;20(4):242–9.

33. Pivarnik JM. Potential effects of maternal physical activity on birth weight: brief review. Med Sci Sports Exerc 1998;30(3):400–6.

34. Ehrman JK, ed. ACSM's Resource manual for guidelines for exercise testing and prescription, 6th edn. Philadelphia: Lippincott Williams & Wilkins, 2010.

35. Wang TW, Apgar BS. Exercise during pregnancy. Am Fam Physician 1998 15;57(8): 1846–52, 57.

36. Wolfe LA, Brenner IK, Mottola MF. Maternal exercise, fetal well-being and pregnancy outcome. Exerc Sport Sci Rev 1994;22:145–94.

37. Pivarnik JM. Maternal exercise during pregnancy. Sports Med 1994;18(4):215–17.

38. Snapp CA, Donaldson SK. Gestational diabetes mellitus: physical exercise and health outcomes. Biol Res Nurs 2008;10(2):145–55.

39. Cramp AG, Bray SR. A prospective examination of exercise and barrier self-efficacy to engage in leisure-time physical activity during pregnancy. Ann Behav Med 2009;37(3):325–34.

40. Chang MW, Nitzke S, Guilford E, et al. Motivators and barriers to healthful eating and physical activity among low-income overweight and obese mothers. J Am Diet Assoc 2008;108(6):1023–8.

41. Mudd LM, Nechuta S, Pivarnik JM, et al. Factors associated with women's perceptions of physical activity safety during pregnancy. Prev Med 2009;49(2–3): 194–9.

42. Pivarnik J, Mudd LM. Oh baby! Exercise during pregnancy and the postpartum period. Health Fit 2009;13(3):8–13.

43. American College of Sports Medicine; Thompson WR, Gordon NF, Pescatello LS. ACSM's guidelines for exercise testing and prescription, 8th edn. Philadelphia: Lippincott Williams & Wilkins, 2010.

44. Canadian Society of Exercise Physiology. Physical activity readiness medical examination for pregnancy. http://uwfitness.uwaterloo.ca/PDF/parmed-xpreg_000.pdf. Accessed August 31, 2010.

45. Davenport MH, Steinback CD, Mottola MF. Impact of pregnancy and obesity on cardiorespiratory responses during weight-bearing exercise. Respir Physiol Neurobio. 2009;167(3):341–7.

46. Mottola MF, Davenport MH, Brun CR, et al. VO2peak prediction and exercise prescription for pregnant women. Med Sci Sports Exerc 2006;38(8):1389–95.

47. Davenport MH, Charlesworth S, Vanderspank D, et al. Development and validation of exercise target heart rate zones for overweight and obese pregnant women. Appl Physiol Nutr Metab 2008;33(5):984–9.

48. Brankston GN, Mitchell BF, Ryan EA, et al. Resistance exercise decreases the need for insulin in overweight women with gestational diabetes mellitus. Am J Obstet Gynecol 2004;190(1):188–93.

49. Avery ND, Stocking KD, Tranmer JE, et al. Fetal responses to maternal strength conditioning exercises in late gestation. Can J Appl Physiol 1999;24(4):362–76.

50. Davies GA, Wolfe LA, Mottola MF, et al. Joint SOGC/CSEP clinical practice guideline: exercise in pregnancy and the postpartum period. Can J Appl Physiol 2003;28(3): 330–41.

51. ACOG Committee Opinion. Exercise during pregnancy and the postpartum period. Number 267, January 2002. American College of Obstetricians and Gynecologists. Int J Gynaecol Obstet 2002;77(1):79–81.

52. Campbell MK, Mottola MF. Recreational exercise and occupational activity during pregnancy and birth weight: a case-control study. Am J Obstet Gynecol 2001;184(3): 403–8.

53. Perkins CC, Pivarnik JM, Paneth N, et al. Physical activity and fetal growth during pregnancy. Obstet Gynecol 2007;109(1):81–7.

54. Dempsey JC, Butler CL, Sorensen TK, et al. A case-control study of maternal recreational physical activity and risk of gestational diabetes mellitus. Diabetes Res Clin Pract 2004;66(2):203–15.

55. Dye TD, Knox KL, Artal R, et al. Physical activity, obesity, and diabetes in pregnancy. Am J Epidemiol 1997;146(11):961–5.

56. Hawley JA. Exercise as a therapeutic intervention for the prevention and treatment of insulin resistance. Diabetes Metab Res Rev 2004;20(5):383–93.

57. Dempsey JC, Sorensen TK, Williams MA, et al. Prospective study of gestational diabetes mellitus risk in relation to maternal recreational physical activity before and during pregnancy. Am J Epidemiol 2004;159(7):663–70.

58. Houmard JA, Tanner CJ, Slentz CA, et al. Effect of the volume and intensity of exercise training on insulin sensitivity. J Appl Physiol 2004;96(1):101–6.

59. Artal R, Catanzaro RB, Gavard JA, et al. A lifestyle intervention of weight-gain restriction: diet and exercise in obese women with gestational diabetes mellitus. Appl Physiol Nutr Metab 2007;32(3):596–601.

60. Mottola MF. The role of exercise in the prevention and treatment of gestational diabetes mellitus. Curr Diab Rep 2008;8(4):299–304.

61. Thorsdottir I, Birgisdottir BE. Different weight gain in women of normal weight before pregnancy: postpartum weight and birth weight. Obstet Gynecol 1998;92(3): 377–83.

62. Amorim AR, Rossner S, Neovius M, et al. Does excess pregnancy weight gain constitute a major risk for increasing long-term BMI? Obesity (Silver Spring) 2007; 15(5):1278–86.

63. Greene GW, Smiciklas-Wright H, Scholl TO, et al. Postpartum weight change: how much of the weight gained in pregnancy will be lost after delivery? Obstet Gynecol 1988;71(5):701–7.

64. Kinnunen TI, Pasanen M, Aittasalo M, et al. Reducing postpartum weight retention – a pilot trial in primary health care. Nutr J 2007;6:21.

65. Leermakers EA, Anglin K, Wing RR. Reducing postpartum weight retention through a correspondence intervention. Int J Obes Relat Metab Disord 1998;22(11): 1103–9.

66. Lombard C, Deeks A, Jolley D, et al. Preventing weight gain: the baseline weight related behaviors and delivery of a randomized controlled intervention in community based women. BMC Public Health 2009;9:2.

67. Olson CM, Strawderman MS, Hinton PS, et al. Gestational weight gain and post-partum behaviors associated with weight change from early pregnancy to 1 y post-partum. Int J Obes Relat Metab Disord 2003;27(1):117–27.

68. Olson CM, Strawderman MS, Reed RG. Efficacy of an intervention to prevent excessive gestational weight gain. Am J Obstet Gynecol 2004;191(2):530–6.

69. Mottola MF. Exercise in the postpartum period: practical applications. Curr Sports Med Rep 2002;1(6):362–8.

70. Mottola MF, Campbell MK. Activity patterns during pregnancy. Can J Appl Physiol 2003;28(4):642–53.

CHAPTER 11

Obesity Co-morbid Conditions in Pregnancy: Diabetes and Hypertension

Eran Hadar and Yariv Yogev

Helen Schneider Hospital for Women, Rabin Medical Center, Petach Tikva and Sackler Faculty of Medicine, Tel Aviv University, Tel Aviv, Israel

Obesity has reached endemic proportions, with an increased overall prevalence in the population, as well as a similar increase in the subgroup of women of reproductive age. Thus, there is an increased proportion of obesity complicating pregnancy. The negative impact of obesity on overall morbidity and mortality is tremendous, with a parallel increase in poor pregnancy outcome. Therefore, it is considered to be one of the major health issues in the Western world, both economically and clinically.

Diabetes mellitus, essential hypertension, ischemic heart disease, stroke, sleep apnea, certain types of cancer, and osteoarthritis are some common obesity-related diseases. These related conditions inflict an increased morbidity and mortality, and when they complicate pregnancy have a negative impact on both maternal and neonatal outcome. The impact of obesity is distributed throughout all stages of gestation, with effects on fertility, pregnancy, labor, delivery, and the postpartum period. Some of the well-established consequences include hypertensive disorders, gestational diabetes mellitus (GDM), macrosomia, and complications during cesarean delivery and anesthesia.

This chapter will outline issues concerning obesity and gestational co-morbid conditions that may arise during pregnancy that are associated with obesity, with a special emphasis on hypertensive complications. Additive effects on overall morbidity when hypertension or diabetes co-exist in obese pregnant women will be discussed. Special considerations in terms of the epidemiology, pathogenesis, diagnosis, and management of diabetes and hypertension in the obese gravida will be reviewed.

Gestational diabetes and gestational hypertension in the obese gravida: the metabolic syndrome of pregnancy

Reaven, in his novel work [1], suggested that insulin resistance underlies the pathogenesis of some of the chief chronic diseases of the Western world: ischemic heart disease, type 2 diabetes mellitus, and essential hypertension. The occurrence of these diseases, along with central/abdominal obesity, was termed the metabolic syndrome. It entails abnormalities that increase the risk for cardiovascular morbidity and mortality, including glucose intolerance, hyperinsulinemia, increased triglyceride levels, and decreased high-density lipoprotein-cholesterol levels. Insulin resistance and hyperinsulinemia may be the basic common ground for the overt clinical conditions of elevated blood pressure and diabetes mellitus. Both of these diseases predispose to long-term cardiovascular complications, including death. In addition, aside from insulin resistance, the metabolic syndrome and its components are also associated with endothelial dysfunction, oxidative stress, and attenuated inflammatory responses [2]. In women of reproductive age, the metabolic syndrome may precede or develop along the duration of pregnancy. As such, obesity, along with hypertensive disorders and GDM, are central attributes of the metabolic syndrome that may occur during pregnancy.

The World Health Organization (WHO) criteria, published in 1999, require the presence of diabetes mellitus, impaired glucose tolerance, impaired fasting glucose, or insulin resistance plus any two of the following: elevated blood pressure (>140/90 mmHg), dyslipidemia, central obesity (defined by a waist:hip ratio over 0.90 for males or above 0.85 for females), or a body mass index (BMI) higher than 30kg/m^2, microalbuminuria, or an albumin:creatinine ratio higher than 30. Overweight and obesity, mainly central obesity, are a paramount feature of the syndrome It is controversial whether obesity and insulin resistance are the causes or the consequences of the pathway leading to metabolic derangement. Other important factors involved in the complex pathophysiology of the syndrome include genetic predisposition, aging, sedentary lifestyle, stress, insulin resistance, coronary heart disease, and an inflammatory systemic reaction.

The prevalence of the metabolic syndrome during pregnancy varies with the presence of various types of pregnancy complication. Using WHO definitions, the incidence is estimated to be 3.3% in women with GDM, 35% in those with gestational hypertension, and 30% within the preeclampsia group [3]. In a recent study by Horváth et al. [4], the metabolic syndrome was shown to have a negative impact on pregnancy outcome.

The study followed 5,869 pregnant women, 172 of whom met the criteria for the metabolic syndrome. Several outcome measures were more prevalent in this group of women. These included preterm delivery (odds ratio [OR] 1.52; 95% confidence interval [CI] 0.996–2.33), fetal growth restriction (OR 6.38; 95% CI 4.24–9.61), and pre-eclampsia (OR 7.93; 95% CI 5.54–11.33).

Obesity, gestational diabetes, and metabolic syndrome

Obesity is the most important risk factor for metabolic syndrome. The National Health and Nutrition Examination Survey study [5] showed that the metabolic syndrome presents in 4.6%, 22.4%, and 59.6% of normal-weight, overweight, and obese men, respectively, with a similar distribution in women. Weight gain and obesity induce glucose intolerance, which is related to insulin resistance and a deterioration in pancreatic beta-cell function [6–8].

Pregnancy exerts a physiological decline in the sensitivity to insulin, which is manifested by elevated postprandial glycemia, and increased triglycerides, low-density lipoprotein, and free fatty acids. In a pathological manner, some patients demonstrate higher degrees of insulin resistance and develop full-blown GDM, along with pancreatic beta-cell dysfunction, higher BMI, central obesity, and exaggerated hyperlipidemia. All of these suggest that GDM is a transient manifestation of long-standing metabolic dysfunction [2]. Noussitou et al. [9], retrospectively studying 5,788 deliveries, identified 159 (2.7%) patients with GDM out of the total study population. In 26% of these women, some aspects of the metabolic syndrome were identified prior to the index pregnancy (obesity, 84%; hypertension, 38%; dyslipidemia, 22%). In the postpartum follow-up, 11% had type 2 diabetes and 16% impaired fasting glucose. Consequently, GDM is accompanied and preceded by metabolic abnormalities compatible with the metabolic syndrome.

Noussitou's study confirmed that women with GDM have a higher risk for developing metabolic syndrome and type 2 diabetes in the years after delivery. Several studies have investigated the relationship of GDM and obesity to a future diagnosis of the metabolic syndrome. Bo et al. [10] reported that the prevalence of the metabolic syndrome and its components was 2–4-fold higher in women with prior gestational hyperglycemia. In women who were also obese, this risk was 10-fold higher. Pallardo et al. [11], studying 788 Caucasian women with GDM 3–6 months after delivery, found that 3.7% had been diagnosed with overt diabetes. The area under the postpartum glucose curve was positively associated with BMI, waist circumference, waist:hip ratio, triglyceride levels, and systolic and diastolic blood pressures. It was concluded that postpartum glucose intolerance predicts a high-risk cardiovascular profile that includes risk factors besides type 2 diabetes. These findings suggest that women who manifest GDM, especially in combination with pre-pregnancy obesity, carry a high lifetime cardiovascular risk.

Of perhaps even greater concern, data are emerging suggesting that fetal exposure to this adverse environment also confers a lifetime risk for metabolic syndrome for the offspring. Verma et al. [12] confirmed this finding, reporting that 27% of 106 children born to mothers diagnosed with GDM developed features of insulin resistance by age 11 years, compared to 8.2% of 101 controls. If pre-pregnancy maternal obesity was also present, the cumulative hazard for the offspring to develop the metabolic syndrome in the next 2 years was 26 times higher compared to controls.

Gestational hypertension, pre-eclampsia, eclampsia, and the metabolic syndrome

The pathogenesis of hypertensive disorders during pregnancy, such as gestational hypertension and pre-eclampsia, and the metabolic syndrome are similar in some aspects and share similar risk factors and common pathological pathways. However, it is unknown whether the abnormal lipid and inflammatory pathways observed in pre-eclampsia are present prior to pregnancy and cause hypertension and other disease manifestations later in gestation, or whether these develop secondary to the disease process of pre-eclampsia.

Srinivas et al. [13] reported that, in 101 patients with metabolic syndrome, there was a higher risk for pre-eclampsia (adjusted OR [AOR] 2.71; 95% CI 1.1–6.67). In addition, the odds of pre-eclampsia were nearly four times higher when the level of C-reactive protein (CRP), a marker of inflammation, was over 8 mg/l (AOR 3.61; 95% CI 2.14–6.12); in this study, cases were recruited when diagnosed with a hypertensive disorder, and controls were recruited at labor. At delivery, controls were on average 39 weeks' gestation, and cases on average 36 weeks. Studies have also confirmed that the metabolic syndrome is a risk factor for additional hypertensive disorders. In 45 patients with eclampsia compared against healthy controls, the risk for intrapartum eclampsia was significantly increased for women with hypercholesterolemia (OR 6.9; 95% CI 2.5–20.7), hypertriglyceridemia (OR 5.0; 95% CI 1.79–14.32), and hyperuricemia (OR 35.3; 95% CI 9.6–14.3) [14].

Erez-Weiss et al. [15], in a retrospective study of 131 non-diabetic patients with gestational hypertension or pre-eclampsia and 131 normal controls, demonstrated that the women with hypertensive disorders tended to be of higher maternal age (28 ± 5.8 versus 26.5 ± 5.3 years), and had higher glucose challenge test (GCT) values (5.8 ± 1.4 versus 5.1 ± 1.1 mmol/l) and an elevated BMI (26 ± 5.1 versus 23 ± 4.0 kg/m^2), with a lower gestational age (38.5 ± 2.1 versus 39.4 ± 1.7 days) and lower birthweight (2,929 ± 614.7 versus 3,225 ± 461.1 g).

It seems that elevated pre-gestational BMI is an independent risk factor for the development of gestational hypertension, and that glucose intolerance has a role in the pathogenesis of pre-eclampsia in obese patients. Sermer et al. [16] investigated mid-pregnancy anthropometry, blood pressure, microalbuminuria, fasting lipids, inflammatory and endothelial damage markers, and family disease history among 184 women with GDM. For the 22 patients who developed pre-eclampsia, there was an increased mid-pregnancy BMI, blood pressure, fasting glucose, fasting insulin, CRP level, and microalbuminuria, and a higher prevalence of family history of hypertension and gestational diabetes. This may suggest that the presence of several metabolic syndrome components is a risk factor for pre-eclampsia. However, fasting dyslipidemia was not found to be an independent predictor for pre-eclampsia.

Still other studies have found a correlation between elevated maternal triglyceride levels and the risk for pre-eclampsia [13, 17]. Wendland et al. [18], in a prospective cohort study of 4,766 pregnant women, found that both GDM and pre-eclampsia were associated with advanced maternal age (OR 2.07; 95% CI 1.65–2.23 versus OR 1.55; 95% CI 1.08–2.23, respectively), pre-pregnancy BMI (OR 1.62; 95% CI 1.40–3.53 versus OR 1.83; 95% CI 1.52–4.80, respectively), and weight gain in early pregnancy (OR 1.28; 95% CI 1.12–1.4 versus OR 1.27; 95% CI 1.06–1.52, respectively). These results imply that GDM and pre-eclampsia share a comparable pattern of risk factors, suggesting the possibility of a common etiology, with obesity and weight gain being key players in the pathogenesis of these pregnancy morbidities.

Insulin resistance: the underlying common pathological explanation for the association between obesity, diabetes, and hypertension

Aside from insulin resistance, endothelial activation and low-grade inflammation play an integral role in pre-eclampsia–eclampsia, obesity, and gestational diabetes. Insulin resistance with secondary hyperinsulinemia is suspected to be the link between hypertension and diabetes. The hypertensive effect of hyperinsulinemia is postulated to be due to weight gain, as well as extracellular volume expansion. This volume expansion is thought to result from renal sodium retention caused by insulin's effect of increasing sympathetic activity [19].

Several studies have suggested that gestational hypertension, but not pre-eclampsia, is associated with insulin resistance [20, 21], while others have illustrated that the association is true for the entire spectrum of hypertensive disorders [16, 22–25], and other studies do not concur with either of these conclusions. Caruso et al. [20] examined 16 women with hypertension during the third trimester using a euglycemic–hyperinsulinemic clamp. Women with gestational hypertension demonstrated a 40% reduction in the steady-state insulin sensitivity index compared to the control subjects; moreover, this reduction did not occur with pre-eclampsia. These findings suggest that insulin resistance contributes to late pregnancy gestational hypertension and not to pre-eclampsia.

In another cohort of 320 normal-weight women without GDM or any history of hypertension or thyroid disease, insulin and C-peptide levels were measured at the time of the routine GCT. The data showed that fasting C-peptide and glucose-stimulated C-peptide concentrations (which served as surrogate markers for insulin resistance) were significantly associated with the later development of gestational hypertension (OR 1.7; 95% CI 1.1–2.7 versus OR 3.8; 95% CI 1.5–9.6, respectively). This association suggests that insulin resistance, even in the absence of obesity, is closely related to gestational hypertension [21].

In contrast, Kajaa et al. [22] report that pre-eclampsia is a state of increased insulin resistance, which persists for at least 3 months after pregnancy. They measured insulin sensitivity using the minimal model technique in 22 pre-eclamptic women and 16 healthy controls, demonstrating that insulin sensitivity was 37% lower in pre-eclamptic women. Similar results were obtained in another study, where 572 normotensive pregnant women were followed with fasting plasma glucose (FPG) and insulin concentrations. Women who subsequently developed either gestational hypertension or pre-eclampsia had higher levels of insulin resistance (OR 3.13; 95% CI 0.41–6.94) [23].

Wolf et al. [24], in a nested case-control study, examined first-trimester sex hormone-binding globulin levels (which are inhibited by insulin and serve as a surrogate marker of insulin resistance) and second-trimester GCT values among 45 women diagnosed with either pre-eclampsia or eclampsia, comparing them to 90 normotensive controls. Women who developed pre-eclampsia were found to have lower sex hormone-binding globulin levels (302 ± 130 versus 396 ± 186 nmol/l) and higher GCT values (122.4 ± 25.2 versus 111.6 ± 23.4 mg/dl). The association of sex hormone-binding globulin with pre-eclampsia reached statistical significance only among women with BMI values over $25 \, kg/m^2$, suggesting an obesity-related threshold effect and an overall association between insulin resistance, obesity, and pre-eclampsia.

Additionally, among non-diabetic gravid women, mid-pregnancy post-prandial glycemia has been noted to be positively associated with the odds of subsequent gestational hypertension and pre-eclampsia. A retrospective case-control study of 97 women with new-onset hypertension in late pregnancy and 77 normotensive control gravidas demonstrated that GCT values were significantly higher among those developing hypertension, after adjusting for BMI and baseline blood pressure [25]. The Toronto Tri-Hospital Gestational Diabetes Project cohort study has found similar correlation between pre-eclampsia and oral glucose tolerance test (OGTT) values in 3,836 women. Postprandial glucose but not fasting glucose values showed an association with the probability for subsequent pre-eclampsia, with the most significant being the 2-hour value [16].

Montoro et al. [26] compared the degree of insulin resistance in GDM patients with and without pre-eclampsia, using not just OGTT values, but also intravenous glucose tolerance tests and glucose clamp studies in the early third trimester and 15 months postpartum. Those who developed pre-eclampsia were significantly taller (61.5 ± 2.4 versus 60.1 ± 2.3 inches), more often nulliparous (38% versus 16%), and had higher systolic (112 ± 10 versus $103 \pm 6.9 \, mmHg$) and diastolic blood pressure (64 ± 9 versus $59 \pm 5 \, mmHg$). However, no significant differences between the groups were found in any measures of the OGTT levels, insulin sensitivity index, glucose effectiveness, acute response to glucose, or disposition index, nor were there any differences found in the euglycemic clamp measures of basal or steady-state levels of glucose, insulin, free fatty acids, hepatic glucose output, peripheral glucose clearance, C-peptide, or glucagon. At 15 months postpartum, blood pressure levels remained significantly higher in the pre-eclamptic group ($n = 19$) compared to the non pre-eclamptic group ($n = 70$). Thus, women with GDM were uniformly insulin resistant, and those who developed pre-eclampsia were not more insulin resistant in either the third trimester or 15 months postpartum.

Level of maternal obesity and hypertensive complications in pregnancy

Numerous studies have shown that obese pregnant women are at a significantly increased risk for various antepartum, intrapartum, and postpartum complications, as summarized in Table 11.1. These studies lack uniformity in the allocation of BMI categories, as well as the definition of obesity by other parameters, such as absolute weight, waist circumference,

Table 11.1 The Impact of obesity on pregnancy outcome: summary of selected studies

Study	Seibre [29]	Cedergren [34]
Study design	Retrospective	Prospective
n	287,213	16,178
Definition of obesity	BMI > 30	BMI > 40
Odds ratio for outcome measures		
Gestational diabetes	3.6	
Hypertensive disorders	2.14	4.82
Cesarean section	1.83	2.69
Postpartum hemorrhage	1.39	
Genital tract infection	1.3	
Urinary tract infection	1.99	
Wound infection	2.24	
Large for gestational age/macrosomia	2.35	3.82
Intrauterine fetal death	1.4	2.79
Shoulder dystocia		3.14
Instrumental delivery		1.4
Meconium aspiration		2.85
Fetal distress		2.52
Fetal growth restriction		
Induction of labor		

BMI, body mass index (kg//m^2).

and others. Edwards et al. [27], in one of the earliest such studies, in 1978, examined the effect of obesity on pregnancy. His findings suggested a significant increase in the incidence of hypertensive disorders, gestational diabetes, large-for-gestational-age (LGA) infants, and wound and episiotomy infections. Garbaciak et al. [28], in another early study, from 1985, similarly concluded that obesity increases mean birthweight. He was one of the first to report that the likelihood of a cesarean delivery is increased in obese laboring women.

To date, one of the largest studies of the effect of maternal obesity on pregnancy was presented by Sebire et al. [29]. In 287,213 gravid women, it was shown that overweight (defined as a BMI of 25–30 kg/m^2) and obese (BMI over 30 kg/m^2) women are at an increased risk for several gestational and puerperal complications when judged against normal-weight women (BMI 20–24.9 kg/m^2). These complications included GDM and pre-eclampsia, as well as other adverse maternal and neonatal outcome meas-

Weiss [32]	Kumari [35]	Perlow [31]	Schrauwers [37]
Prospective	Retrospective	Retrospective	Retrospective
	188	111	370
BMI > 35	BMI > 40	> 300 lb	All BMI classes
4.0	11.1		8.82–27.38
3.2–3.3	9.9	30	2.38–3.75
2.29	1.63	2.26	2.2–5.47
1.9–4	3.5	2.6	4.04
			2.2–5.47
		9.0	
			3.17

ures. Compared to women with a BMI of less than 25 kg/m², overweight women had a higher risk for pre-eclampsia (0.97% versus 0.7%; OR 1.44) and GDM (1.7% versus 0.75%; OR 1.68). Importantly, they also demonstrated that the correlation between maternal weight and adverse outcomes was of a linear nature: as maternal BMI increased, the associated outcomes were more likely. Compared to women with a BMI of less than 25 kg/m², obese women had a higher risk for pre-eclampsia (1.43% versus 0.7%; OR 2.14) and GDM (3.5% versus 0.75%; OR 3.6).

Isaacs et al. [30] showed that women weighing over 300 lb have a higher incidence of chronic hypertension (33% versus 5%, $p < 0.05$) and diabetes complicating pregnancy (15% versus 3.3%, $p < 0.05$) compared to a non-obese control group. Perlow et al. [31], who also defined obesity as maternal weight over 300 lb, found that these women were more likely to suffer from pre-pregnancy chronic hypertension (27.0% versus 0.9%, $p < 0.0001$) and type 2 diabetes (19.8% versus 2.7%, $p < 0.0001$). Weiss et al. [32], in a large prospective study, showed that obesity (BMI 30–35 kg/m^2) and morbid obesity (BMI > 35 kg/m^2) had a statistically significant association with gestational hypertension, pre-eclampsia, GDM, macrosomia, and cesarean section. Baeten et al. [33] also showed that overweight and obese nulliparas were at an increased risk for gestational diabetes, pre-eclampsia, eclampsia, cesarean delivery, and delivery of a macrosomic infant.

Cedergren and Kumari, in two different studies, examined the effect of morbid obesity (defined as BMI over 40 kg/m^2) on pregnancy outcome. Cedergren [34] found that there was an increased risk for the following outcome measures: pre-eclampsia, cesarean delivery, instrumental delivery, shoulder dystocia, meconium aspiration, fetal distress, early neonatal death, LGA infants, and intrauterine fetal death. Kumari [35] found similar risks, including hypertensive disorders, cesarean section, and macrosomia. He also added a finding of a higher risk for GDM, which was not demonstrated in the study by Cedergren. Bianco et al. [36] also studying morbid obesity (defined as a BMI over 35 kg/m^2) found an increased risk for diabetes, hypertension, pre-eclampsia, arrested/protracted labor, fetal distress, meconium, and cesarean delivery than their non-obese counterparts. Even when morbid obesity is defined by a lower threshold (BMI > 35 kg/m^2), similar adverse pregnancy outcomes are shown, but to a lesser extent [34,35]. This again suggests the direct relationship between degree of obesity and frequency of adverse pregnancy outcome.

In the most recent study of obesity outcome, Schrauwers et al. [37] retrospectively studied 370 Australian women with all BMI subclasses – overweight (BMI 25.1–30 kg/m^2), obese (BMI 30.1–40 kg/m^2), and morbidly obese women (BMI > 40 kg/m^2). Pregnancy hypertension occurred significantly more in women with a BMI in the two highest categories (OR 2.38 and 3.75, respectively), as did GDM (OR 8.82 and 27.38, respectively).

Obesity as a risk factor for hypertensive disorders during pregnancy

Hypertension is the most common medical complication of pregnancy, affecting 8–10% of pregnancies [38–40]. Risk factors for the development of pre-eclampsia include diabetes, obesity, nulliparity, age extremities (younger than 18, older than 35), renal insufficiency or chronic renal disease, pre-existing hypertension, a personal history of pre-eclampsia, a family history of pre-eclampsia, molar pregnancy, multifetal gestation, fetal hydrops, and thrombophilia [41–44].

With regard to obesity as a risk factor, it is now well accepted, and has been demonstrated by multiple studies, that there is a higher proportion of hypertensive disorders during pregnancy in obese and overweight women. The risk for pre-eclampsia and gestational hypertension is increased by 2–3-fold for obese women. Moreover, there is up to a 10-fold increase in the prevalence of chronic hypertension in obese pregnant women [45,46]. Sebire et al. [29], in a previously mentioned study, found that overweight women (BMI 25–30 kg/m^2) are at an increased risk for pre-eclampsia (OR 1.44; 95% CI 1.28–1.62), as are overweight women (OR 2.14; 95% CI 1.85–2.47). Cedregen [34] added knowledge of women who are morbidly obese, demonstrating that a BMI over 40 kg/m^2 poses an increased risk for pre-eclampsia (OR 4.82; 95% CI 4.04–5.74). Additionally, Kumari [35], in a population of morbidly obese women (also defined as BMI > 40 kg/m^2) showed that the overall rate of hypertensive complications was 28.8%, compared to a rate of 2.9% in a non-obese population. In a meta-analysis of over 1.4 million women, the pre-eclampsia risk was doubled with each 5–7 kg/m^2 increase in pre-pregnancy BMI. This relation persisted in studies that excluded women with chronic hypertension, diabetes mellitus, or multiple gestations, and other confounders [47].

How to improve pregnancy outcome in obese diabetic patients

Several studies have found that weight loss prior to pregnancy in obese women can improve pregnancy outcome and may reduce maternal and neonatal complications. Weight reduction can be achieved by a variety of methods combining modalities such as physical activity, diet, pharmacological therapy, and operative interventions (see Chapter 3).

As for obese women with pre-existing diabetes, the approach should be multidisciplinary and begin prior to conception. Preconception counseling should focus on patient education, glycemic control, and pre-pregnancy weight loss. Dedicated prenatal management with tight glycemic control and screening for possible obesity-related complications is needed. In addition, postpartum follow-up is desirable to minimize the medical, social, and economic consequences of pregnancies in overweight and obese women.

Pre-pregnancy weight loss

Obese diabetic and hypertensive patients should be encouraged to undertake a weight-reduction program before attempting pregnancy. As the numerous studies previously discussed have shown that pre-pregnancy obesity is a risk factor for several gestational and perinatal complications, it seems only extremely logical that weight reduction prior to pregnancy is beneficial [48]. There is also direct proof from several studies which have found significant weight loss prior to pregnancy in obese women to be important in reducing poor pregnancy outcome [49,50]. Deitel et al. [51] studied 139 morbidly obese women who lost at least half of their weight post bariatric surgical procedures. A subset of women from this study population had had several medical complications during past pregnancies. The complications included hypertension (26.7%), pre-eclampsia (12.8%), diabetes (7.0%), and deep vein thrombosis (7.0%). After weight loss stabilization by bariatric surgery, none of these obstetric adverse events took place.

Controlled gestational weight gain

The 1990 report of nutrition during pregnancy from the Institute of Medicine (IOM) is pivotal in the management of weight gain during pregnancy [52]. However, this report was written with a focus on small-for-gestational-age babies, related to insufficient weight gain during pregnancy, especially in underweight women. Available data suggest lower thresholds for weight gain during pregnancy than those proposed in the 1990 IOM monograph (Table 11.2) [52].

Cedergren [53] reported an optimal weight gain of 5–22 lb in women with a pregravid BMI between 20 and 24.9, less than 20 lb for a BMI

Table 11.2 Recommendations for weight gain during pregnancy, according to pre-pregnancy body mass index (BMI)

Pre-pregnancy BMI (kg/m²)	Recommended weight gain (lb)
Institute of Medecine recommendations [52]	
BMI < 19.8	28–40
BMI 19.8–36	25–35
BMI 26–29	15–25
BMI > 29	>15
Cedergren [53]	
BMI 20–24.9	5–22
BMI 25–29.9	<20
BMI > 30	<13
Devader [54] and Keil [55]	
BMI 20–24.9	<25
BMI 25–29.9	<15
BMI > 30	<15

between 25 and 29.9, and less than 13 lb with a BMI greater than or equal to 30 kg/m^2. Again, a decrease in adverse obstetric and neonatal outcomes was observed with lower weight gain among obese women. DeVader et al. [54], studying women with a normal pre-pregnancy BMI, compared those gaining 25–35 lb against women gaining less than 25 lb during pregnancy. He found lower odds for pre-eclampsia (AOR 0.56; 95% CI 0.49–0.64), cephalopelvic disproportion (AOR 0.64; 95% CI 0.55–0.75), failed induction (AOR 0.68; 95% CI 0.59–0.78), cesarean delivery (AOR 0.82; 95% CI 0.78–-0.87), LGA infants (AOR 0.40; 95% CI 0.37–0.44), and increased odds for small-for-gestational-age infants (AOR 2.14; 95% CI 2.01–2.27). Similarly, Kiel et al. [55], using the same birth registry, report that in overweight and obese women, gaining less than the recommended 15 lb (only 31%) was associated with a significantly lower risk for pre-eclampsia, cesarean delivery, and LGA births.

In a randomized controlled trial by Wolff et al. [56], 50 non-diabetic obese pregnant women were randomized into intervention group (restriction of gestational weight gain to 6–7 kg [13–15 lb]) and a control group. They showed that women in the intervention group not only successfully limited their energy intake, and restricted the gestational weight gain to 6.6 kg (14.6 lb) versus a gain of 13.3 kg (29.3 lb) in the control group ($p = 0.002$; 95% CI 2.6–10.8 kg [5.7–23.8 lb]). Both serum insulin and serum leptin were reduced by 20% in the intervention group compared to the control group at week 27.

Achieving desired level of glycemic control

Non-diabetic pregnant women have been the population examined in most of the studies in which the relationship between maternal pre-pregnancy weight and perinatal outcome has been addressed, and there are scant data on pregnancy outcome in obese or overweight patients with GDM. At the same time, numerous studies have shown that strict glycemic control in diabetic pregnancies reduces the risk for macrosomia [57], but it remains unclear whether this applies in the same manner and magnitude for obese diabetic women. The few studies reporting obesity in gestational diabetes lack information on the effect of achieving targeted levels of glycemic control and on choice of treatment modalities on pregnancy outcome [58,59]. These studies had small sample sizes, failed to provide information on glycemic control, and only evaluated single outcome variables. Higher maternal age and parity, as well as obesity, are over-represented among women with GDM. These variables need to be controlled for in any study in order to draw accurate conclusions. Therefore, it is not clear if obesity, level of glycemia, or treatment modalities are independently or cumulatively responsible for fetal growth abnormalities and perinatal outcome in the setting of diabetes in pregnancy [60].

Leikin et al. [61] found that non-obese GDM women with fasting hyperglycemia treated with diet and insulin had a frequency of macrosomia no different from that of non-diabetic women, while diet and insulin did not prevent excess macrosomia in women who were obese. However, no information regarding the degree of glycemic control in the obese group was provided, thus limiting the interpretation of the results of this study. Similarly, Schaefer-Graf et al. [62] concluded that, in obese women, the high rate of fetal macrosomia does not appear be normalized by therapy based on maternal euglycemia. In contrast, Langer et al. [63] found that obese and overweight patients with GDM achieving established levels of glucose control with insulin therapy showed no increased risk for composite outcome, macrosomia, and LGA in comparison to normal-weight patients with GDM. In contrast, even when diet-treated obese patients achieved good glycemic control, there was no improvement in pregnancy outcome in comparison to normal-weight patients. Poorly controlled overweight and obese patients, regardless of treatment modality, had significantly higher rates of composite outcome, metabolic complications, macrosomia, and LGA. Although obesity in itself is related to adverse outcome in pregnancy, gestational diabetic women treated with insulin and possibly oral antidiabetic drugs who achieve targeted levels of glycemic control will have pregnancy outcomes equivalent to those of normal-weight women. The improved outcome in the insulin-treated overweight and obese women may be due to an unidentified effect of insulin itself on the fetus or activation of other metabolic fuel pathways.

Yogev et al. [64] found no significant difference between diabetic obese and morbidly obese women in pregnancy outcome when targeted levels of glycemic control were achieved. Nevertheless, it should be noted that adequate glycemic control in morbidly obese women may be more difficult to achieve. Only two-thirds of the morbidly obese patients achieved the desired level of glycemic control, and 69% were treated with insulin. In addition to constitutional risk factors such as previous macrosomia and parity, level of glycemic control, obesity, and treatment modality were found to be independent contributors to the outcome variable. These findings support the premise that treatment with insulin and achievement of the established level of glycemic control in obese patients will result in improved pregnancy outcome.

The treatment of diabetes was also studied in respect to hypertensive disorders. The majority of studies have found an association between hypertensive disorders and obesity. Regardless of achieving established levels of glycemic control, the rate of pre-eclampsia was not significantly different between diet-treated overweight and obese subjects. The relatively low rate of GDM severity in diet-treated patients (FPG < 95 mg/dl) may account for this difference. In insulin-treated subjects, an approximately threefold higher risk for pre-eclampsia was found in the patients who failed to achieve established levels of glycemic control. Insulin-treated overweight/obese patients in all BMI categories who achieved established levels of glycemic control had similar rates of pre-eclampsia [64,65].

In a study by Yogev et al. [65], the rate of pre-eclampsia was tested against the severity of GDM by level of glycemic control. A total of 1,813 patients with GDM were enrolled, and they were stratified after treatment initiation by level of glycemic control (good control being defined as a mean blood glucose < 95 mg/dl). Severity of GDM was categorized using FPG on a 3-hour OGTT by 10 mg/dl increments. Overall, pre-eclampsia was diagnosed in 9.6% (174 of 1,813) of diabetic patients. The subjects with GDM who developed pre-eclampsia were significantly younger, had a higher nulliparity rate, were more obese, and gained significantly more weight during pregnancy. However, no difference was found in glycemic profile characteristics between the groups. A comparison between patients with an FPG below and above 105 g/dl revealed that the rate of pre-eclampsia increased significantly: 7.8% versus 13.8%, respectively (OR 1.81; 95% CI 1.3–2.51). Pre-eclampsia rate was further evaluated in relation to level of glycemic control; for the well-controlled patients (mean blood glucose < 95 mg/dl, $n = 994$), similar rates of pre-eclampsia were found between each category of FPG severity. In contrast, in poorly controlled patients (mean blood glucose > 95 mg/dl, $n = 819$), a comparison between severity threshold of FPG below 115 and FPG above 115 mg/dl revealed that the pre-eclampsia rate was 9.8% versus 18% (OR 2.56; 95% CI 1.5–4.3). In a logistic regression model, only pre-pregnancy BMI (OR 2.3; 95% CI 1.16–2.30) and severity of GDM (OR 1.7; 95% CI 1.21–2.38) were independently and significantly associated with an increased risk for pre-eclampsia. The authors concluded that the rate of pre-eclampsia was influenced by the severity of GDM and pre-pregnancy BMI, and optimizing glucose control during pregnancy may decrease the rate of pre-eclampsia, even in those with a greater severity of GDM.

Summary

The alarming rates of obesity are impacting women of reproductive age, with implications for pregnancy outcome. Obesity in pregnancy leads to a multitude of antepartum, intrapartum, and postpartum complications – hypertension and diabetes being the two most common. It is important to emphasize not only that pregestational obesity is a risk factor, but also that exaggerated weight gain during pregnancy is a major risk factor for hypertensive and diabetic complications. Although poorly defined, gestational diabetes and gestational hypertensive disorders in the obese gravida may represent a variant or a predictor of the metabolic syndrome, all of which share the common link of insulin resistance. In order to improve pregnancy outcome in obese diabetic patients, a multidisciplinary approach of preconception counseling, pre-pregnancy weight loss, controlled gestational weight gain, and proper glycemic control is needed.

References

1. Reaven GM. Banting Lecture 1988. Role of insulin resistance in human disease. Diabetes 1988;37(12):1595–607.
2. Carpenter MW. Gestational diabetes, pregnancy hypertension, and late vascular disease. Diabetes Care 2007;30(Suppl. 2):S246–50.
3. Bartha JL, González-Bugatto F, Fernández-Macías R, et al. Metabolic syndrome in normal and complicated pregnancies. Eur J Obstet Gynecol Reprod Biol 2008;137(2): 178–84.
4. Horváth B, Kovács L, Riba M, et al. The metabolic syndrome and the risks of unfavorable outcome of pregnancy. Orv Hetil 2009;150(29):1361–5.
5. Ford ES, Giles WH, Dietz WH. Prevalence of the metabolic syndrome among US adults: findings from the third National Health and Nutrition Examination Survey. JAMA 2002;287(3):356–9.
6. Reaven GM. Role of insulin resistance in human disease (syndrome X): an expanded definition. Annu Rev Med 1993;44:121–31.
7. Felber JP, Acheson KJ, Tappy L. From obesity to diabetes. New York: John Wiley, 1993.
8. Rondinone CM. Adipocyte-derived hormones, cytokines, and mediators. Endocrine 2006;29(1):81–90.
9. Noussitou P, Monbaron D, Vial Y, et al. Gestational diabetes mellitus and the risk of metabolic syndrome: a population-based study in Lausanne, Switzerland. Diabetes Metab 2005;31(4 Pt 1):361–9.
10. Bo S, Monge L, Macchetta C, et al. Prior gestational hyperglycemia: a long-term predictor of the metabolic syndrome. J Endocrinol Invest 2004;27(7):629–35.
11. Pallardo F, Herranz L, Garcia-Ingelmo T, et al. Early postpartum metabolic assessment in women with prior gestational diabetes. Diabetes Care 1999;22(7):1053–8.
12. Verma A, Boney CM, Tucker R, et al. Insulin resistance syndrome in women with prior history of gestational diabetes mellitus. J Clin Endocrinol Metab 2002;87(7): 3227–35.
13. Srinivas SK, Sammel MD, Bastek J, et al. Evaluating the association between all components of the metabolic syndrome and pre-eclampsia. J Matern Fetal Neonatal Med 2009;22(6):501–9.
14. Isezuo SA, Ekele BA. Comparison of metabolic syndrome variables among pregnant women with and without eclampsia. J Natl Med Assoc 2008;100(9):1059–62.
15. Erez-Weiss I, Erez O, Shoham-Vardi I, et al. The association between maternal obesity, glucose intolerance and hypertensive disorders of pregnancy in nondiabetic pregnant women. Hypertens Pregnancy 2005;24(2):125–36.
16. Sermer M, Naylor CD, Gare DJ, et al. Impact of increasing carbohydrate intolerance on maternal-fetal outcomes in 3637 women without gestational diabetes: the Toronto Trihospital Gestational Project. Am J Obstet Gynecol 1995;173:146–56.

17. Ray JG, Diamond P, Singh G, et al. Brief overview of maternal triglycerides as a risk factor for pre-eclampsia. Br J Obstet Gynaecol 2006;113(4):379–86.

18. Wendland EM, Duncan BB, Belizán JM, et al. Gestational diabetes and pre-eclampsia: common antecedents? Arq Bras Endocrinol Metabol 2008;52(6):975–84.

19. Howard G, O'Leary DH, Zaccaro D, et al. Insulin sensitivity and atherosclerosis. Circulation 1996;93(10):1809–17.

20. Caruso A, Ferrazzani S, De Carolis S, et al. Gestational hypertension but not pre-eclampsia is associated with insulin resistance syndrome characteristics. Hum Reprod 1999;14(1):219–23.

21. Yasuhi I, Hogan JW, Canick J, et al. Midpregnancy serum C-peptide concentration and subsequent pregnancy-induced hypertension. Diabetes Care 2001;24(4):743–7.

22. Kaaja R, Laivuori H, Laakso M, et al. Evidence of a state of increased insulin resistance in preeclampsia. Metabolism 1999;48(7):892–6.

23. Sierra-Laguado J, García RG, Celedón J, et al. Determination of insulin resistance using the homeostatic model assessment (HOMA) and its relation with the risk of developing pregnancy-induced hypertension. Am J Hypertens 2007;20(4): 437–42.

24. Wolf M, Sandler L, Munoz K, et al. First trimester insulin resistance and subsequent preeclampsia: a prospective study. Clin Endocrinol Metab 2002;87(4):1563–8.

25. Solomon CG, Graves SW, Green MF, et al. Glucose intolerance as a predictor of hypertension in pregnancy. Hypertension 1994;23(6 Pt 1):717–21.

26. Montoro MN, Kjos SL, Chandler M, et al. Insulin resistance and preeclampsia in gestational diabetes mellitus. Diabetes Care 2005;28(8):1995–2000.

27. Edwards LE, Dickes WF, Alton IR, et al. Pregnancy in the massively obese: course, outcome, and obesity prognosis of the infant. Am J Obstet Gynecol 1978;131(5): 479–83.

28. Garbaciak JA, Jr., Richter M, Miller S, et al. Maternal weight and pregnancy complications. Am J Obstet Gynecol 1985:15;152(2):238–45.

29. Sebire NJ, Jolly M, Harris JP, et al. Maternal obesity and pregnancy outcome: a study of 287,213 pregnancies in London. Int J Obes Relat Metab Disord 2001;25(8): 1175–82.

30. Isaacs JD, Magann EF, Martin RW, et al. Obstetric challenges of massive obesity complicating pregnancy. J Perinatol 1994;14(1):10–4.

31. Perlow JH, Morgan MA, Montgomery D, et al. Perinatal outcome in pregnancy complicated by massive obesity. Am J Obstet Gynecol 1992;167(4 Pt 1):958–62.

32. Weiss JL, Malone FD, Emig D, et al. FASTER Research Consortium. Obesity, obstetric complications and cesarean delivery rate – a population-based screening study. Am J Obstet Gynecol 2004;190(4):1091–7.

33. Baeten JM, Bukusi EA, Lambe M. Pregnancy complications and outcomes among overweight and obese nulliparous women. Am J Public Health 2001;91:436–40.

34. Cedergren MI. Maternal morbid obesity and the risk of adverse pregnancy outcome. Obstet Gynecol 2004;103(2):219–24.

35. Kumari AS. Pregnancy outcome in women with morbid obesity. Int J Gynaecol Obstet 2001;73(2):101–7.

36. Bianco AT, Smilen SW, Davis Y, et al. Pregnancy outcome and weight gain recommendations for the morbidly obese woman. Obstet Gynecol 1998;91(1):97–102.

37. Schrauwers C, Dekker G. Maternal and perinatal outcome in obese pregnant patients. J Matern Fetal Neonatal Med 2009;22(3):218–26.

38. Sibai BM. Diagnosis and management of gestational hypertension and preeclampsia. Obstet Gynecol 2003;102:181–92.

39. Coppage KH, Sibai BM. Treatment of hypertensive complications in pregnancy. Curr Pharm Des 2005;11(6):749–57.

40. Roberts JM, Pearson GD, Cutler JA, et al. National Heart Lung and Blood Institute. Summary of the NHLBI Working Group on Research on Hypertension During Pregnancy. Hypertens Pregnancy 2003;22(2):109–27.

41. Sibai BM, Gordon T, Thom E, et al. Risk factors for preeclampsia in healthy nulliparous women: a prospective multicenter study. The National Institute of Child Health and Human Development Network of Maternal-Fetal Medicine Units. Am J Obstet Gynecol 1995;172(2 Pt 1):642–8.

42. Griffith J, Conway DL. Care of diabetes in pregnancy. Obstet Gynecol Clin North Am 2004;31(2):243–56.

43. Coustan DR. Gestational diabetes. In National Institutes of Diabetes and Digestive and Kidney Diseases. Diabetes in America, 2nd edn. NIH Publication No. 95-1468. Bethesda, MD: NKKD, 1995, pp. 703–17.

44. Sibai BM. Chronic hypertension in pregnancy. Obstet Gynecol 2002;100(2):369–77.

45. Livingston JC, Maxwell BD, Sibai BM. Chronic hypertension in pregnancy. Minerva Ginecol 2003;55(1):1–13.

46. Sibai BM, Ewell M, Levine RJ, et al. Risk factors associated with preeclampsia in healthy nulliparous women. The Calcium for Preeclampsia Prevention (CPEP) Study Group. Am J Obstet Gynecol 1997;177(5):1003–10.

47. O'Brien TE, Ray JG, Chan WS. Maternal body mass index and the risk of preeclampsia: a systematic overview. Epidemiology 2003;14(3):368–74.

48. Saldana TM, Siega-Riz AM, Adair LS, et al. The relationship between pregnancy weight gain and glucose tolerance status among black and white women in central North Carolina. Am J Obstet Gynecol 2006;195(6):1629–35.

49. American College of Obstetricians and Gynecologists. Obesity in Pregnancy. ACOG Committee Opinion. No. 315. Washington, DC: ACOG, 2005.

50. Galtier-Dereure F, Boegner C, Bringer J. Obesity and pregnancy: complications and cost. Am J Clin Nutr 2000;71(5 Suppl.):1242S–8S.

51. Deitel M, Stone E, Kassam HA, et al. Gynecologic-obstetric changes after loss of massive excess weight following bariatric surgery. J Am Coll Nutr 1988;7:147–53.

52. Institute of Medicine of the National Academies. Committee on Nutritional Status during Pregnancy and Lactation, Institute of Medicine. Nutrition during pregnancy. Part I: Weight gain. Part II: Nutrient supplements. Washington, DC: National Academies Press, 1990.

53. Cedergren MI. Optimal gestational weight gain for body mass index categories. Obstet Gynecol 2007;110:759–64.

54. DeVader SR, Neeley HL, Myles TD, et al. Evaluation of gestational weight gain guidelines for women with normal prepregnancy body mass index. Obstet Gynecol 2007;110:745–51.

55. Kiel DW, Dodson EA, Artal R, et al. Gestational weight gain and pregnancy outcomes in obese women: how much is enough? Obstet Gynecol 2007;110:752–8.

56. Wolff S, Legarth J, Vangsgaard K, et al. A randomized trial of the effects of dietary counseling on gestational weight gain and glucose metabolism in obese pregnant women. Int J Obes (Lond) 2008;32(3):495–501.

57. Chaudry R, Gilby P, Carroll PV. Pre-existing (type 1 and type 2) diabetes in pregnancy. Obstet Gynaecol Reprod Med 2007;17:339–44.

58. Lucas MJ, Lowe TW, Bone L. Class A1 gestational diabetes: a meaningful diagnosis? Obstet Gynecol 1993;82(2):260–5.

59. Casey BM, Lucas MJ, Mcintire DD, et al. Pregnancy outcomes in women with gestational diabetes compared with the general obstetric population. Obstet Gynecol 1997;90(6):869–73.

60. Yogev Y, Visser GH. Obesity, gestational diabetes and pregnancy outcome. Semin Fetal Neonatal Med 2009;14(2):77–84.
61. Leikin E, Jenkins JH, Graves WL. Prophylactic insulin in gestational diabetes. Obstet Gynecol 1987;70(4):587–92.
62. Schaefer-Graf UM, Heuer R, Kilavuz O, et al. Maternal obesity not maternal glucose values correlates best with high rates of fetal macrosomia in pregnancies complicated by gestational diabetes. J Perinat Med 2002;30:313–21.
63. Langer O, Yogev Y, Xenakis EM, et al. Overweight and obese in gestational diabetes: the impact on pregnancy outcome. Am J Obstet Gynecol 2005;192(6):1768–76.
64. Yogev Y, Langer O. Pregnancy outcome in obese and morbidly obese gestational diabetic women. Eur J Obstet Gynecol Reprod Biol 2008;137(1):21–6.
65. Yogev Y, Xenakis EMJ, Langer O. The association between preeclampsia and the severity of gestational diabetes: the impact of glycemic control. Am J Obstet Gynecol 2004;191:1655–60.

CHAPTER 12

Obstetric Management of the Obese Parturient

James M. Alexander

University of Texas Southwestern Medical Center, Dallas, Texas, USA

Obesity has increased in the population to a point that it is now endemic. Its prevalence has increased at a steady rate for decades and is now encountered in one out of three pregnancies [1,2]. Unfortunately, once a woman is pregnant, little can be done to modify the presence of obesity as it is recommended that women do not pursue weight loss during pregnancy; instead, women are advised to modify their weight gain.

Obstetric management of the obese parturient presents many challenges, and marked obesity is without question a hazard to the woman and her fetus. All aspects of obstetric management are affected due to co-morbidities often associated with obesity, such as hypertension and diabetes, fetal macrosomia, an increased risk for pre-eclampsia, higher rates of cesarean delivery, difficulty encountered with anesthesia for labor and delivery, and postpartum complications [3–9]. Many of these factors are interrelated and somewhat additive in risk. For example, a woman with type 2 diabetes, a not uncommon medical diagnosis associated with obesity, who becomes pregnant is at increased risk for macrosomia and may require a cesarean delivery for cephalopelvic disproportion. Postoperative recovery from a cesarean delivery in such a patient is more likely to be complicated by morbidities such as wound infection or even a thromboembolic event when compared to the normal-weight woman. Chu et al. have demonstrated an increased use of healthcare services in obese women, including increased prenatal fetal tests, ultrasonographic examinations, medication use, prenatal visits, and increased lengths of hospital stays related to cesarean delivery and obesity-related high-risk conditions [10].

Pregnancy in the Obese Woman, 1st edition. Edited by Deborah L. Conway.
© 2011 Blackwell Publishing Ltd.

Intrapartum management of the obese parturient

Co-morbidities

Diabetes, especially gestational diabetes, is commonly encountered in obese women, and its incidence is rising [11]. In general, women with diet-controlled gestational diabetes who do not require insulin can avoid early delivery or other interventions and can expect an excellent pregnancy outcome. Macrosomia, however, is a risk in these women, especially with poor glucose control, and can lead to birth trauma and its associated neonatal morbidity. The American College of Obstetricians and Gynecologists has suggested that a primary cesarean be performed for an estimated fetal weight of 4,500 g or more as a strategy to limit the risk for birth trauma [12]. This recommendation acknowledges that the risk for birth trauma increases with birthweight and that brachial plexus injury is greatly reduced by cesarean delivery.

The clinical effectiveness of offering prophylactic cesarean delivery is not established, however, and data supporting this strategy have been questioned. Gonen et al. implemented a policy of recommending cesarean delivery for macrosomia (estimated fetal weight >4,500 g). Of the 16,416 deliveries in the study, 133 had confirmed macrosomia (0.8% of the population); however, accurate antenatal diagnosis of these cases was poor, with fewer than 20% being correctly identified [13]. More importantly, the policy had a negligible impact on the incidence of brachial plexus injury despite a liberal use of cesarean delivery in the cases of suspected macrosomia. Rouse et al. performed a cost analysis of the impact of a policy of prophylactic cesarean delivery for suspected macrosomia [14]. They estimated that 3,695 cesarean sections would need to be performed to prevent one permanent injury, at a cost of $8.7 million dollars for each injury avoided [15]. Similarly, electively inducing labor to prevent shoulder dystocia is controversial, and the routine use of this intervention is not currently endorsed [16,17].

Women with gestational diabetes who require insulin for fasting hypoglycemia and overt diabetics require additional intervention to minimize morbidity and the risk for fetal loss. Unexplained stillbirth occurs in as many as 1% of these pregnancies, and fetal testing is employed in the third trimester to minimize this risk [18]. This frequently leads to labor induction. Unfortunately, success rates are low and cesarean delivery rates are as high as 50–80% [19–23]. It is recommended that labor induction should be attempted only in those women whose fetus is not excessively large or whose cervix is favorable so that the risk for prolonged labor can be avoided unless there is significant concern about fetal well-being.

Insulin treatment in diabetic women requires that intrapartum glucose levels be carefully managed, and careful consideration should be given to the type and amount of insulin used during labor. Long-acting insulin should be either reduced or not given at all on the day of delivery, and short-acting insulin should be given in response to frequent blood glucose level determination. A constant low-dose insulin infusion administered by a calibrated pump can be very helpful and allows a quick response to glucose values. Normoglycemia should be maintained, and intravenous fluids with glucose should be administered as needed. Postpartum insulin requirements are often quite low and may not be needed at all during the first 24 hours or so postpartum.

Several studies have shown an association between obesity and hypertension in pregnancy [24,25]. Pre-existing hypertension is 3–10 times more common in obese compared to lean women [24]. Sebire et al. correlated the rate of chronic hypertension with the degree of obesity. Women with a body mass index (BMI) of 20–24.9 kg/m^2 had an incidence of chronic hypertension of 3.8%, those with a BMI of 25–29.9 had an incidence of 6.6%, and women with a BMI over 30 had an incidence of 12.5%, threefold greater than the lean group [25]. The increased risk for chronic hypertension places the pregnancy at increased risk for fetal growth restriction, abruption, preterm delivery, prenatal death, and superimposed pre-eclampsia.

In addition to the association with chronic hypertension, obesity is independently associated with pregnancy-related hypertension. In the above-referenced study, Sebire et al. demonstrated a twofold increase in the risk for pre-eclampsia after controlling for several confounders including chronic hypertension. Weiss et al. showed an increased risk for gestational hypertension in morbidly obese women (12.3% versus 4.8%) as well as pre-eclampsia (6.3% versus 2.1%) [26]. Several others have demonstrated similar results [27,28]. O'Brien et al. provide a systemic review of 13 studies comprising nearly 1.4 million women [29]. As shown in Figure 12.1, there was a strong correlation between BMI and risk for pre-eclampsia. The authors state that the risk for pre-eclampsia typically doubled with each 5–7 kg/m^2 increase in BMI. The relationship persisted when chronic hypertension and other confounders were adjusted for.

These co-morbidities, as well as the more difficult and sometimes long labors encountered in the obese parturient, lead to intrapartum management difficulties. External monitoring of contractions as well as obtaining the fetal heart rate can be challenging due to the thickness of adiposity, and in some extreme cases is not possible. Likewise, estimation of the fetal weight and determination of the fetal lie can be very challenging. Often the fetus cannot be palpated on abdominal examination in the obese woman. Sonography can be helpful with these cases, but ironically is most challenging in the obese patient because the probe is far away from the fetus due to the adipose tissue, thus limiting resolution.

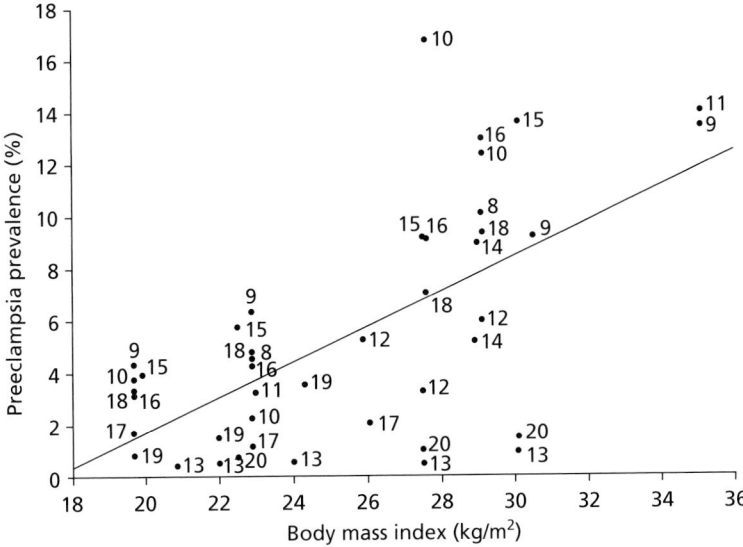

Figure 12.1 Relation between body mass index and pre-eclampsia from 13 cohort studies. (Reproduced from O'Brien et al. [29], with permission from Wolters Kluwer Health.)

Dysfunctional labor

Obesity is related to dysfunctional labor. This relationship is unfortunately most often manifested in the increased cesarean rates seen in obese women. Zhang and colleagues studied the impact of obesity on uterine contractility using clinical and laboratory markers of uterine function [30]. Clinical evidence of decreased uterine contractility included an increased risk for first-stage cesarean section independent of birthweight, increased need for labor argumentation, and increased risk for blood loss in women experiencing spontaneous labor. The *in vitro* part of their study showed that the myometrium contracted with less force and less frequently at term in obese women than in non-obese women at term.

Others have proposed that the physical characteristics of the obese may also impact labor progression. Vahratrian et al. demonstrated that labor progression is slower in overweight and obese women when compared to normal-weight women between 4 and 10 cm dilated, suggesting that the uterus is less effective in these women [31]. This effect persisted after adjustment for several variables, including oxytocin use. The authors hypothesized that more force is needed to overcome added soft tissue deposits in overweight and obese women, and that this, coupled with a larger fetus, necessitates a stronger and longer duration of contractions to effect delivery.

Roy points out that dystocia in labor may reflect that women may be poorly adapted to the affluence of the modern diet [32]. He proposed

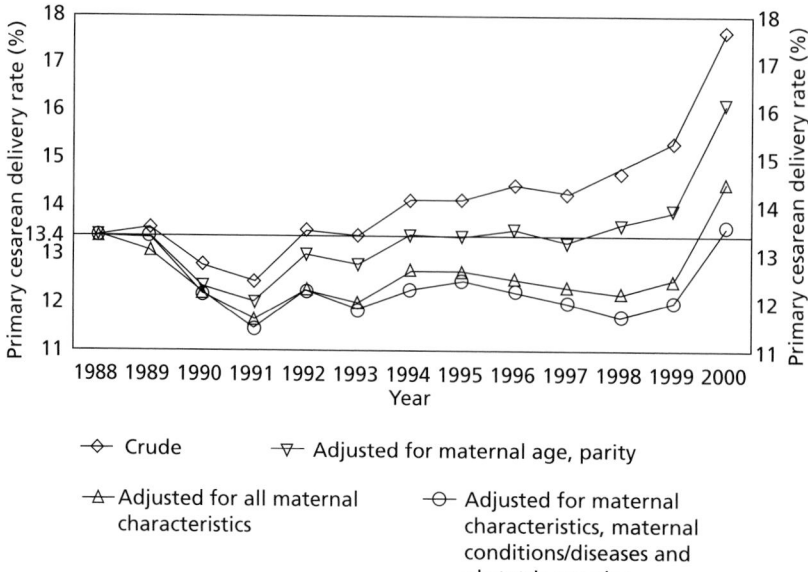

Figure 12.2 Observed rates of primary cesarean delivery in Nova Scotia, 1988–2000, and rates adjusted sequentially for changes in maternal characteristics, maternal conditions or diseases, and obstetric practice. (Reproduced from Joseph et al. [33], with permission from Wolters Kluwer Health.)

that the high frequency of dystocia diagnosed in modern times may be due to the inability of natural selection to keep up with the rather rapid change in our food sources. His theory states that dystocia has resulted from the ready availability of calories in the modern world compared to the relatively caloric-starved past. Fetuses are larger now than before, and the pelvis has not had time to increase in size in response. Joseph et al. provide evidence supporting this view [33]. As seen in Figure 12.2, maternal characteristics including obesity played a significant role in the experience in Nova Scotia from 1988 to 2000, accounting for the majority of the increase in primary cesarean deliveries seen during this time.

The increased risk for labor dystocia has many consequences for the obese parturient. Cesarean delivery is more common. Chorioamnionitis, postpartum endometritis, and wound infections are all increased. The evidence of excessive blood loss and the need for blood transfusion are elevated as well.

Cesarean delivery

Cesarean delivery rates in the USA reached an all-time high in 2007 of 31.9%, reflecting a trend that began in 1996 when rates were 31.8% [34].

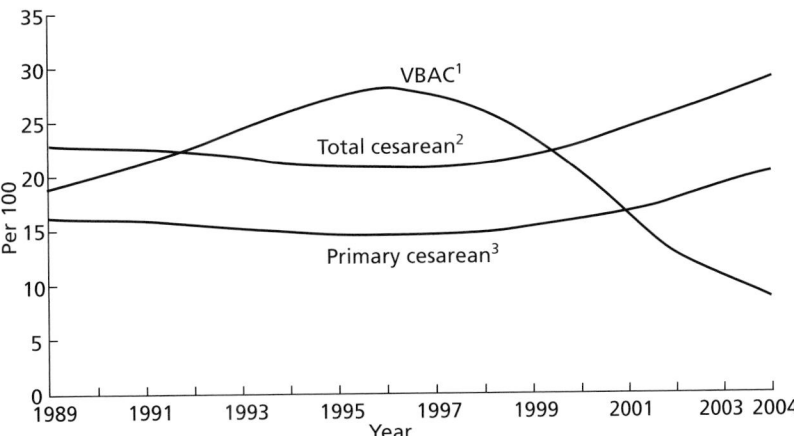

[1]Number of vaginal births after cesarean (VBAC) per 100 live births to women with a previous cesarean delivery.
[2]Percentage of all live births by cesarean delivery.
[3]Number of primary cesarean deliveries per 100 live births to women who have not had a previous cesarean.

Figure 12.3 Total and primary cesarean rate and vaginal birth after cesarean rate: USA, 1989–2004. (Reproduced from Martin et al. [69], with permission from Wolters Kluwer Health.)

This recent increase is due to many complex and sometimes interrelated factors and represents an increase in both the primary and the repeat cesarean delivery rate. The increase in the overall cesarean delivery rate exactly parallels the rise in the primary cesarean rate, which has increased from 15% to 20.6% between the years 1996 and 2004 (Figure 12.3). Factors that have influenced the primary cesarean rate include the overuse of labor induction, elective cesareans, concern over malpractice litigation, abandonment of vaginal breech delivery, and increased intervention for suspected fetal distress due to the increased and widespread use of electronic fetal monitoring and other antepartum tests of fetal well-being. Concomitant to the rise in the primary cesarean rate, vaginal birth after cesarean rates have fallen dramatically. After reaching a peak of 26% in 1996, rates have steadily declined and by 2007 had fallen to 8.5%.

There is increasing evidence that obesity has a direct impact on the cesarean rate. This effect is directly proportional to the degree of obesity, with rates of cesarean in morbidly obese women double that of those women with a BMI in the normal range. Barau and colleagues examined 16,952 consecutive singleton live births and correlated the mothers' BMIs with the rate of cesarean delivery [35]. As shown in Figure 12.4, the cesarean rate in women with a BMI of 20–24.9 kg/m^2 (normal) was 16% compared to 23% in obese women and greater than 30% in morbidly obese women with a BMI greater than 40 kg/m^2. This association was seen in women with and without a prior cesarean and was still present after

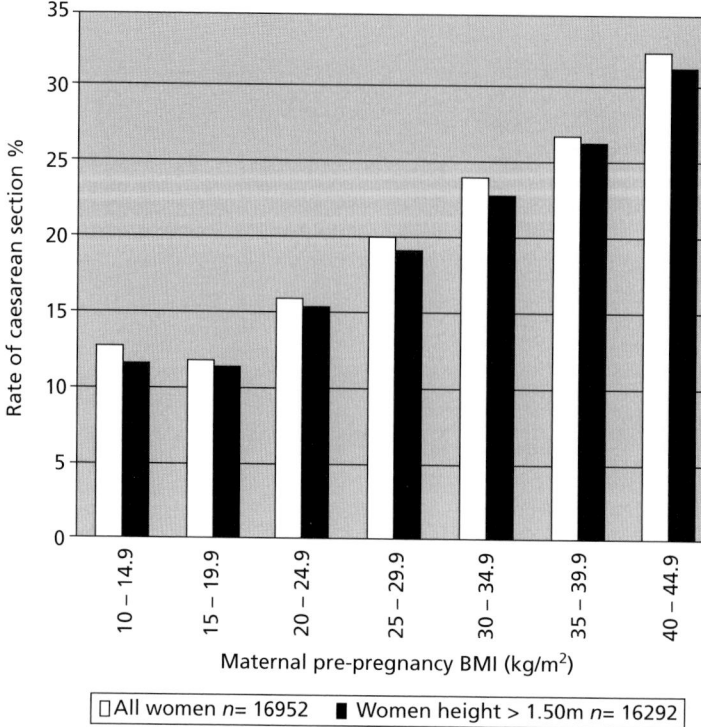

Figure 12.4 Caesarean section rate and pre-pregnancy maternal body mass index (BMI). (Reproduced from Barau et al. [35], with permission from Blackwell Publishing Ltd.)

adjusting for gestational diabetes, term pregnancies, maternal height, parity, and maternal age.

Lynch et al. reported spontaneous vaginal delivery rates in obese primigravid and multigravid women [36]. Spontaneous vaginal delivery rates decreased from 50% in normal-weight primigravid women to 38% in morbidly obese primigravid women, and from 78% to 61% in morbidly obese multigravid women. Conversely, cesarean rates were elevated in the morbidly obese woman primarily due to an almost threefold increase in emergent cesareans. Burstein et al. conducted a prospective cohort study comparing cesarean rates in obese and non-obese women [37]. As shown in Table 12.1, the two groups had similar rates of labor induction, preterm delivery, and baby outcomes, but the obese group had a dramatically increased rate of cesarean delivery. Adjustments for parity, gestational diabetes, and macrosomia did not significantly modify this risk. These reports are consistent with the now extensive literature that associates obesity with cesarean delivery [38–40].

BMI also correlates with the outcome of a trial of labor after a previous cesarean delivery, as shown by Hibbard et al. in a secondary analysis of

Table 12.1 Obstetric risk factors in obese and non-obese patients.

Characteristics	Obese (n = 79)	Nonobese (n = 297)	p Value
Labor induction (%)	1.3	1.4	0.65
Placental abruption (%)	8.9	9.1	0.57
Failed induction (%)	0.0	0.3	0.84
Meconium-stained amniotic fluid (%)	14.0	19.2	0.13
Cesarean delivery (%)	32.9	18.9	0.006
Apgar at 1 min <7 (%)	11.4	7.4	0.29
Apgar at 5 min <7 (%)	3.8	1	0.18
Birth weight (g)	3121 ± 816.5	3040 ± 610	0.38
Birth weight			
<2500 g (%)	5.1	3.4	0.44
>4000 g (%)	11.4	3.4	0.006
Gender			
Male (%)	47.8	48.8	
Female (%)	52.2	51.4	0.72
Postpartum hemorrhage (%)	0.0	0.3	0.84
Postpartum fever (%)	1.3	2.0	0.69

Reproduced from Burstein et al. [37], with permission from Thieme.

the Maternal–Fetal Medicine Units (MFMU) Network cesarean registry [41]. This registry was a result of a prospective cohort observational study conducted at 19 centers that were part of the National Institute of Child Health and Human Development (NICHD)-funded MFMU Network. A total of 14,142 women who underwent a trial of labor after previous cesarean and 14,304 women who underwent elective repeat cesarean delivery were included in Hibbard et al.'s secondary analysis. A failed trial of labor directly correlated with the BMI, ranging from 15.2% in normal-weight women to 39.3% in morbidly obese women. Morbidly obese women who failed a trial of labor also experienced a sixfold increase in maternal morbidity compared to those who had a successful trial of labor. This morbidity included a prolonged hospital stay, endometritis, and neonatal intensive care unit admission.

The risk for cesarean delivery due to obesity can be modified from one pregnancy to another. Paramsothy et al. estimated the effect of interpregnancy weight gain on the risk for cesarean delivery in women with gestational diabetes [42]. The risk for cesarean delivery increased 70% in women who experienced 10 lb of weight gain or more between pregnancies. This risk was proportional to the amount of interpregnancy weight gain, with women gaining more than 27 lb of weight at the greatest risk for a cesarean (odds ratio [OR] 2.36 compared to women with a stable interpregnancy weight). Conversely, women who experienced interpregnancy weight loss demonstrated a 50% decrease in the risk for cesarean delivery when compared to women who had a stable interpregnancy weight (OR 0.55; 95% confidence interval 0.28–1.10). Although weight loss during pregnancy is not advised, preconceptual weight loss should be strongly encouraged to modify the greatly increased risk for cesarean in the obese woman.

Bariatric surgery is being increasingly used to treat obesity. Over 150,000 procedures were performed in the USA in 2007, half of which occurred in women of reproductive age [43]. The three most commonly employed procedures include vertical gastroplasty, gastric banding, and Roux-en-Y gastric bypass. The improvement in pregnancy outcomes after these procedures is remarkable. Buchwald and associates showed that surgical procedures that treat morbid obesity can improve or even resolve diabetes, hyperglycemia, and hypertension [44]. Wax et al. have demonstrated that obstetric outcomes including cesarean rates are similar in women who have undergone gastric bypass surgery to those in the general obstetric population [45]. Although there is no evidence of a decrease in the risk for cesarean section after bariatric surgery, morbidity from cesareans is certainly reduced by the decrease in co-morbidities seen.

Anesthetic concerns

The pregnant woman faces increased morbidity from anesthesia when compared to the non-pregnant individual. This is primarily due to aspiration of the gastric contents sometimes associated with a difficult intubation. This risk for failed intubation in the obstetric patient is well recognized and is reported to be 1 in 280 compared to 1 in 2,230 in the general population [46]. This risk is primarily due to the soft tissue changes that occur during pregnancy. The capillaries of the nasopharynx and larynx are engorged, and edema of the soft tissue of the larynx occurs [47,48]. This soft tissue edema is even more pronounced in pre-eclampsia and is not always present on initial evaluation of the airway. The risk for failed intubation, although rare, has not decreased over time and in fact has slightly increased [49].

Obesity further increases the risk for failed intubation due to increased soft tissue mass, the short neck often seen in these women and its associated decrease in motility, and the added weight in the breasts, which further decreases lung volumes. Juvin et al. demonstrated that difficult tracheal intubation is more common in obese patients (15.3%) compared to lean patients (2.2%) using the Intubation Difficulty Score [50]. Obese women were more likely to have a difficult airway, as demonstrated by a Mallampati Score of class III or IV, had less motility of the neck, and had an elevated risk for oxygen desaturation during intubation. In addition to the increased risk for failed intubation, there is increased difficulty in maintaining adequate mask ventilation [51]. Desaturation is more common, and preoxygenation is crucial and can provide important time to remedy a difficult situation.

The increased risk for failed intubation and desaturation and the difficulties encountered with masked ventilation demand that a second pair of hands is present during the administration of a general anesthesia in the obese patient [52]. The second person can help with mask ventilation and the jaw thrust maneuver, and provide positive-pressure ventilation and cricoid pressure. Awake intubation, fiberoptic techniques, the use of the laryngeal mask airway, and even cricothyrotomy may be required in some circumstances, and the appropriate equipment to perform these techniques should be available. One should not proceed with rapid-sequence induction of general anesthesia if intubation is expected to be difficult without appropriate preparation, and some of these alternative techniques may be performed primarily when rapid sequence induction is too risky. In addition, the case should not be started until effective anesthesia has been established.

A regional anesthetic is preferred for cesarean delivery as it helps to avoid the increased risk for failed intubation altogether. Furthermore, in laboring women who require a cesarean, an epidural is often already in place and can usually be dosed adequately for surgery. The American College of Obstetricians and Gynecologists has concluded that the increased morbidity and mortality of general anesthesia suggests that regional anesthesia is the preferred method of anesthesia in the pregnant patient [53]. Regional analgesia, however, is more difficult in the obese parturient because anatomical landmarks are obscured. Failure rates as high as 42% have been reported [26]. Jordan et al., in 1994, noted that over 70% of obese women needed more than one attempt, and 14% required more than attempts [54]. Others have noted that the incidence of dural puncture is much higher than in the non-obese patient, likely secondary to the increase in number of attempts [55,56]. Several investigators have demonstrated an increased distance from the skin to the epidural space based on BMI [18,57]. Proper positioning of the patient can decrease this distance. Grau et al. demonstrated a benefit of ultrasound in aiding epidural placement [58–60]. The number of puncture attempts, catheter adjustments, and side effects such as headaches were decreased in these studies. Others, however, have shown the limitations of these techniques in the morbidly obese [61]. Once placed, the risk for epidural catheter dislodgement is increased in the obese parturient [62,63].

One of the most concerning complications of regional anesthesia in the obese parturient is the unpredictable and exaggerated spread of anesthetic, resulting in excess motor blockade and a high spinal block [64]. Increased abdominal compression and pressure may be the cause of this effect. Greene attributed this to decreased cerebrospinal fluid volume due to compression of the dural sac caused by compression of the vena cava [65]. Awareness of this risk can help avoid an emergent general anesthetic.

Postpartum management of the obese parturient

The obese parturient is at risk for several complications after delivery, including hemorrhage, thromboembolism, infectious morbidity, prolonged hospital stay, and in some cases difficulty with lactation. These complications are both direct and indirect consequences of obesity. For example, abnormal labor increases the risk for undergoing cesarean delivery as well as infectious morbidity, both of which impact the postpartum recovery. A more direct effect of obesity on postpartum recovery is the decreased mobility that is often seen, which prolongs hospitalization and can lead to several problems including thromboembolism and other pulmonary complications.

Usha Kiran and colleagues demonstrated an increased incidence of postpartum hemorrhage in obese patients [66]. Although cesarean delivery and associated blood loss were contributory, excessive blood loss was also seen in vaginal delivery. Sebire reported a 44% increased risk for major hemorrhage in women with a BMI greater than $30 kg/m^2$ that persisted after correcting for confounders [25]. The risk was related to the degree of obesity, with those considered grossly obese having a 70% increased risk compared to normal-weight women. The authors hypothesized that this might be due to a larger placenta and its associated implantation site, but felt the finding was more likely due to the decreased uterine contractility and increase in labor dystocia previously discussed.

Postoperative atelectasis and pneumonitis is increased, especially in the woman who undergoes a cesarean and/or general anesthesia. The length of time required to perform the cesarean can be longer than average due to the technical difficulties encountered, further increasing these risks. Early ambulation and incentive spirometry should be strongly encouraged to minimize these complications.

Deep vein thrombosis and pulmonary embolism are more common, and measures should be taken to prevent these complications. The use of thromboembolic deterrent devices until ambulation is established and the administration of low molecular weight heparin are proven measures to minimize these risks, especially in the postoperative patient. Although not generally used after vaginal delivery, they should be considered in the woman who does not ambulate quickly, especially if she is morbidly obese.

Infectious morbidity, including endometritis, urinary tract infections, and wound infections, is common. Wound infection is a particular concern as these infections often present in a delayed manner, require prolonged treatment, may require closure by secondary intention, and further limit patient mobility. Good surgical technique, use of prophylactic antibiotics, meticulous hemostasis, and closure of the subcutaneous fascia reduce the incidence of postoperative wound infections [67]. Early identification of seromas and hematomas can prevent more complicated infections later, and these can often be closed quickly after evacuation if no infection is present. Treatment of wound infections is evolving, and the use of the "wound vac" is now common and greatly speeds recovery. Some hospitals employ wound care teams in an effort to facilitate recovery and hospital discharge.

Obesity is associated with decreased use of breastfeeding and an overall shorter duration in those who do. The reasons for this observation are unclear but may be simply related to difficulties with infant positioning and latching on [68].

References

1. Pleis JR, Schiller JS, Benson V. Summary health statistics for US adults: National Health Interview Survey, 2000. Vital Health Stat 10 2003;(215):1–132.
2. Mokdad AH, Ford ES, Bowman BA, et al. Prevalence of obesity, diabetes, and obesity-related health risk factors, 2001. JAMA 2003;289:76–9.
3. Kiran TS, Hemmadi S, Bethel J, et al. Outcome of pregnancy in a woman with an increased body mass index. Br J Obstet Gynaecol 2005;112:768–72.
4. Dixit A, Girling JC. Obesity and pregnancy. J Obstet Gynaecol 2008;28:14–23.
5. Yu CKH, Teoh TG, Robinson S. Obesity in pregnancy. Br J Obstet Gynaecol 2006;113:1117–25.
6. Stotland NE. Obesity and pregnancy. Br Med J 2008;338:107–10.
7. Weiss JL, Malon FD, Emig D, et al. Obesity, obstetric complications and cesarean delivery rate – a population based screening study. FASTER Research Consortium. Am J Obstet Gynecol 2004;190:1091–7.
8. Castro LC, Avina RL. Maternal obesity and pregnancy outcomes. Curr Opin Obstet Gynecol 2002;14:601–6.
9. Andreasen KR, Andersen ML, Schantz AL. Obesity and pregnancy. Acta Obstet Gynecol Scand 2004;83:1022–9.
10. Chu SY, Bachman DJ, Callaghan WM, et al. Association between obesity during pregnancy and increased use of health care. N Engl J Med 2008;358:1444–52.
11. Geiss LS, Pan L, Cadwell B, et al. Changes in incidence of diabetes in U.S. adults, 1997–2003. Am J Prev Med. 2006;30:371–7.
12. American College of Obstetricians and Gynecologists. Fetal macrosomia. Practice Bulletin No. 22, November 2000. Washington, DC: ACOG.

13. Gonen R, Bader D, Ajami M. Effects of policy of elective cesarean delivery in cases of suspected fetal macrosomia on the incidence of brachial plexus injury and the rate of cesarean delivery. Am J Obstet Gynecol 2000;183:1296–300.

14. Rouse DJ, Owen J. Prophylactic cesarean delivery for fetal macrosomia diagnosed by means of ultrasonography – a Faustian bargain? Am J Obstet Gynecol 1999;181: 332–8.

15. Rouse DJ, Owen J, Goldenberg RL, et al. The effectiveness and costs of elective cesarean delivery for fetal macrosomia diagnosed by ultrasound. JAMA 1996;276: 1480–6.

16. Combs CA, Singh NB, Khoury JC. Elective induction versus spontaneous labor after sonographic diagnosis of fetal macrosomia. Obstet Gynecol 1993;81:492–6.

17. Adashek JA, Lagrew DC, Iriye BK, et al. The influence of ultrasound examination at term on the rate of cesarean section. Abstract No. 66. Presented at Society of Perinatal Obstetricians 16th Annual Meeting, February 4–10, 1996. Am J Obstet Gynecol 1996;174:328.

18. Hamza J, Smida M, Benhamous D, et al. Parturient's posture during epidural puncture affects the distance from skin to epidural space. J Clin Anesth 1995;7:1–4.

19. Gabbe SG, Mestman JH, Freeman RO, et al. Management and outcome of diabetes mellitus, classes B–R. Am J Obstet Gynecol 1977;129:723–32.

20. Kitzmiller JL, Coloherty JP, Younger MD, et al. Diabetic pregnancy and perinatal morbidity. Am J Obstet Gynecol 1978;131:560–80.

21. Leveno KJ, Hauth JC, Gilstrap LC III, et al. Appraisal of "rigid" blood glucose control during pregnancy in the overtly diabetic woman. Am J Obstet Gynecol 1979; 135:853.

22. Martin FR, Health P, Mountain KR. Pregnancy in women with diabetes. Fifteen years' experience: 1973–1985. Med J Aust 1987;146:187.

23. Schneider JM, Curet LB, Olson RW, et al. Ambulatory care of the pregnant diabetic. Obstet Gynecol 1980;56:144–9.

24. Kumari AS. Pregnancy outcome in women with morbid obesity. Int J Gynecol Obstet 2001;73:101–7.

25. Sebire NJ, Jolly M, Harris JP, et al. Maternal obesity and pregnancy outcome: a study of 287,213 pregnancies in London. Int J Obes 2001;25:1175–82.

26. Weiss JL, Malon FD, Emig D, et al. Obesity, obstetric complications and cesarean delivery rate – a population based screening study. FASTER Research Consortium. Am J Obstet Gynecol 2004;190:1091–7.

27. Cedergren MI. Maternal morbid obesity and the risk of adverse pregnancy outcome. Obstet Gynecol 2004;103:219–24.

28. Jensen DM, Damm P, Sorensen B, et al. Pregnancy outcome and prepregnancy body mass index in 2459 glucose-tolerant Danish women. Am J Obstet Gynecol 2003;189: 239–44.

29. O'Brien TE, Ray JG, Chan W. Maternal body mass index and the risk of preeclampsia: a systematic overview. Epidemiology 2003;14:368–74.

30. Zhang J, Bricker L, Weay S, et al. Poor uterine contractility in obese women. Br J Obstet Gynaecol 2007;114:343–8.

31. Vahratian A, Zhang J, Troendle JF, et al. Maternal prepregnancy overweight and obesity and the pattern of labor progression in term nulliparous women. Obstet Gynecol 2004;104:943–51.

32. Roy RP. A Darwinian view of obstructed labor. Obstet Gynecol 2003;101:397–401.

33. Joseph KS, Young DC, Dodds L, et al. Changes in maternal characteristics and obstetric practice and recent increases in primary cesarean delivery. Obstet Gynecol 2003;102:791–800.

34. Hamilton BE, Martin JA, Ventura SJ. Births: preliminary data for 2007. National vital statistics reports, Web release; vol. 57 no 12. Released March 18, 2009. Hyattsville, MD: National Center for Health Statistics.

35. Barau G, Robillard P-Y, Hulsey TC, et al. Linear association between maternal pre-pregnancy body mass index and risk of caesarean section in term deliveries. Br J Obstet Gynaecol 2006;113:1173–7.

36. Lynch CM, Sexton DJ, Hession RM, et al. Obesity and mode of delivery in primigravid and multigravid women. Am J Perinatol 2008;25:163–7.

37. Burstein E, Levy A, Mazor M, et al. Pregnancy outcome among obese women: a prospective study. Am J Perinatol 2008;25:561–6.

38. Crane SS, Wojtowycz MA, Dye TD, et al. Association between pre-pregnancy obesity and the risk of cesarean delivery. Obstet Gynecol 1997;82:213–16.

39. Chu SY, Kim SY, Schmid CH, et al. Maternal obesity and risk of cesarean delivery: a meta-analysis. Obes Rev 2007;8:385–94.

40. Sherrard A, Platt RW, Vallerand D, et al. Maternal anthropometric risk factors for caesarean delivery before or after onset of labour. Br J Obstet Gynaecol 2007;114:1088–96.

41. Hibbard JU, for the National Institute of Child Health and Human Development Maternal-Fetal Medicine Units Network. Trial of labor or repeat cesarean delivery in women with morbid obesity and previous cesarean delivery. Obstet Gynecol 2006;108:125–33.

42. Paramsothy P, Lin YS, Kernic MA, et al. Interpregnancy weight gain and cesarean delivery risk in women with a history of gestational diabetes. Obstet Gynecol 2009;113:817–23.

43. Catalano PM. Management of obesity in pregnancy. Obstet Gynecol 2007;109:419–33.

44. Buchwald H, Estok R, Fahrbach K, et al. Trends in mortality in bariatric surgery: a systematic review and meta-analysis. Surgery 2007;142:621–32.

45. Wax JR, Cartin A, Wolff R, et al. Pregnancy following gastric bypass surgery for morbid obesity: maternal and neonatal outcomes. Obes Surg 2008;18:540–4.

46. Barnardo PD, Jenkins JG. Failed tracheal intubation in obstetrics: a 6-year review in a UK region. Anaesthesia 2000;55:685–94.

47. King TA, Adams AP. Failed tracheal intubation. Br J Anaesth 1984;39:1105–16.

48. Hawthorne L, Wilson R, Lyons G, et al. Failed intubation revisited: 17-yr experience in a teaching maternity unit. Br J Anaesth 1996;76:680–4.

49. Hawkins JL. Anesthesia-related maternal mortality. Clin Obstet Gynecol 2003;46:679–87.

50. Juvin P, Lavaut E, Dupont H, et al. Difficult tracheal intubation is more common in obese than in lean patients. Anesth Analg 2003;97:595–600.

51. Rocke DA, Murray WB, Route CC, et al. Relative risk analysis of factors associated with difficult intubation in obstetric anesthesia. Anesthesiology 1992;77:67–73.

52. D'Angelo R, Dewan DD. Obesity. In Chestnut DH (ed.), Obstetric Anesthesia: principles and practice, 3rd edn. Philadelphia: Elsevier Mosby, 2004, pp. 893–903.

53. American College of Obstetricians and Gynecologists. Obstetric analgesia and anesthesia. Practice Bulletin No. 36, July 2002. Washington, DC: ACOG.

54. Jordan H, Perlow MD, Mark A, et al. Massive maternal obesity and perioperative cesarean morbidity. Am J Obstet Gynecol 1994;170:560–5.

55. Faure E, Moreno R, Thisted R. Incidence of postural puncture headache in morbidly obese parturients. Reg Anesth 1994;19:361–3.

56. Hood DD, Dewan DM, Kashtan K. Anesthesia outcome in the morbidly obese parturient. Anesthesiology 1993;79:1210–18.

57. Bahk JH, Kim JH, Lee JS, et al. Computed tomography study of the lumbar (L3–4) epidural depth and its relationship to physical measurements in young adult men. Reg Anesth Pain Med 1998;23:262–5.

58. Grau T, Bartusseck E, Contadi R, et al. Ultrasound imaging improves learning curves in obstetric epidural anesthesia. A preliminary study. Can J Anaesth 2003;50: 1047–50.

59. Grau T, Liepold RW, Conradi R, et al. Efficacy of ultrasound imaging in obstetric epidural anesthesia. J Clin Anesth 2002;14:169–75.

60. Grau T, Leipold RW, Conradi R, et al. Ultrasound control for presumed difficult epidural puncture. Acta Anesthesiol Scand 2001;45:766–1.

61. Whitty RJ, Maxwell CV, Carbalho JCA. Complications of neuraxial anesthesia in an extreme morbidly obese patient for cesarean section. Int J Obstet Anesth 2007; 16:139–44.

62. Faheem M, Sarwar N. Sliding of the skin over subcutaneous tissue is another important factor in epidural catheter migration. Can J Anesth 2002;49:634.

63. Iwama H, Katayama T. Back skin movement also causes "walking" epidural catheter. J Clin Anesth 1999;11:140–41.

64. Hodgkinson R, Hussain FJ. Obesity and the cephalad spread of analgesia following epidural administration of bupivacaine for cesarean section. Anesth Analg 1980;59: 89–92.

65. Greene NM. Distribution of local anesthetic solutions within the subarachnoid space. Anesth Analg 1985;64:715–30.

66. Usha Kiran TS, Hemmadi S, Bethel J, et al. Outcome of pregnancy in a woman with an increased body mass index. Br J Obstet Gynaecol 2005;112:768–72.

67. Naumann RW, Hauth JC, Owen J, et al. Subcutaneous tissue approximation in relation to wound disruption after cesarean delivery in obese women. Obstet Gynecol 1995;85:412–16.

68. Donath SM, Amir LH. Does maternal obesity adversely affect breastfeeding initiation and duration? J. Paediatr Child Health 2000;36:482–6.

69. Martin JA, Hamilton BE, Sutton PD, et al. National Vital Statistics Reports 2006;55: 1–102.

CHAPTER 13

Abdominal Surgery in the Morbidly Obese Patient

Ashley Parker and Deborah L. Conway
University of Texas School of Medicine, San Antonio, Texas, USA

It has been well documented in the literature and discussed elsewhere in this text that maternal obesity increases the risk for cesarean delivery in both the primigravid and the multigravid woman. In general, cesarean delivery is associated with increased maternal risk compared to vaginal delivery, but it poses an even greater threat to the morbidly obese parturient. Morbidly obese patients are at higher risk for infectious complications, and have a higher likelihood of co-existing diseases such as hypertensive disorders and diabetes mellitus, as well as of other independent risk factors for infection and postoperative complications. Longer surgical procedure times should be expected, and higher rates of wound separation and other postoperative morbidity have also been well documented. This chapter intends to discuss helpful techniques and special considerations in the approach to abdominal surgery, primarily cesarean section, in the morbidly obese patient.

Preparation for surgery

In preparation for cesarean delivery in the morbidly obese patient, most of the accepted preoperative standards of care apply. However, certain considerations for additional equipment and instruments should be made in advance of the surgery whenever possible. For example, plans for an operating table that will accommodate the weight of the patient may need to be arranged in advance of the scheduled cesarean delivery. Typical operating room tables hold a weight of 500–800 lb, and some can be adjusted in terms of length and width. It is prudent for an obstetric care provider to know the capacity of the operating tables in his or her delivery suites. In addition, mechanical lifting devices may be necessary to assist in moving the patient from the bed or gurney to the operating table, as

Pregnancy in the Obese Woman, 1st edition. Edited by Deborah L. Conway.
© 2011 Blackwell Publishing Ltd.

might unique instruments with long handles for the surgical procedure [1]. Special attention should be taken to place the patient in a secure and stable position on the table. Once the patient seems adequately positioned on the operating table, operating room personnel should look for and pad any pressure points to prevent injury [1].

Anesthetic considerations

Preoperative evaluation by the anesthesia team should take place as far in advance as feasible, whether upon arrival to the hospital in labor or for a planned surgical procedure, or, preferably, prior to the day of surgery. This preparation is necessary because both regional and general anesthesia can be problematic in morbidly obese patients. In fact, even routine procedures such as obtaining intravenous access can become challenging. Although regional anesthesia is typically the preferred approach to surgical analgesia and muscle relaxation for cesarean delivery, successful regional anesthesia may be hampered in the morbidly obese by an inability to palpate crucial landmarks [2,3]. On the other hand, failed endotracheal intubation for general anesthesia is a risk in morbidly obese patients due to excessive tissue and thick neck circumference, with the potential for significant morbidity and even mortality. Towels and shoulder rolls can be useful in extending the neck for ease of intubation, but equipment for fiberoptic visualization of the vocal cords should be readily available, as well as anesthesia personnel with knowledge and experience in its use.

Higher rates of intraoperative complications such as hypotension and inadequate anesthesia have also been documented in obese parturients. Obese patients have an increased volume of distribution and may require that medications be administered in higher doses [1,2,4]. There are not many studies involving anesthetic outcomes in obese pregnant patient populations, but most studies show a higher failure rate of epidural pain control in obese parturients when compared to patients with a lower body mass index (BMI) [2]. In a study of 1,477 parturients undergoing cesarean delivery, 54% of patients were obese and 7% were morbidly obese. Regional anesthesia was used in 73% of the patients, with a 3–4% failure rate, and with progressively more difficulty in placement with increased BMI. General anesthesia with intubation was used in 26% of the patients, but the authors report no notable association between laryngoscopy grades and obesity. This study also reported similar results in patient satisfaction in their anesthesia when comparing obese and non-obese study participants [5]. Other studies demonstrate an increased incidence of complications such as hypotension, shivering, and inadequate anesthesia as reported by patients [6].

Extubation and postanesthetic recovery are to be undertaken carefully as well. Postoperatively, the patient's oxygenation status should be monitored closely, as many morbidly obese patients also suffer from obstructive sleep apnea and are unable to adequately protect their airway in a semi-conscious state.

Antibiotics and other preoperative infection control considerations

It is a well-established standard care for pregnant and non-pregnant patients to receive preoperative antibiotics to reduce the risk for infectious morbidity related to the surgical procedure. Antibiotics should be given within a 30-minute window prior to skin incision. Cephalosporins such as cefazolin are dosed as 1 g for the first 80 kg (176 lb) body weight and 2 g for weights above 80 kg; clindamycin 900 mg is a recommended alternative for patients allergic to cephalosporins and/or penicillins. The long-standing practice of withholding prophylactic antibiotics until after umbilical cord clamping at cesarean delivery has been shown to result in less reduction of postoperative infection than antibiotics given before skin incision [7]. Morbidly obese patients may have different pharmacokinetics and might therefore require more antibiotics and have subtherapeutic effects postoperatively. Obesity has been proven to be an independent risk factor for postoperative wound infection in spite of prophylactic antibiotics. Several theories to explain this include decreased oxygen tension, immune impairment, and ischemia of suture lines [4,8–12].

Every effort should be made to employ evidence-based techniques whenever possible to reduce this increased burden of infectious complications. However, in a Cochrane review, no difference in postoperative infectious morbidity could be detected between patients who had preoperative hair removal and those who did not. Different methods commonly employed include razors, clippers, and chemical creams. Electric clippers are thought to cause less trauma to the skin. Chemical creams require allergy testing prior to their use. Interestingly, the same Cochrane review failed to show any method as being superior [13]. If hair removal is employed, the timing of hair removal should be as close to operating time as possible [14]. It should be noted that we lack data to say whether this lack of difference holds true in a population consisting exclusively of morbidly obese patients, much less in an obstetric cohort of morbidly obese patients.

Another important aspect of skin preparation is abdominal washing. Body washing is a way to remove transient organisms and inhibit the growth of new organisms. In one commonly endorsed method, patients are instructed to use an antiseptic wash, such as chlorhexidine, for several consecutive days leading up to a planned surgical procedure. A Cochrane review showed no clear evidence that this method of patient showering or bathing was better at preventing surgical site infections than use of other washing products, nor was it better than no preparatory self-washing in the days before surgery [15]. However, as with hair removal, the data available pertain to all surgical patients and not solely to obstetric or obese populations.

As not all surgical procedures are planned, there is clearly a need for some form of preoperative abdominal prep that takes place immediately preoperatively. Scrubbing the abdominal wall with a soap scrub and antimicrobial agent to adequately remove dirt and oil and aid in the reduction of bacteria should be a regular practice [16]. In the morbidly obese patient, doing this skin preparation adequately may require additional time and extra personnel to assist with lifting the abdominal panniculus.

Approach to the skin incision

The anatomy of the abdominal wall in the morbidly obese patient can be quite distorted, and the surgeon may not be able to rely on typical landmarks to correctly place the abdominal incision to gain access to the lower uterine segment (Plate 13.1). The Pfannenstiel skin incision is the most commonly used skin incision for cesarean delivery, but access to the suprapubic region may be impossible without displacing the heavy abdominal tissue upward onto the chest. This poses problems for both patient ventilation and effective retraction by surgical assistants. On the other hand, midline incisions can also be difficult to place correctly, and infraumbilical incisions often pass through the thickest portion of the subcutaneous fat.

Unfortunately, no studies exist to definitively prove either a transverse or a vertical incision superior in an obese population of patients. A cohort study by Wall et al. included 239 women with a BMI over 35kg/m^2 and looked at rates of surgical site infections and other complications between patients who had transverse versus vertical incisions for primary cesarean delivery. Vertical incisions were associated with an odds ratio of 12 for wound complication, defined as anything that required the incision to be reopened [17]. In a report of four massively obese patients undergoing cesarean section via Pfannenstiel skin incisions, there was no incidence of postoperative wound infection or other major complications [18]. Reports such as these suggest that a Pfannenstiel incision, when feasible, may result in less problematic healing.

Among midline skin incision types, there is also a surgical decision to be made between supra- versus infraumbilical placement of the incision. The patient's abdominal tissue can be manually displaced, in either a caudad or a cephalad direction, to help ensure abdominal entry close to the lower uterine segment (Plate 13.2). Surgeons should be aware of and exercise appropriate caution in terms of the distorted anatomy that may become evident only upon surgical entry to the peritoneal cavity. It is not uncommon to extend the initial midline skin incision above the umbilicus to create an appropriate visual field that includes the portion of the uterus to be entered. Careful attention should be paid to avoid the tissue under a large panniculus, which is the most anaerobic region on the abdomen and hence at great risk for infection and postoperative breakdown [1]. One should also consider that assistance from retracting devices may be necessary to help in visualization of the sterile field, and to help reduce physician fatigue during the operative course [1]. Anticipating the need for such a device can allow operating personnel to best prepare the room for the case.

Tixier et al. describe their experience with using infra- or supraumbilical transverse incision for cesarean delivery in women with large, pendulous abdominal walls. There were 18 patients with average BMI of $47\,kg/m^2$. Infraumbilical and supraumbilical incisions were used as deemed appropriate, and both were found to result in no difficulty in fetal extraction from the incision. Direct access to the lower uterine segment was noted in all cases. In order to determine the ideal placement of the incision, a point 2 cm above the symphysis pubis was identified and projected anteriorly through the abdominal wall; in 28% of the patients in this series, this projection placed the incision above the umbilicus. The authors reported two small wound hematomas that resorbed spontaneously, and no wound infections [19]. This approach might be used in selected patients to avoid midline incision.

Following skin and peritoneal entry, the uterine incision and delivery of the fetus typically proceeds without an increased incidence of complications compared to non-obese patients, assuming an adequate visual field following skin and abdominal entry. However, the surgeon should anticipate a larger than average infant, and plan the uterine incision accordingly [20].

The technique of panniculectomy is well described in the literature and surgical texts, and has been described in conjunction with both benign [21] and cancer-related [22] gynecological surgery. Although it may help with visualization and exposure, the procedure will generally result in increased operative time and blood loss (500–700 ml), in addition to other postoperative morbidity such as hypovolemia, increased hospitalization time, and higher rates of thrombotic events. Cesarean section is not an appropriate time for this additional procedure.

Closure of fascia

Careful attention must be paid to fascial closure in the obese woman due to an increased likelihood of incisional hernia [23], particularly when employing a midline incision (Plate 13.3). Using a mass closure technique (i.e. incorporating the peritoneal and rectus fascial layers together in the closure) has been shown to reduce the short-term complication of fascial dehiscence, and the long-term complication of ventral hernia formation [24,25]. Sutures should be placed approximately 1–2 cm apart from one another and should be carefully placed 1–2 cm back from the incised edge of the fascia. A delayed-absorbable suture, such as polydioxanone, is recommended because it retains its tensile strength for longer than rapidly absorbed material, such as polyglactin 910. Sutures can either be interrupted or running, in a non-locked fashion. Careful attention should be paid such that tension seems to spread evenly throughout the repair of the fascia. Herniation has generally been thought to be associated with lack of sufficient suture length as the incision expands postoperatively. Few data are available looking at hernia rates specifically in post-cesarean populations.

Upon closure of the fascia, attention is next turned to the subcutaneous tissue.

Closure of subcutaneous tissue and skin

It is well known that the significant amount of adipose tissue in patients with higher BMIs is less vascular and likely has less penetration of prophylactic antibiotics, leading to a higher incidence of wound infection and wound breakdown postoperatively. Also, it is again important to consider the difference in distorted landmarks that makes surgical closure more difficult and less cosmetic and structurally sound in morbidly obese surgical patients [26].

There are different types of wound complications that can occur after any surgical procedure (Box 13.1). Obesity is a dominant independent risk factor for major postoperative wound complications, and the greater the depth of subcutaneous fat tissue, the greater the risk for wound disruption [11]. Two of the main issues addressed throughout the literature are whether closure of the subcutaneous layer "dead space" affects infection and wound disruption rates, and whether or not subcutaneous drain

> **Box 13.1 Types of surgical wound complications described in studies**
>
> Infection
>
> Superficial
>
> Deep
>
> Fascial dehiscence
>
> Wound seroma
>
> Wound hematoma
>
> Necrotizing fasciitis

placement into this a space affects infection/disruption rates. A study by Chelmow et al. looked at wound infection and disruption rates following cesarean delivery, comparing closure of the subcutaneous space with a plain running suture versus an unclosed space. The study population was not specifically limited to obese patients. Among the two groups of approximately 160 participants each, there was noted to be no difference in wound infection rates in closed versus open subcutaneous tissue. There was a statistical difference in skin separation and seroma formation: 2% in the patients with subcutaneous tissue closure versus 4% in those whose subcutaneous tissue was not reapproximated [27].

Specifically for our purposes, it would be best to address the effectiveness of these interventions in a population of obese pregnant women, and several randomized studies are available for this. In a study by Naumann et al., obese women, defined as subcutaneous fat depth of at least 2 cm, who were undergoing cesarean section were randomized to either closure or no closure of the Camper fascia [26]. The mean BMI in both groups was approximately 37 kg/m^2. Similar to the findings of the study in the general obstetric population [27], there was found to be no difference in wound infection rates but a significant difference in wound disruption rates in these two sets of patients. Patients whose subcutaneous tissue was closed had a 14.5% wound disruption rate versus 26.6% in those without subcutaneous tissue closure [26].

Other studies have not only involved subcutaneous tissue reapproximation, but also included placement of a subcutaneous drain. A study by Magann and colleagues randomized 964 pregnant patients with a subcutaneous tissue depth of greater than 2 cm at the time of cesarean delivery, allocating them into three groups: those with no closure of subcutaneous tissue, those with suture closure, and those with both placement of drain and suture closure. Following their cesarean sections, each group was found to have an approximately 10% wound disruption rate, with no statistical difference between closure techniques [28]. Conversely, Allaire et al. [29] and Al-Inany et al. [30] conducted randomized trials that suggested that subcutaneous fat closure or placement of a suction drain might slightly reduce the overall incidence of major wound complications, such as infection or separation, but not to the extent of other measures such as antibiotic prophylaxis.

Ramsey et al. conducted a multicenter randomized trial of women with 4 cm or more of subcutaneous tissue who were undergoing cesarean delivery. Women with this degree of subcutaneous adipose thickness had a mean BMI of over 45 kg/m². They had two groups of approximately 150 patients each who had their incisions closed with either suture alone or suture plus drain. Their outcomes of interest were rates of dehiscence, seromas, abscesses, and similar wound disruptions. The composite wound morbidity rate in incisions closed with a suture only was 17.4%, versus 22.7% in those with closure plus drain placement, a non-significant difference [31]. This study did not include a group with no subcutaneous layer intervention. However, there appears to be little scientific evidence to support an improvement in outcome for obese women undergoing cesarean delivery when subcutaneous tissue is closed, with or without drain placement.

Finally, there is the decision of whether to close the skin with suture or staples (Plate 13.4). There has also been a significant amount of literature pertaining to this issue, although not all obstetric in nature or specific to obese populations. In the obese patient, staples have been shown to demonstrate anywhere from a slight increase in wound infection rates to double the risk for surgical site infection compared to suture closure. Cosmesis and postoperative pain are judged to be similar between the two skin closure methods [9, 12].

Complications of wounds

When wound complications do arise, it is important to know how best to address them. Wound infection is one of the most common postoperative complications, occurring in anywhere from 2% to 26% of cases depending on the obstetric population under study. Wound infections are primarily caused by microorganisms that grow on the skin and in the genital tract. Antibiotics for postoperative wound infections should be directed at the most common organisms, including *Staphylococcus, Escherichia coli, Proteus,* and *Ureaplasma*. Reasonable choices to cover these organisms include, but are not limited to, oral clindamycin or bactrim, and vancomycin if the intravenous route is indicated. Modern medical care mandates coverage of methicillin-resistant *Staphylococcus aureus* for nearly any wound infection.

Wound hematomas and seromas are common with cesarean incisions, and occur with increased frequency in obese patients. Studies show that when subcutaneous tissue is greater than 2 cm in depth, there is a 27% incidence of wound disruption rate, compared to 18.7% in control populations. When wound seromas or hematomas are encountered, they should be opened and allowed to drain. In this instance, healing by secondary intent should be undertaken either with daily wet to dry dressing changes, or with secondary closure [32]. If secondary closure is to be performed, it is best to wait 1–4 days following the opening of the wound. A polypropylene suture is then used to perform a mattress stitch and may be removed 7 days following placement. Two studies have shown an average healing time for wounds to be approximately 15–17 days when allowed to heal in this manner. This healing time is significantly less than the average of 61 days for wounds allowed to heal by secondary intent with dressing changes [33,34]. Those wounds left open to heal by secondary intent should be dressed carefully with wet dressings filling the entire incision. Wet dressings have been shown to reduce healing times and causes less trauma to tissue [32]. Patients should be advised that materials such as hydrogen peroxide and alcohol should be avoided as they damage valuable materials in the cellular healing process. Normal saline and sterile water are generally sufficient to help cleanse surface areas.

More modern approaches to wound care include negative-pressure wound therapy and vacuum-assisted wound closure. These function by not only reducing the exposure to bacterial elements, but also reducing edema in the infected area. The resultant increase in tissue oxygenation and angiogenesis helps promote healthy granulation tissue. A polyurethane foam is first placed over the wound, which is attached to tubing used for suction and evacuation. An occlusive adhesive dressing is finally placed over the top of the entire site for security, and the tubing is connected to a vacuum pump that collects fluid into a canister. Dressing changes are still needed, but less often and with a significantly reduced healing time. This device is more costly than dressing materials for a secondary wound healing process, but has proven to help improve wound healing for obese patients, and may succeed in reducing the overall cost of home health assistance and time to complete healing [32].

Other postoperative considerations

Abdominal surgery in any patient should include careful planning for the postoperative recovery period. This planning should include goals for recovery from anesthesia, resumption of normal oral intake and bowel function, resumption of mobility, and wound healing. Obstetric providers should be aware that postoperative healing and recovery may take longer in obese women who are also recovering from pregnancy. Obese patients generally will have some degree of sleep apnea, which could be exacerbated by the effects of anesthetics. Oxygen saturation levels should be closely monitored, and there should be high suspicion for atelectasis, especially if fever ensues in the days immediately postoperatively. Obese patients have a reduced compliance in their chest wall, leading to increased breathing effort and atelectasis with subsequent desaturation, especially following intubation. Atelectasis generally occurs in the first 3 postoperative days following abdominal surgery and is the most common cause of postoperative fever. For patients with signs of respiratory distress in the postoperative period, a high suspicion for pulmonary embolism should be entertained [3].

All postoperative patients, especially obese patients and patients undergoing intra-abdominal surgery, are also at increased risk for venous thromboembolic events, due in part to venous stasis and in part to hypercoagulable states. Prevention of these events begins preoperatively, sometimes with the use of heparin or low molecular weight heparin for prevention of thrombi. Sequential compression devices should be used throughout the surgical procedure and immediately postoperatively to prevent venous thromboembolism. Patients in the recovery period should be encouraged to ambulate early in the hours and days of the postoperative period. Again, anticoagulation therapy may be necessary until the patient is fully ambulatory, and high suspicion should always be maintained for subsequent events such as pulmonary embolism.

Postoperative ileus is a rare complication after cesarean delivery, and it is generally safe for patients to eat within several hours of their surgery. The most common side effects in the gastrointestinal system are nausea, typically of brief duration, and abdominal distension, usually as a result of anesthetic effect. Antiemetics and slow advancement of diet generally prove to be helpful during this time.

Postoperative pain management is essential, because excessive postoperative pain can impede a woman's efforts at ambulation and deep breathing. Surgeons and anesthesiologists should take care to avoid narcotics where possible, as these depress both respiratory function and bowel function. Better pain control, conversely, will encourage better ambulation and, in turn, more expeditious recovery. Obese patients in particular may benefit from epidural pain management with drugs such as bupivacaine and marcaine, and favorable data are emerging on intra-incisional local anesthetic devices.

Conclusions

This chapter has served as a brief overview of the many pre-, intra-, and postoperative considerations necessary in the approach to obese parturi-

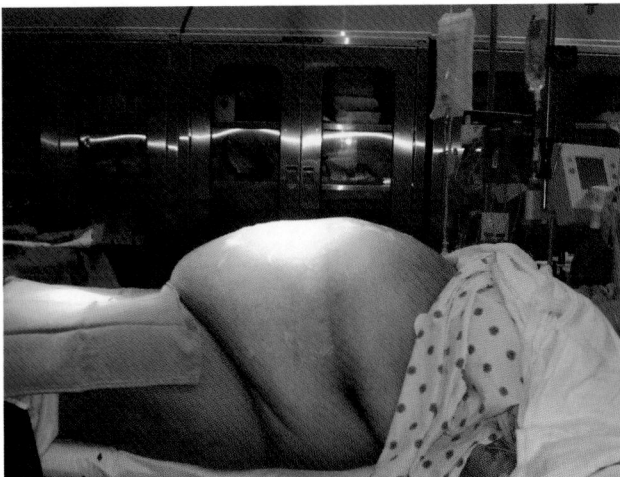

Plate 13.1 Pre-surgical view of a morbidly obese pregnant patient. (Plate courtesy of Dr Luke Newton.)

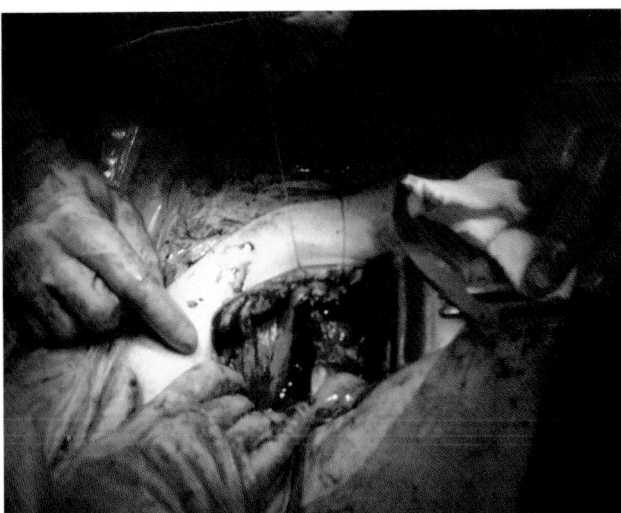

Plate 13.2 A supraumbilical vertical incision 12 cm in length for cesarean delivery resulted in entry to the peritoneum over the lower uterine segment. The hysterotomy is visible after delivery of the fetus and placenta. Note the relatively shallow depth of the subcutaneous fat at this level. (Plate courtesy of Dr Luke Newton.)

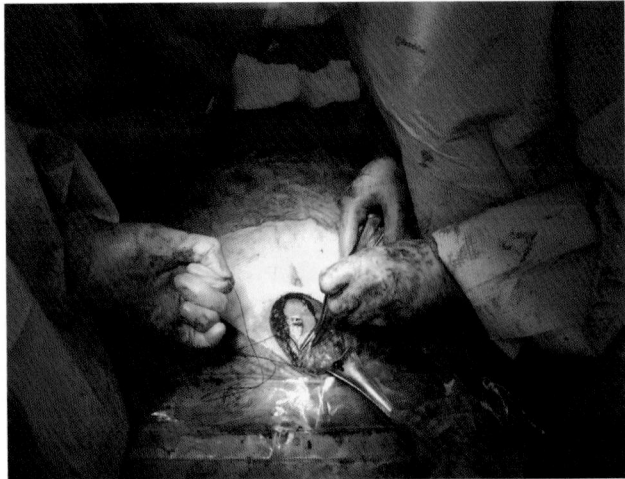

Plate 13.3 Subcutaneous tissue closure of the supraumbilical vertical incision. Again, note the relatively thin subcutaneous tissue at this level. (Plate courtesy of Dr Luke Newton.)

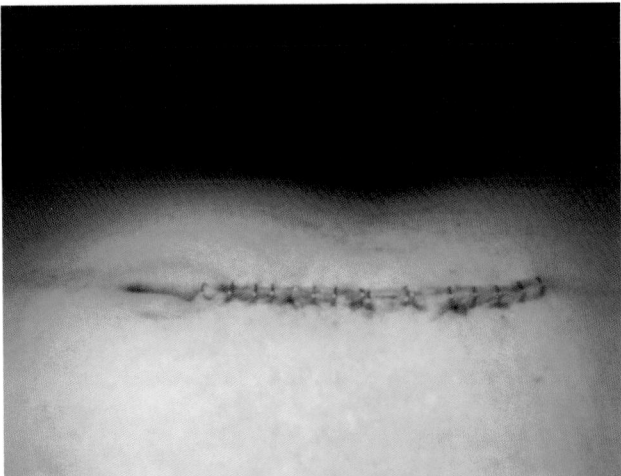

Plate 13.4 Completed incision closure of the supraumbilical skin incision following cesarean section, approximately 6–7 cm at completion. (Plate courtesy of Dr Luke Newton.)

ents undergoing abdominal surgery. Although the focus was primarily on cesarean delivery, the most common surgical procedure performed in modern times, it is important to also keep in mind that obese pregnant females may also require other abdominal surgical procedures, including, but not limited to, ovarian cystectomy, cholecystectomy, appendectomy, and emergent exploratory trauma surgery. The main points are that careful planning leads to the most successful surgical approach and management, while keeping in mind that surgical emergencies occur often and should be anticipated whenever possible. Upon completion of the surgical procedure, there are still the important days and weeks of postoperative care that lie ahead of the responsible surgeon and his or her team.

References

1. Shenkman Z, Shir Y, Brodsky, JB. Perioperative management of the obese patient. Br J Anaesth 1993;70:349–59.
2. Hood DD, Dewan DM. Anesthetic and obstetric outcome in morbidly obese parturients. Anesthesiology 1993;79(6):1210–18.
3. Roofthooft E. Anesthesia for the morbidly obese parturient. Curr Opin Anaesthesiol 2009;22(3):341–6.
4. DeMaria EJ, Carmody BJ. Perioperative management of special populations: obesity. Surg Clin N Am 2005;85(6):1283–9, xii.
5. Bamgbade OA, Khalaf WM, Ajai O, et al. Obstetric anesthesia outcome in obese and non-obese parturients undergoing cesarean delivery: an observational study. Int J Obstet Anesth 2009;18(3):221–5.
6. Edomwonyi NP, Osaigbovo PE. Incidence of obesity in parturients scheduled for cesarean section, intra-operative complications, management and outcome. East Afr Med J 2006;83(4):112–19.
7. Sullivan SA, Smith T, Chang E, et al. Administration of cefazolin prior to skin incision is superior to cefazolin at cord clamping in preventing postcesarean infectious morbidity: a randomized, controlled trial. Am J Obstet Gynecol 2007;196(5):455 e1–5.
8. Gould D. Cesarean section, surgical site infection and wound management. Nurs Stand 2007;21(32):57–8.
9. Johnson A, Young D, Reilly J. Cesarean section surgical site infection surveillance. J Hosp Infect 2006;64(1):30–5.
10. Mead PB, Pories SE, Hall P. Decreasing the incidence of surgical wound infections: validation of a surveillance-notification program. Arch Surg 1986;121:458–61.
11. Myles TD, Gooch J, Santolaya J. Obesity as an independent risk factor for infectious morbidity in patients who undergo cesarean delivery. Obstet Gynecol 2002; 100(5 Pt 1):959–64.
12. Olsen MA, Butler AM, Willers DM, et al. Risk factors for surgical site infection after low transverse cesarean section. Infect Control Hosp Epidemiol 2008;29(6): 477–84.
13. Tanner J, Woodings D, Moncaster K. Preoperative hair removal to reduce surgical site infection. Cochrane Database Syst Rev 2006;(3):CD004122.
14. Alexander JW, Fischer JE, Boyajian M, et al. The influence of hair removal methods on wound infections. Arch Surg 1983;118: 347.

15. Webster J, Osborne S. Preoperative bathing or showering with skin antiseptics to prevent surgical site infection. Cochrane Database Syst Rev 2007;(2):CD004985.

16. Tanner J, Khan D. Surgical site infection, preoperative body washing and hair removal. J Perioper Pract 2008;18(6):232, 237–43.

17. Wall PD, Deucy EE, Glantz JC, et al. Vertical skin incisions and wound complications in the obese parturient. Obstet Gynecol 2003;102(5 Pt 1):952–6.

18. Ahern JK, Goodlin RC. Cesarean section in the massively obese. Obstet Gynecol 1978;51(4):509–10.

19. Tixier H, Thouvenot S, Coulange L, et al. Cesarean section in morbidly obese women: Supra or subumbilical transverse incision? Acta Obstet Gynecol Scand 2009;88(9):1049–52.

20. Lynch CM, Sexton DJ, Hession M, et al. Obesity and mode of delivery in primigravid and multigravid women. Am J Perinatol 2008;25(3):163–7.

21. Powell JL, Kasparek DK, Connor GP. Panniculectomy to facilitate gynecologic surgery in morbidly obese women. Obstet Gynecol 1999;94(4):528–31.

22. Pearl ML, Valea FA, Disilvestro PA, et al. Panniculectomy in morbidly obese gynecologic oncology patients. Int J Surg Investig 2000;2(1):59–64.

23. Sugerman HJ, Kellum JM, Jr, Reines HD, et al. Greater risk of incisional hernia with morbidly obese than steroid-dependent patients and low recurrence with prefascial polypropylene mesh. Am J Surg 1996;171(1):80–4.

24. Seid MH, McDaniel-Owens LM, Poole GV, et al. A randomized trial of abdominal incision suture technique and wound strength in rats. Arch Surg 1995;130(4): 394–7.

25. Ceydeli A, Rucinski J, Wise L. Finding the best abdominal closure: an evidence-based review of the literature. Curr Surg 2005;62(2):220–5.

26. Naumann RW, Hauth JC, Owen J, et al. Subcutaneous tissue approximation in relation to wound disruption after cesarean delivery in obese women. Obstet Gynecol 1995;85(3):412–6.

27. Chelmow D, Huang E, Strohbehn K. Closure of the subcutaneous dead space and wound disruption after cesarean delivery., J Matern Fetal Neonatal Med 2002;11(6): 403–8.

28. Magann EF, Chauhan SP, Rodts-Palenik S, et al. Subcutaneous stitch closure versus subcutaneous drain to prevent wound disruption after cesarean delivery: a randomized clinical trial. Am J Obstet Gynecol 2002;186(6):1119–23.

29. Allaire AD, Fisch J, McMahon MJ. Subcutaneous drain versus suture in obese women undergoing cesarean delivery. A prospective randomized trial. J Reprod Med 2000;45(4):327–31.

30. Al-Inany H, Youssef G, Abd El Maguid A, et al. Value of subcutaneous drainage system in obese females undergoing cesarean section using pfannenstiel incision. Gynecol Obstet Invest 2002;53(2):75–8.

31. Ramsey PS, White AM, Guinn DA, et al. Subcutaneous tissue reapproximation, alone or in combination with drain, in obese women undergoing cesarean delivery. Obstet Gynecol 2005;105(5 Pt 1):967–73.

32. Sarsam SE, Elliott JP, Lam GK. Management of wound complications from cesarean delivery. Obstet Gynecol Surv 2005;60(7):462–73.

33. Dodson MK, Magann EF, Meeks GR. A randomized comparison of secondary closure and secondary intention in patients with superficial wound dehiscence. Obstet Gynecol 1992;80(3 Pt 1):321–4.

34. Walters MD, Dombroski RA, Davidson SA, et al. Reclosure of disrupted abdominal incisions. Obstet Gynecol 1990;76(4):597–602.

CHAPTER 14

Breast Feeding and Contraception

Elizabeth Reifsnider
University of Texas Medical Branch, Galveston, Texas, USA

Obesity is a common problem encountered in the care of women, and it is increasing in prevalence [1,2]. Many obese women are of reproductive age, and, as noted earlier in this book, pregnancy in obese women carries greater risks for perinatal complications for mother and child than it does for normal-weight women. Therefore, many obese women, their partners, and their healthcare providers are interested in effective contraception. However, obesity has effects on contraception, and various contraceptives have effects on a woman's weight. At the termination of an obese woman's pregnancy, she faces questions of how to feed her infant. Obesity can affect a woman's ability to breastfeed, and breastfeeding can in turn have an effect on a woman's weight. Postpartum contraceptive and breastfeeding counseling are intensive for most women; when issues of obesity add difficulties, careful counseling and planning take on added significance.

Impact of obesity on fertility

Obesity can have effects on a woman's fertility. The impact depends partly on the presence or absence of hormonal irregularities. Polycystic ovarian syndrome, which produces clinical hyperandrogenism, as shown by hirsutism, acne, and occasionally male pattern alopecia [3], is often associated with obesity, infertility, and hormonal and metabolic abnormalities such as insulin resistance, hyperinsulinemia, and disrupted gonadotropin levels [4]. Even obese women without polycystic ovarian syndrome have lower levels of sex hormone-binding globulin, which allows higher levels of free testosterone to circulate [5]. In addition, higher levels of androgens are present in women with central obesity than in those with peripheral obesity [6].

Women who are overweight or obese but have regular menses, indicating fertility, on average take longer to conceive when not using contraception

Pregnancy in the Obese Woman, 1st edition. Edited by Deborah L. Conway.
© 2011 Blackwell Publishing Ltd.

than do women with normal weight [7]. Gesink Law et al. found the median time to conception to be 1 month longer for overweight women and 3 months longer for obese women. Nevertheless, obese women need effective contraception despite possible decreased fecundity.

Impact of obesity on breastfeeding

The first report of an association between obesity and reduced breastfeeding incidence and duration came in 1992 [8], and since then, many studies have found lower rates of breastfeeding among women who are overweight or obese [9]. The reasons suggested for the association are physiological, medical/physical, and sociocultural. Data from the Third National Health and Nutrition Examination Survey [10], and the Pediatric Nutrition Surveillance System and Pregnancy Nutrition Surveillance System [11] show that obese women are less likely to have ever breastfed. Higher maternal BMI before pregnancy and higher gestational weight gain are both independently associated with reduced breastfeeding incidence.

Data from the Longitudinal Study of Australian Children [9] revealed a dose–response situation, with increasing rates of obesity among women associated with a reduced incidence of breastfeeding. Obese women with a body mass index (BMI) of over $40 \, \text{kg/m}^2$ were the least likely to breastfeed. This dose–response relationship between increased obesity and a lower incidence of breastfeeding was also found in a large sample of Danish women [12]. Finding this association in societies that are very supportive of breastfeeding (Denmark and Australia) suggests that the association may be due to physiological factors, in addition to psychological or cultural factors.

Physiological factors

The postpartum onset of copious lactation is lactogenesis II, also known colloquially as when the milk "comes in," and usually occurs between 48 and 72 hours postpartum. Delayed lactogenesis II is said to occur when copious milk is not available more than 72 hours after delivery. Delayed lactogenesis II has been associated with a high maternal pre-pregnancy BMI, and this delay in copious milk production can lead to a shorter breastfeeding duration. However, if in-depth breastfeeding support is present, the negative effects of greater maternal BMI can be overcome [13].

Several factors have been proposed to explain the discrepancy in the onset of lactogenesis II between obese women and normal-weight women. First, obese new mothers have lower levels of prolactin in the first 48 hours after delivery [14]. Release of prolactin is connected to the numerous hormonal changes that occur postpartum, but its release is reduced in obese individuals compared to lean controls [15]. The prolactin response to the infant's sucking is lower in obese women at 2 and 7 days postpartum; this can reduce the mother's confidence that her milk is sufficient for her child and lead to early cessation of breastfeeding. In addition, the decline in insulin concentrations that occurs from the end of pregnancy to the initiation of lactation is less in obesity, perhaps leading to less glucose being available for milk synthesis [16]. Higher leptin levels have also been described in obese women postpartum. This can inhibit oxytocin's effect on muscle contractions *in vitro*, leading to an increased incidence of dysfunctional labor and higher cesarean section rates among obese women [17].

Finally, poor mammary development during pregnancy may occur due to overfeeding during childhood [15]. Numerous studies in domesticated animals have shown that a high-energy intake during early development and gestation can lead to reduced growth of the mammary glands and reduced milk yield. This has been extensively studied in dairy cows, and has the "fat cow syndrome" label [18]. This also occurs in pigs and sheep, as well as experimental animals such as laboratory rats and mice. However, the ways in which early feeding contributes to the development of connective, adipose, and epithelial tissue, all of which comprise human breasts, remains unclear. It is not yet known whether breast development in obese women mimics the reduced mammary development that occurs in overfed animals.

Medical/physical factors

As described in earlier chapters, obese women are more likely to have co-morbid conditions and to develop certain pregnancy-related diseases, leading to higher rates of complicated labor, higher rates of cesarean delivery, and more postpartum complications such as hemorrhage [19,20]. Recovery is longer after difficult labors and/or cesarean deliveries than after spontaneous labors and vaginal deliveries, and women experience more wound, genital tract, and urinary tract infections, more pain, and greater delay in putting the infant to the breast [20]. The delay in putting the infant to breast may be due to pain from the wound, from separation of the newborn and mother for observation in the newborn nursery, or from the need to attend to the health of the mother after the complicated delivery. It is also more difficult to hold an infant in the traditional "Madonna" position after a cesarean section because of abdominal pain. Furthermore, the mechanical difficulties of latching an infant onto a large breast with excess periareolar adipose tissue may require specialized lactation expertise [21]. This unique challenge for obese nursing mothers is discussed in greater detail in a following section.

Sociocultural factors

While physiological or medical factors among obese women can have direct effects on lactation, sociocultural factors may exert an indirect effect on lactation. The National Immunization Survey conducted by the Centers for Disease Control and Prevention [22] revealed that rates of exclusive breastfeeding were lowest among the infants of mothers who were under the age of 20 years, with a high-school education or less, unmarried, living in rural areas, and at or below the federal poverty level [22]. In population-based studies, obese women have been found more likely to have a lower income, less education, and a higher smoking rate than women of normal weight [9,23]. Although obesity has been found to be an independent risk factor for low rates of breastfeeding [24], the combination of obesity, low levels of education, rural residence, poverty, smoking, and being unmarried predict a high risk for not breastfeeding. Women with this combination of variables will need special lactation education, counseling, and support to overcome the risk for failing to breastfeed.

The impact of breastfeeding on obesity

Breastfeeding can have short- and long-term effects on the weight of postpartum women [25]. Breast milk contains varying amounts of calories based on the child's age, the mother's diet, and the amount of milk produced by the mother. Calories in milk can range from 53 to 75 kcal/100 ml, also depending on the mother's dietary intake. Mothers in developed countries produce breast milk with higher calories than mothers in developing countries [26], probably because women in developed countries are better nourished. The mother whose infant consumes a liter of breast milk a day may use 600 kcal per day in milk production. Postpartum weight loss can result if the breastfeeding woman does not increase her dietary intake by a corresponding number of calories. In studies in Brazil [27], postpartum weight retention was lowest in women who breastfed for 4–12 months, and was highest for mothers who breastfed for less than 1 month or more than 12 months. However, 5 years after the birth of their children, BMI did not significantly differ between women who had breastfed and those who had not [28]. Breastfeeding did not have a significant effect on postpartum weight retention in obese women, although it did on women with a normal pre-pregnancy BMI [29].

Studies from the Danish National Birth Cohort have shown that if obese women breastfeed as recommended (exclusively to 6 months, and continuing in addition to solid food to 12 months), this would eliminate postpartum weight retention and reduce BMI by 18 months postpartum [30]. The Stockholm Pregnancy and Weight Development Study provided

15 years of follow-up in women who delivered in 1984–85. Women with a higher BMI at the 15-year follow-up had a higher BMI before pregnancy and gained more weight during pregnancy [31]; women who remained of normal weight had breastfed longer and more exclusively than women who became overweight over the 15 years.

The long-term impact of lactation on BMI was examined in the Women's Health Initiative. Thirty-five years after childbearing, women who had breastfed for a cumulative lifetime duration of 12 months or longer were less likely to have hypertension, diabetes, hyperlipidemia, or cardiovascular disease [32]. In summary, breastfeeding can promote postpartum weight loss depending on breastfeeding intensity (exclusive or supplemental), duration in months, and the woman's dietary intake. Breastfeeding can thus be beneficial, not only for the infant, but also for the breastfeeding mother.

Recommendations for postpartum care of obese women

Given the findings that breastfeeding is beneficial to women's and infants' health, that obese women are at more risk for developing cardiovascular disease, and that obese women are less likely to breastfeed, it is important for obstetric care providers to assist obese postpartum women to breastfeed. Many clinicians are unaware of the research showing that obese women have lower rates of breastfeeding, or the reasons for the lower rates [33]. Thus, clinicians need to be aware of the risks of lactation failure in obese women and target these women for additional education and support during pregnancy and after delivery (Box 14.1). Latching on of

---

Box 14.1 Clinical lactation support for obese postpartum women

Encourage skin-to-skin contact

Limit maternal–newborn separation, and encourage mother and baby care in same room

Put the newborn to the breast as soon after birth as possible

Encourage frequent sucking and ad lib newborn feeding at the breast

Demonstrate a variety of nursing positions to relieve pressure on the nipples

Assist mothers with flat or inverted nipples to use shields to allow for nipple protrusion

Demonstrate correct latch-on to mothers, and assist with latch-on until the mother is competent

Support large breasts with a towel placed under the breast

Teach mothers how to use a breast pump and encourage pumping between feedings to increase the milk supply

Teach mothers how to wake a "sleepy baby" and encourage the neonate to nurse

Teach mothers how to recognize neonate swallowing of breast milk

Refer to a lactation specialist if needed

the infant to the breast can be more difficult for obese women, and they will benefit from specific counseling on latching on and from breast support with a towel placed under the breast [21,33]. Pumping from both breasts using a double-pump system between infant feedings can increase milk production and promote the woman's sense of accomplishment in feeding her infant [21].

In a study of exclusively breastfed neonates during the first 2 weeks of life, neonates who had up to 5–6 stools per day and had the first appearance of yellow stool by day 6 lost the least amount of birthweight (2–4%) and had the earliest return to birthweight (4–5 days). Conversely, neonates who had 2–3 stools per day and did not have yellow stool until day 12 lost up to 14% of their birthweight [34]. Teaching the mother to recognize signs of adequate infant intake through stooling can reassure her that her milk is sufficient for her infant; this can promote breastfeeding duration and exclusivity.

Oral contraceptives

Efficacy of oral contraceptives in obesity

Oral contraceptives with both estrogen and progestin (OCs) are the most popular form of hormonal contraception for all women, including obese women, and the most popular form of reversible contraception in the USA [35,36]. OCs may be less effective in obese women than in normal-weight women because of dilution in the larger blood volume and fat mass, or inadequate suppression of the hypothalamic–pituitary–ovarian axis [37]. Other proposed mechanisms for the effects of obesity on drug metabolism include alterations of steroid metabolism due to increased basal metabolic rate, increased hepatic enzyme metabolism, and increased drug sequestration in the fat mass [38].

The metabolism of ethinyl estradiol (EE), the most commonly used synthetic estrogen in OCs, and levonorgestrel (LNG) was studied in a prospective cohort study of 20 obese and normal-weight women. The clearance of EE and LNG was altered in obese women, and this resulted in higher levels of follicle-stimulating hormone and luteinizing hormone, indicating a greater potential for ovulation to occur with low-dose OCs or missed pills. The half-life of LNG was significantly longer, and concentrations were lower in obese women [37].

Population-based studies of the effects of obesity on OC effectiveness have had conflicting outcomes. Using the 2002 National Survey of Family Growth sample of 7,643 women aged 15–44 years, the outcome of unintended pregnancy was studied by BMI. No significant differences in rates of unintended pregnancy were found between women in the normal-weight, overweight, or obese BMI categories, even with adjustments for age, marital status, and race/ethnicity [39].

A case-cohort study using data from the 1999 Behavioral Risk Factor Surveillance System (BRFSS) and the 2000 Pregnancy Risk Assessment Monitoring System (PRAMS) examined the association between BMI and OC failure [40]. The sample included 358 women, 153 of whom were cases of unintended pregnancy from the PRAMS dataset, and 205 of whom were women who had responded to the BRFSS and represented the population at risk for unintended pregnancy (the cohort). Cases of overweight were 35.5% with 16% obese, compared to 22.4% and 9.1% respectively for the cohort. The odds ratio (OR) for OC failure showed a dose–response by BMI, with an OR of 2.54 (95% confidence interval [CI] 1.18–5.50) for overweight (BMI 25–29.9 kg/m^2) and of 2.82 (95% CI 1.05–7.58) for obese (BMI > 30 kg/m^2) women. When the results were stratified by race/ethnicity, white overweight and obese women had 2.64 times the risk for OC failure (95% CI 1.16–6.05) compared to normal-weight women. However, the risk for OC failure in overweight or obese African-American women was no longer significant when compared to normal-weight African-American women (OR 1.29; 95% CI 0.43–3.88).

In the 1999 PRAMS survey [41], the researchers also examined unintended pregnancy among women using (cases) and not using (controls) contraception. There was no association between BMI and unintended pregnancy among women who were not using contraception at the time of conception. Conversely, among the women using contraception, the OR of having an unintended pregnancy increased with increasing BMI. Women with a BMI of 25–29.9 kg/m^2 had an OR of 1.73 (95% CI 1.26–2.36), and women with a BMI over 30 kg/m^2 had an OR of 1.75 (95% CI 1.21–2.52) for unintended pregnancy compared to normal-weight women. One limitation of this study was a lack of information about the type of contraception being used at the time of unintended conception, as well as any measure of compliance with a chosen method.

A recent review of the literature on BMI and OC failure [42] found two studies which concluded that obesity increases the risk for OC failure, and six studies which concluded that obesity does not increase the risk for OC failure. The authors of the review did not find convincing evidence that obese women are at higher risk for OC failure with perfect use, but noted that imperfect use may result in OC failure since the metabolism of OCs in obese women provides a smaller "margin of error." Thus, when initiating OCs for overweight and obese women, it is essential that they are made aware of their increased potential for ovulation and unintended pregnancy with missed or delayed doses.

Weight changes with oral contraceptives

Women may complain about weight gain when taking OCs, but a systematic review of 40 studies that compared contraceptives found no differences in weight among participants [43]. The three randomized controlled trials included in the review did not find evidence to support the view that OCs cause weight gain. A recent comparison of depot medroxyprogesterone acetate (DMPA) injection, OCs, and non-hormonal contraceptives found that women using OCs did not gain weight but increased their percentage of body fat and decreased their percentage of lean body mass [44]. The authors of the systematic study observed that, over the 3 years of observation, the women became less active, which could have accounted for the loss of lean body mass. Most women gain weight as they age, and they may mistakenly attribute their weight gain to OCs instead of a change in activity levels. Given the findings of these studies, it is reasonable to counsel an obese woman that initiating OCs will have no impact on her weight or her efforts to lose weight, as long as her eating habits and activity levels do not worsen.

Safety of oral contraceptives in obese women

There is also controversy concerning the safety of OC for obese women [45]. One of the well-known adverse effects of OC is an increased risk for venous thrombosis, especially during the first year of use [46]. Obesity also is associated with increased risk for deep venous thrombosis (DVT) and pulmonary embolism (PE) in women, and this appears to be a stronger risk factor in women under 40 years of age than in older women. One reason for the increased risks of DVT and/or PE among obese women may be higher levels of plasminogen activator inhibitor-1, which is also present in diabetes and the metabolic syndrome [47].

The number of patients discharged from hospitals from 1979 to 1999 with the diagnoses of obesity and DVT or PE were examined using the International Classification of Diseases, Ninth Revision, Clinical Modification (ICD-9-CM) to classify obesity, DVT, and PE [48]. Of the obese hospitalized patients, 0.76% had PE and 2.02% had DVT. The corresponding percentages of non-obese hospitalized patients with these conditions were 0.34% and 0.80%. The relative risk for a DVT in obese women under the age of 40 compared to non-obese women of the same age was 6.10 (95% CI 6.04–6.17), and the relative risk for a PE in obese women of the same age compared to non-obese women was 5.19 (95% CI 5.11–5.28). Among obese women compared to women whose BMI was less than 25kg/m^2 who took OCs, the OR of DVT increased to 9.8 (95% CI 3.0–31.8) [49]. The absolute risk (rate per 10,000 woman–years) for DVT among all women who take OCs varies from 1.84 to 7.84 depending on age, socioeconomic status, and type of estrogen and progestin used

[46], and all sources cite increased odds for DVT for obese women who take contraceptives. At this time, we lack data to quantify the additive risks of obesity and OC use on DVT rates, although there is no evidence of increased DVT with progestin-only contraception [38].

The use of OCs in women with obesity has been rated as generally safe by the World Health Organization when the benefits of contraception outweigh the risks of use, that is, when the risks of pregnancy in obese mothers are greater than the risks of contraception [50]. Prescribers in the USA generally follow the World Health Organization guidelines and do not consider obesity alone a contraindication to OC use [50]. In the UK, the use of OC by women who have a BMI of 30–34.9 kg/m^2 is viewed as generally safe, but their use is discouraged when the BMI is 35–39 kg/m^2 because the risks of use are judged to outweigh the benefits, and OCs are viewed as an unacceptable health risk with a BMI of 40 kg/m^2 or more [50,51].

The type of OC, specifically the type of progestin, and the risks of DVT and PE have been examined for several decades. EE is the most common estrogen used, but the progestin component can be one of eight progestins, not all of which are available in the USA. Several studies in the past decade have examined the rates of thrombosis with use of OC-containing desogestrel, norgestimate, or gestodene (often considered "third-generation" progestins) and have found increased thrombotic risk [52]. Recent case-control and cohort studies have re-examined the risks of thrombosis, specifically with the use of third-generation progestins. A recent study compared exposure to progestins in OCs in 1,524 women with thrombosis and 1,760 control women without thrombosis. The risk for thrombosis was approximately five times higher for OC users than for non-users. Importantly, the authors found a 6–7-fold risk for thrombosis in users of OC containing desogestrel and drospirenone than in non-users, compared to a 3–4-fold risk with LNG-containing OC use [53]. A Danish national cohort study [46], encompassing 10.4 million woman–years and including over 4,000 venous thrombotic events, demonstrated that OCs with desogestrel, gestodene, or drospirenone were associated with approximately 86% higher risks of thrombosis than OCs containing LNG or norgestrel.

Recommendations for use of oral contraceptives in obese women

A family history of thromboembolism is an important risk factor to note when considering the use of OCs in obese women [54]. Age, smoking, and risks of pregnancy are other factors to consider when advising obese women about contraceptive choices. The risks of thrombosis increase with age, and smoking is an independent risk factor for thrombosis. Obesity, smoking, and age over 35 years may be a lethal combination that should be avoided. If an OC is the chosen contraceptive, a low estrogen dose combined with a low dose of LNG appears to be the first choice [46].

Although progestins in the combined OC pill contribute to a higher risk for thrombosis, especially in obese women, no similar risk exists for obese women who take the progestin-only pill (POP). Numerous studies have shown that the POP does not increase the risk for thrombosis or cardio-vascular disease [55], so a POP may be a safe alternative for an obese woman who is concerned about the risks of thromboembolism and cardio-vascular disease. Unfortunately, for women who are at risk for developing type 2 diabetes or who had gestational diabetes during their pregnancies, progestin-only contraceptives have been associated with increased risks of developing diabetes [56–58]. This association has been seen with the POPs [58] and with injectable progestins [56,58]. The reasons for the increased risk remain to be elucidated, but may be due to the increased weight gain that accompanies injectable contraceptives, increased insulin resistance associated with progesterone [36], or other factors still unidentified.

Contraceptive vaginal ring

The contraceptive vaginal ring (CVR) on the market contains 15 μg EE and 120 μg etonogestrel (related to desogestrel), although a formulation with a new progestin is currently in clinical trial [59]. The CVR is inserted by the user and remains in place for 21 days; it is removed for 7 days to allow for withdrawal bleeding, which is similar to the OC pill and transdermal patch. Women who use the CVR are exposed to lower doses of EE than women who use OC or the transdermal patch [60], but the exposure is more stable and precise. However, the same contraindications exist for use of the CVR as for any estrogen-containing contraceptive, specifically current or historical DVT, migraine with aura, current breast or reproduc-tive cancer, etc. [61]. No adequate information exists on the impact of the CVR on lipid metabolism, coagulation, or fibrinolysis factors [62]. A pro-spective clinical trial compared 31 overweight or obese women who used OCs to 34 similar women who used the CVR, and at the conclusion of the study 6 months later, the OC group had greater insulin resistance than the CVR group [36]. The CVR may thus be a preferred method for obese women since it exposes them to lower doses of EE, has fewer side effects related to insulin sensitivity, and is not affected by body weight [63].

The transdermal patch

The transdermal patch contains EE and norelgestromin (related to norg-estimate). One fresh patch is placed by the user weekly for 3 weeks any-where on the body except the breasts. Then one week is patch-free to allow for withdrawal bleeding. A systematic review [64] found that the patch produced more side effects than the OC or CVR, and a cohort study revealed twice the risks of DVT and PE among patch users as among OC users [65]. Obesity appears to reduce the effectiveness of the patch [66], and the patch has been found to be less effective in women weighing more than 90 kg (198 lb) [67], who may or may not be obese depending on their height. For obese women, other methods are more effective and should be recommended over the transdermal patch.

Depot medroxyprogesterone acetate (injection)

DMPA is given intramuscularly 150 mg/1 ml every 12 weeks. It is a highly effective contraceptive, resulting in a typical usage failure rate of 3% [68] and is as effective in obese women as in normal-weight women. Increased body weight does not decrease the effectiveness of DMPA, and in one open-label study of DMPA, no pregnancies were observed regardless of body weight [63,69]. It does not contain estrogen, so for obese women who may be at risk for DVT or PE, DMPA is safer than contraceptives containing estrogen [63].

The side effect of DMPA that causes most concern is weight gain. Berenson and Rahman [44] found that DMPA users gained on average 4.4 kg (9.7 lb) in 2 years and 5.1 kg (11.2 lb) in 3 years. For women who are already obese, this level of weight gain can be a significant deterrent. In addition, DMPA users had an increase in visceral fat, which is most metabolically active in promoting dyslipidemia. In a study comparing insulin-sensitive normal-weight and obese women, and insulin-resistant normal-weight and obese women, visceral fat was the most important predictor of insulin sensitivity/resistance [70]. More insulin-resistant women used DMPA than did insulin-sensitive subjects. DMPA may promote weight gain through its suppression of endogenous estrogen since hypoestrogenemia (e.g. menopause) has been linked to visceral fat and weight gain [71].

Intrauterine devices

IUDs have not been shown to affect weight in women [72]. When women who are using IUDs complain of weight gain, it is most likely due to aging, since the basal metabolic rate decreases 2% each decade after 18 years of age. IUDs can be an effective contraception for obese women, especially those who want to avoid weight gain and estrogen-related side effects. The LNG-releasing IUD may be the preferred choice for obese women as the progestin protects the endometrium from the development of hyperplasia from long-term exposure to excess estrogen related to obesity [73]. The impact of obesity on an IUD is primarily on the difficulty of insertion. Determining the size and direction of the uterus and completely visualizing the cervix can be more difficult in obese women. Using a larger speculum or ultrasound could help [45], along with insertion by a skilled practitioner with experience inserting IUDs.

Barrier contraceptives

Obesity does not have any impact on barrier contraceptives, and barrier contraceptives do not have any effect on weight in obese women, other than their lower level of effectiveness, which can be problematic for women who should avoid pregnancy for health reasons. It has been a common practice to instruct women to have their diaphragms refitted with a 5–10 lb or greater loss or gain of weight, but this advice has not been shown to be evidenced-based. Women who gained or did not gain weight had the same proportion of diaphragm refitting or retention of their original size [74].

Sterilization

Sterilization has an effectiveness rate similar to that of IUDs, but obesity is a risk factor for complications [75]. The types of sterilization procedures in use at present include laparoscopy, minilaparotomy, and transcervical sterilization (with the Essure microinsert device, which is inserted into the fallopian tubes; Conceptus, Inc., Mountain View, CA, USA). Obesity can complicate each type of procedure. The Centers for Disease Control and Prevention's collaborative review of sterilization reported that, in women who had sterilization by laparoscopy, obesity increased the risk for surgical complications by 70% (relative risk 1.7; 95% CI 1.2–2.6) [76]. Obesity caused the increased risk by increasing operative time and causing more difficulty in providing general anesthesia, more difficult visualization of tubes, unintended major surgery, and longer hospitalization. However, with skilled providers, complications from sterilization are low (1.6 per 100 procedures in the Centers for Disease Control and Prevention review), and sterilization can be a safe and effective contraceptive for obese women who do not want additional children.

Recommendations for contraception for obese women

The evaluation for contraception for an obese woman should include a personal, social, family, and medical history that includes noting the presence of contraindications to hormonal contraceptives (specifically the contraindications to use of estrogens) and IUDs. If no contraindications are present based on history, a woman's risk for pregnancy should be noted, based on frequency of intercourse, prior fertility, and her own desires for avoiding conception. After a complete physical examination, along with appropriate laboratory studies as indicated by the history and physical findings, the full range of contraception that is appropriate for the woman should if possible be offered to her. The obese woman should be encouraged to make her decision about contraception based on her own circumstances after all the risks and benefits of all the methods have been fully and appropriately addressed. Obese women should be made aware of the benefits of improving overall health and reducing their BMI prior to conceiving in order to have safer pregnancies and deliveries, improved lactation, and reduced risks associated with contraceptives. Recommendations and strategies for optimizing health prior to conception are discussed in Chapter 3.

References

1. Centers for Disease Control. US obesity trends. Trends by state 1985–2008. http://www.cdc.gov/obesity/data/trends.html. Updated August 19, 2008. Accessed August 28, 2009.
2. Ogden CL, Carroll MD, McDowell MA, et al. Obesity among adults in the United States – no change since 2003–2004. NCHS Data Brief No. 1. Hyattsville, MD: National Center for Health Statistics, 2007.
3. Venturoli S, Porcu E, Fabbri R, et al. Longitudinal evaluation of the different gonadotropin pulsatile patterns in anovulatory cycles of young girls. J Clin Endocrinol Metab 1992;74(4):836–41.
4. Pasquali R. Obesity, fat distribution and infertility. Maturitas 2006;54(4):363–71.
5. Norman RJ, Clark AM. Obesity and reproductive disorders: a review. Reprod Fertil Dev 1998;10(1):55–63.
6. Evans DJ, Hoffmann RG, Kalkhoff RK, et al. Relationship of androgenic activity to body fat topography, fat cell morphology, and metabolic aberrations in premenopausal women. J Clin Endocrinol Metab 1983;57(2):304–10.
7. Gesink Law DC, Maclehose RF, Longnecker MP. Obesity and time to pregnancy. Hum Reprod 2007;22(2):414–20.
8. Rutishauser IH, Carlin JB. Body mass index and duration of breast feeding: a survival analysis during the first six months of life. J Epidemiol Community Health 1992;46(6):559–65.
9. Donath SM, Amir LH. Maternal obesity and initiation and duration of breastfeeding: data from the longitudinal study of Australian children. Maternal Child Nutr 2008; 4(3):163–70.
10. Li R, Ogden C, Ballew C, et al. Prevalence of exclusive breastfeeding among US infants: the Third National Health and Nutrition Examination Survey (Phase II, 1991–1994). Am J Public Health 2002;92(7):1107–10.
11. Li R, Jewell S, Grummer-Strawn L. Maternal obesity and breast-feeding practices. Am J Clin Nutr 2003;77(4):931–6.

12 Baker JL, Michaelsen KF, Sorensen TI, et al. High prepregnant body mass index is associated with early termination of full and any breastfeeding in Danish women. Am J Clin Nutr 2007;86(2):404–11.

13. Chapman DJ, Perez-Escamilla R. Maternal perception of the onset of lactation is a valid, public health indicator of lactogenesis stage II. J Nutr 2000;2972–80.

14. Rasmussen KM, Kjolhede CL. Prepregnant overweight and obesity diminish the prolactin response to suckling in the first week postpartum. Pediatr 2004;113(5): e465–71.

15. Rasmussen KM. Association of maternal obesity before conception with poor lactation performance. Annu Rev Nutr 2007;27:103–21.

16. Lovelady CA. Is maternal obesity a cause of poor lactation performance? Nutr Rev 2005;63(10):352–5.

17. Moynihan AT, Hehir MP, Glavey SV, et al. Inhibitory effect of leptin on human uterine contractility in vitro. Am J Obstet Gynecol 2006;195(2):504–9.

18. Morrow DA. Fat cow syndrome. J Dairy Sci 1976;87:672–9.

19. Rasmussen KM, Kjolhede CL. Maternal obesity: a problem for both mother and child. Obes 2008;16(5):929–31.

20. Sebire NJ, Jolly M, Harris JP, et al. Maternal obesity and pregnancy outcome: a study of 287,213 pregnancies in London. Int J Obes Related Metab Disord 2001; 25(8):1175–82.

21. Jevitt C, Hernandez I, Groer M. Lactation complicated by overweight and obesity: supporting the mother and newborn. J Midwifery Womens Health 2007;52(6): 606–13.

22. Centers for Disease Control and Prevention. Breastfeeding trends and updated national health objectives for exclusive breastfeeding – United States, birth years 2000–2004. MMWR Morb Mortal Wkly Rep 2007;56(30):760–3.

23. Eriksson J, Forsen T, Osmond C, et al. Obesity from cradle to grave. Int J Obes Related Metab Disord 2003;27(6):722–7.

24. Oddy WH, Li J, Landsborough L, et al. The association of maternal overweight and obesity with breastfeeding duration. J Pediatr 2006;149(2):185–91.

25. Walker LO, Freeland-Graves JH, Milani T, et al. Weight and behavioral and psycho-social factors among ethnically diverse, low-income women after childbirth. II: Trends and correlates. Women Health 2004;40(2):19–34.

26. Lauber E, Reinhardt M. Studies on the quality of breast milk during 23 months of lactation in a rural community of the Ivory Coast. Am J Clin Nutr 1979;32(5): 1159–73.

27. Araujo CL, Victora CG, Hallal PC, et al. Breastfeeding and overweight in childhood: evidence from the Pelotas 1993 birth cohort study. Int J Obes 2006;30(3):500–6.

28. Gigante DP, Victora CG, Barros FC. Breast-feeding has a limited long–term effect on anthropometry and body composition of Brazilian mothers. J Nutr 2001; 131(1):78–84.

29. Kac G, Benicio MH, Velasquez-Melendez G, et al. Gestational weight gain and pre-pregnancy weight influence postpartum weight retention in a cohort of Brazilian women. J Nutr 2004;134(3):661–6.

30. Baker JL, Gamborg M, Heitmann BL, et al. Breastfeeding reduces postpartum weight retention. Am J Clin Nutr 2008;88:1543–51.

31. Linne Y, Dye L, Barkeling B, et al. Weight development over time in parous women – the SPAWN study – 15 years follow-up. Int J Obes Related Metab Disord 2003; 27(12):1516–22.

32. Schwarz EB, Ray RM, Stuebe AM, et al. Duration of lactation and risk factors for maternal cardiovascular disease. Obstet Gynecol 2009;113(5):974–82.

33. Rasmussen KM, Lee VE, Ledkovsky TB, et al. A description of lactation counseling practices that are used with obese mothers. J Hum Lact 2006;22(3):322–7.

34. Shrago LC, Reifsnider E, Insel K. The Neonatal Bowel Output Study: indicators of adequate breast milk intake in neonates. Pediatr Nurs 2006;32(3):195–201.

35. Mosher WD, Martinez GM, Chandra A, et al. Use of contraception and use of family planning services in the United States: 1982–2002. Adv Data 2004;350:1–36.

36. Elkind-Hirsch KE, Darensbourg C, Ogden B, et al. Contraceptive vaginal ring use for women has less adverse metabolic effects than an oral contraceptive. Contraception 2007;76:348–56.

37. Edelman AB, Carlson NE, Cherala G, et al. Impact of obesity on oral contraceptive pharmacokinetics and hypothalamic-pituitary-ovarian activity. Contraception 2009; 80:119–27.

38. Teal SB, Ginosar DM. Contraception for women with chronic medical conditions. Obstet Gynecol Clin North Am 2007;34(1):113–26.

39. Kaneshiro B, Edelman A, Carlson N, et al. The relationship between body mass index and unintended pregnancy: results from the 2002 National Survey of Family Growth. Contraception 2008;77(4):234–8.

40. Brunner Huber LR, Hogue CJ, Stein AD, et al. Body mass index and risk for oral contraceptive failure: a case-cohort study in South Carolina. Ann of Epidemiol 2006;16(8):637–43.

41. Brunner Huber LR, Hogue CJ. The association between body weight, unintended pregnancy resulting in a livebirth, and contraception at the time of conception. Maternal Child Health J 2005;9(4):413–20.

42. Trussell J, Schwarz EB, Guthrie K. Obesity and oral contraceptive pill failure. Contraception 2009;79(5):334–8.

43. Gallo MF, Grimes DA, Schulz KF, et al. Combination estrogen-progestin contraceptives and body weight: systematic review of randomized controlled trials. Obstet Gynecol 2004;103:359–73.

44. Berenson AB, Rahman M. Changes in weight, total fat, percent body fat, and central-to-peripheral fat ration associated with injectable and oral contraceptive use. Am J Obstetrics Gynecol 2009;200:329 e1–8.

45. Grimes DA, Shields WC. Family planning for obese women: challenges and opportunities. Contraception 2005;72(1):1–4.

46. Lidegaard Ø, Løkkegaard E, Svendsen AL, et al. Hormonal contraception and risk of venous thromboembolism: national follow-up study. Br Med J 2009;339: b2890.

47. Westrick RJ, Eitzman DT. Plasminogen activator inhibitor-1 in vascular thrombosis. Curr Drug Targets 2007;8(9):966–1002.

48. Stein PD, Beemath A, Olson RE. Obesity as a risk factor in venous thromboembolism. Am J Med 2003;118(9):978–80.

49. Abdollahi M, Cushman M, Rosendaal FR. Obesity: risk of venous thrombosis and the interaction with coagulation factor levels and oral contraceptive use. Thromb Haemost 2003;89(3):493–8.

50. Trussell J, Guthrie KA, Schwarz EB. Much ado about little: obesity, combined hormonal contraceptive use and venous thrombosis. Contraception 2008;77(3):143–6.

51. Poulter NR, Chang CL. Venous thromboembolic disease and combined oral contraceptives: results of international multicentre case-control study. World Health Organization Collaborative Study of Cardiovascular Disease and Steroid Hormone Contraception. Lancet 1995;346:1575–82.

52. Vandenbroucke JP, Rosing J, Bloemenkamp KW, et al. Oral contraceptives and the risk of venous thrombosis. N Engl Med 2001;344(20):1527–35.

53. van Hylckama Vlieg A, Helmerhorst FM, Vandenbroucke JP, et al. The venous thrombotic risk of oral contraceptives, effects of oestrogen dose and progestogen type: results of the MEGA case-control study. Br Med J 2009;339:b2921.

54. Vandenbroucke JP, van der Meer FJ, Helmerhorst FM, et al. Family history and risk of venous thromboembolism with oral contraception. Family history is important tool. Br Med J 2001;323(7315):752.

55. Mansour D. Implications of the growing obesity epidemic on contraception and reproductive health. J Fam Plann Reprod Health Care 2004: 30(4);209–11.

56. Kahn HS, Curtis KM, Marchbanks PA. Effects of injectable or implantable progestin-only contraceptives on insulin-glucose metabolism and diabetes risk. Diabetes Care 2003;26(1);216–25.

57. Kjos SL, Peters RK, Xiang A, et al. Contraception and the risk of type 2 diabetes mellitus in the Latina woman with prior gestational diabetes mellitus. JAMA 1998;280(6):533–8.

58. Xiang AH, Kjos SL, Kawakubo M, et al. Long-acting injectable progestin contraception and risk of type 2 diabetes in Latino women with prior gestational diabetes mellitus. Diabetes Care 2006;29(3):613–17.

59. Population Council, US Agency for International Development, Eunice Kennedy Shriver National Institute of Child Health and Human Development (NICHD), World Health Organization. A multicenter, open-label study on the efficacy, cycle control and safety of a contraceptive vaginal ring delivering a daily dose of 150 ug of Nestorone® and 15 ug of ethinyl estradiol. http://clinicaltrials.gov/ct2/show/NCT00263341. Updated October 1, 2008. Accessed August 30, 2009.

60. van den Heuvel MW, van Bragt AJM, Alnabawy AKM, et al. Comparison of ethinylestradiol pharmacokinetics in three hormonal contraceptive formulation: the vaginal ring, the transdermal patch and an oral contraceptive. Contraception 2005; 72:168–74.

61. Madden T, Blumenthal P. Contraceptive vaginal ring. Clin Obstet Gynecol 2007; 50(4): 878–85.

62. Sukar NN. The combined contraceptive vaginal device (NuvaRing®): a comprehensive review. Eur J Contracept Reprod Health Care 2005;10(2):73–8.

63. Gordon L, Thakur N, Atlas M, et al. Clinical inquiries. What hormonal contraception is most effective for obese women? J Fam Pract 2007;56(6):471–3.

64. Lopez LM, Grimes DA, Gallo MF, et al. Skin patch and vaginal ring versus combined oral contraceptives for contraception. Cochrane Database Syst Rev 2008;(1):CD003552.

65. Cole JA, Norman H, Doherty M, et al. Venous thromboembolism, myocardial infarction, and stroke among transdermal contraceptive system users. Obstet Gynecol 2007;109:339–46.

66. Zieman M, Guillebaud J, Weisberg E, et al. Contraceptive efficacy and cycle control with the Ortho Evra/Evra transdermal system: the analysis of pooled data. Fertil Steril 2002;77(2 Suppl. 2):S13–18.

67. Courtney C. The contraceptive patch: latest developments. AWHONN Lifelines 2006;10(3):2504.

68. Goldberg AB, Grimes DA. Injectable contraceptives. In Hatcher R, Trussell J, Nelson A, Cates W, Stewart F, Kowal D (eds.), Contraceptive technologies, 19th edn. New York: Ardent Media, 2007, pp. 157–80.

69. Jain J, Jakimiuk AJ, Bode RF, et al. Contraceptive efficacy and safety of DMPA-SC. Contraception 2004;70:269–75.

70. Jennings CL, Lambert EV, Collins M, et al. Determinants of insulin-resistant phenotypes in normal-weight and obese black African women. Obes 2008;16(7):1602–9.

71. Clark MK, Dillon JS, Sowers M, et al. Weight, fat mass, and central distribution of fat increase when women use depot-medroxyprogesterone acetate for contraception. Int J Obes 2005;29(10):1252–8.

72. Hassan DF, Petta CA, Aldrighi JM, et al. Weight variation in a cohort of women using copper IUD for contraception. Contraception 2003;68(1):27–30.

73. Bahamondes L, Ribeiro-Huguet P, de Andrade KC, et al. Levonorgestrel-releasing intrauterine system (Mirena) as a therapy for endometrial hyperplasia and carcinoma. Acta Obstet Gynecol Scand 2003;82(6):580–2.

74. Fiscella K. Relationship of weight change to required size of vaginal diaphragm. Nurs Pract 1982;7(7):21, 25.

75. Pollack AE, Thomas LJ, Barone MA. Female and male sterilization. In Hatcher R, Trussell J, Nelson A, Cates W, Stewart F, Kowal D (eds.), Contraceptive technologies, 19th edn. New York: Ardent Media, 2007, pp. 361–401.

76. Jamieson DJ, Hillis SD, Duerr A, et al. Complications of interval laparoscopic tubal sterilization: findings from the United States Collaborative Review of Sterilization. Obstet Gynecol 2000;96(6):997–1002.

Index